OCCUPATIONAL THERAPY WITH CHILDREN

Understanding children's occupations and enabling participation

Edited by

Sylvia Rodger

Head of Division of Occupational Therapy
School of Health and Rehabilitation Sciences
The University of Queensland
Australia

Jenny Ziviani

Associate Professor, Division of Occupational Therapy
School of Health and Rehabilitation Sciences
The University of Queensland
Australia

D0770383

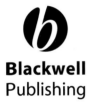

Blackwell
Publishing

© 2006 by Blackwell Publishing Ltd

Editorial offices:
Blackwell Publishing Ltd, 9600 Garsington Road, Oxford OX4 2DQ, UK
    Tel: +44 (0)1865 776868
Blackwell Publishing Inc., 350 Main Street, Malden, MA 02148-5020, USA
    Tel: +1 781 388 8250
Blackwell Publishing Asia Pty Ltd, 550 Swanston Street, Carlton, Victoria 3053, Australia
    Tel: +61 (0)3 8359 1011

The right of the Author to be identified as the Author of this Work has been asserted in
accordance with the Copyright, Designs and Patents Act 1988.

First published 2006 by Blackwell Publishing Ltd

ISBN-10: 1-4051-2456-3
ISBN-13: 978-1-4051-2456-0

Library of Congress Cataloging-in-Publication Data

Occupational therapy with children : understanding children's occupations and
enabling participation / edited by Sylvia Rodger, and Jenny Ziviani.
    p. cm.
  Includes bibliographical references and index.
  ISBN-13: 978-1-4051-2456-0 (pbk.: alk. paper)
  ISBN-10: 1-4051-2456-3 (pbk.: alk. paper)
  1. Occupational therapy for children. I. Rodger, Sylvia. II. Ziviani, Jenny.
  [DNLM: 1. Occupational Therapy – Child. 2. Child Development.
  3. Interpersonal Relations – Child. WS 105 015 2006]
  RJ53.025033 2006
  615.8′515′083–dc22
  2005024030

A catalogue record for this title is available from the British Library

Set in 10/12.5 pt Sabon
by Graphicraft Limited, Hong Kong
Printed and bound in India
by Replika Press Pvt Ltd.

The publisher's policy is to use permanent paper from mills that operate a sustainable
forestry policy, and which has been manufactured from pulp processed using acid-free
and elementary chlorine-free practices. Furthermore, the publisher ensures that the text
paper and cover board used have met acceptable environmental accreditation standards.

For further information on Blackwell Publishing, visit our website:
www.blackwellpublishing.com

CONTENTS

Foreword   ix
Preface   xii
Acknowledgements   xiii
About the editors   xiv
Contributors   xv

**SECTION 1: CHILDREN'S ROLES, OCCUPATIONS
AND PARTICIPATION IN CONTEMPORARY
SOCIETY**

1   **Children, their environments, roles and occupations
    in contemporary society**   3

    Children in contemporary society   3
        Social environment   4
        Physical environment   5
        Cultural environment   5
        Technological environment   6
    International classification of function framework   7
        ICF structure   8
        Reactions to the ICF   10
    Children's roles and occupations   11
        Types of roles   12
        Occupational roles during childhood   13
        Roles, socialization and learning   15
        Role dysfunction and role competence   16
    Summary   18

2   **Families and children's occupational performance**   22

    Families in contemporary society   22
        Changes in family formation and functioning   23
        Diversity of family types   23
        Children in families   24
        Role of society in supporting children   26
    Impact of families on children's roles and occupations 28
        Lien   29
    Working in partnership with families   30

Family-centred practice   30
Collaborative parent and service provider partnerships   32
Family occupations   32
The role of childhood professionals in advocacy   34
Advocating for clients   35
Class advocacy   36
Advocacy skills   37
Summary   37

3   Environmental influences on children's participation   41

The nature of children's environments   42
Home environments   44
Neighbourhood environments   44
Community environments   47
Virtual environments   48
Evaluating children's environments   50
Geographic information systems   51
Evaluating specific environments   52
Collaborative environmental design and advocacy   53
Children as collaborators   56
Children's playgrounds   57
Designing for difference   59
Summary   61

4   Participation of children in school and community   67

Participation   67
Classification of participation   68
Participation: relationship to health, wellbeing and development   70
Participation: relationship to occupation and occupational performance   72
Participation in school   72
Political agenda   73
Physical environment   74
Social environment   75
Participation in community   75
Physical environment   75
Social and cultural environment   76
Economic environment   78
Occupational therapists and participation   79
An ecological approach to facilitating children's participation   80
Enabling participation: a multi-method, multi-level approach   81
Adopting a strengths based approach   82
Advocacy and community building   82
Maximizing person–environment–occupation fit   82

Matthew 83
Research 84
Summary 86

5 Children's occupational time use 91

The division of time 91
Activities of daily living 92
Work 93
Leisure 93
The personal and contextual factors impacting on time use 94
Personal factors 94
Contextual factors 95
The effect of time use on wellbeing 96
Wellbeing 96
Is there occupational balance? 100
How is occupational balance affected by family and
societal change? 102
How is occupational balance affected by technological change? 103
How is occupational balance affected by disability? 105
The occupational therapist's role in the quest for balance 105
Intervention at the individual level 106
Intervention at the family level 106
Intervention at the community and political level 107
Summary 107

SECTION 2: MASTERING OCCUPATIONS, ROLES AND ENABLING CHILDREN'S PARTICIPATION

6 Doing, being and becoming: their importance for children 115

The importance of doing, being and becoming 116
Outcomes of occupational engagement 117
Consequences of not being able to do 119
Approaches to enable doing 122
Motor learning approaches 122
Evidence based practice 123
Client centred practice 123
International classification of functioning, disability and
health (ICF) 123
Matthew 124
Let's not forget being 125
Children and spirituality 127
Palliative care and being 130
Occupational balance 131
Summary 132

7   The occupational development of children   **136**

Occupational development defined   137
    Occupational development: situated among and distinct from
    other forms of development   138
  Micro-occupational development: developing occupational
  competence   139
  Meso-occupational development: developing an occupational life
  course   141
    The interactional model of occupational development (IMOD)   141
  The principles of interactionism   143
    Staged continuity   143
    Multiple determinicity   144
    Multiple patternicity   150
  Macro-occupational development: the evolution of
  human occupations   151
  Implications for practice   153
  Summary   154

8   Communication and social skills for occupational engagement   **158**

Acquisition of communication skills   159
  Some definitions   159
  Social interactional perspective   160
  Stages of communication   161
  Development of socio-dramatic play   163
  Communication skills of the school-age child   164
  Social competence and social skills: inter-professional
  management   165
    Defining social competence and social skills   165
    Friendships   166
    Children with social skills deficits   167
    Ethan   167
    Hannah   167
    Social skills assessment   167
    Social skills intervention   168
  Summary   173

9   Developing as a player   **177**

Definitions of play   178
Valuing play: the functions of play   180
The occupational role of player   181
  Henry   181
Enabling goodness of child–play–environment fit: optimizing
  participation   182
  Using assessment to guide intervention   184

Suzie: assessing development through play 184
Kaisa: assessing and enabling playfulness 186
Ensuring the right conditions for play: assessing barriers and supports 189
Enabling optimal child–environment–play fit 190
Summary 195

10   I can do it: developing, promoting and managing children's self-care needs   200

Children's self-care skills 201
Managing ADL challenges: optimizing children's self-care participation 202
Application of ICF model to paediatric self-care issues 211
Maria 214
The importance of self-care skills 219
Summary 219

11   The transition to school   222

Occupational therapy and preparing children for school 223
Understanding childhood transitions 224
Making the transition to primary school 225
Models of transition 227
The skills only model of transition 227
Developmental model of transition 232
Assisting children to make optimal transitions 232
Goodness of fit 233
Occupational therapy assessment 234
Occupational therapy intervention 234
Summary 236

12   Student participation in the classroom   241

Occupational role of student 242
The student 243
The learning environment 244
The curriculum 249
Occupational therapy to support children's education 250
Occupational therapy evaluation in the schools 251
Occupational therapy intervention in the schools 252
Summary 256

13   Children's participation in physical activity at school   261

Physical activity: definitions, benefits and determinants 261
Definitions 261
Benefits 262
Determinants 262

Current dilemmas surrounding children and physical activity 263
Physical activity within the school curriculum 264
Place and structure of school sport 265
Physical activity: making friends and enemies within the curriculum 266
Physical activity beyond the school curriculum 268
  Recess 268
  Transport to and from school 269
Remedial activity and occupational therapy 271
Summary 273

14 Children's participation beyond the school grounds 280

Defining participation beyond the school grounds 281
  Distribution of out of school time 281
  Balance 284
Leisure 284
  A multidimensional model of time use: the SCOPE-IT model 288
Healthy leisure 290
  Psychosocial benefits 290
  Protective spread of activities 290
  Competence enlargement 291
At-risk leisure 292
  Negative outcomes 292
  Over-committed children 292
  Television viewing 293
  Computer use 294
Summary 294

Index 299

FOREWORD

By Charles H. Christiansen
Professor and Dean
School of Allied Health Sciences, University of Texas Medical Branch

Worldwide, occupational therapy continues to struggle with competing paradigms, characterized by those who prefer to view therapy according to the structural and functional approaches of traditional medicine, versus those who elect to embrace a view of intervention within a paradigm based in activity (occupations) and participation (Christiansen, 1990). The reclamation of occupational therapy's founding principles in practice has been a painfully slow crusade (Kielhofner, 1977; Shannon, 1983). This seems illogical in light of Adolph Meyer's ringing endorsement of occupation as the virtual source of human adaptation and wellbeing (Meyer, 1922). Thus, happily, from my perspective, this book is based on occupational therapy's original founding principles, grounded in the belief that the most effective occupational therapy practice recognizes the inherent developmental and health promoting properties of activity engagement and participation, especially where children are concerned. Accordingly, viewing children as occupational beings is an essential requirement for both occupational therapists and parents, if they hope to be effective in what they do.

My own early experience in the practice arena largely involved adolescents and children but these early years of practice were devoid of the kinds of educational experiences or frameworks that have built on the legacies of the past or that have emerged more recently from occupational science and the new ecological models for understanding health and function in the context of activity and participation. The latest of these models, *The International Classification of Functioning, Disability and Health* (ICF) (WHO, 2001) was used as a key framework for this volume.

Of course, much of what I know that is important and relevant to understanding children and adolescents as individuals with developmental needs has come from the trial and error learning experiences of my role as parent and father to three children who are now young adults. Based on these three unique case studies, I now understand children as emerging 'selves' who are exceptionally influenced by their participation in the world around them. To observe is to participate vicariously and children are keen observers of their worlds. The construction of Carrie, Erik and Kalle's personhoods (my familial case studies) represented a fascinating process of gradual engagement in their worlds, resulting in more confidence and more risk taking and autonomy as they participated in more new activities. Imagine being turned loose in a large clothing store to try on a seemingly endless supply of garments of various colours and styles. This metaphor aptly represents the opportunities children and adolescents have for trying new activities and roles as they develop interests and skills. For my children, this process was a personal quest for each of them to find the most satisfactory fit to complement their emerging identity; a process no doubt motivated by the mental images of their 'possible selves' as described by Hazel Markus and Paul Nurius (1986).

The unfolding of personhood as one moves through every age creates both amazement and anxiety. A US psychologist, Lawrence Kutner (1991), observed: 'Childhood is an adventure both for children and for their parents. There should be freedom to explore and joy in discovery. The important discoveries for both parents and children seldom come at the points where the path is smooth and straight. It is the curves in that path to adventure that make the trip interesting and worthwhile.' (1991, p. 43). Indeed, there is probably little useful progress in identity formation until children encounter new opportunities and challenges. A strong argument can be made that these opportunities and challenges come in the context of role acquisition and development, first in the roles of family membership and later in relationships with others outside the family (as friend, student, team member, classmate, etc.).

Personality psychologist Robert Hogan has asserted that the context of role is necessary as a supporting structure for meaningful interaction. His theory asserts that satisfactory development and maturation throughout the life course depends on an interaction of identity, social roles and a reputation influenced by personality factors (Hogan & Roberts, 2000). As social animals requiring the acceptance of others, humans cannot flourish without an acceptable identity, and this makes the formation of personhood (as defined by roles and activities) an essential and primary task of development. The occupational therapist that understands the important relationships among activities, tasks and roles unlocks the potential of human occupation to use as a powerful therapeutic tool.

Clearly, the chapters in this volume support this perspective. Rodger and Ziviani have laid out a masterful framework for conveying this message in a manner that is logical and well documented. They have assembled a respected and competent group of contributors to examine the influences of environment and individual factors on participation and to illustrate how engagement in occupations leads to the development of skills and mastery necessary for competent role performance and identity formation.

In my opinion, this volume explains ecological approaches to participation exceedingly well, while also providing a useful analysis of developmental perspectives. I am pleased to find that the volume includes chapters on childhood time use, occupational balance (perhaps better understood as a perspective on how to portray the lifestyles of children as more or less beneficial to development), advocacy and leisure; and that it did not neglect a coherent treatment of how learning occurs within various contexts.

It can be argued that the overall view presented is consistent with constructivist approaches to understanding learning as advanced by Vygotsky and others (e.g. Bruner, 1990). Vygotsky (1978) believed that children learned primarily through their social world, which was the source of all their concepts, ideas, facts, skills and attitudes. Constructivism recognizes the unique place of roles in providing a framework for the acquisition of knowledge and skills necessary for assuming a productive and acceptable place in the world. Occupational therapists who understand this will appreciate that they bring a special set of knowledge and skills to the therapeutic setting that will serve them well for interventions with children. They will also find that this book provides a framework that makes planning effective therapy with children practical, relevant, and effective. Rodger and Ziviani should be congratulated for helping occupational therapy reclaim some lost territory in its quest to fully exploit the potential waiting within its heritage. Their contribution to the literature has helped unleash the genie of occupation in the service of improved therapy with children.

References

Bruner, J. (1990). *Acts of Meaning*. Cambridge, MA: Harvard University Press.

Christiansen, C. H. (1991). The perils of plurality. *Occupational Therapy Journal of Research*, 10, 259–265.

Hogan, R. & Roberts, B. W. (2000). A socioanalytic perspective on person/environment interaction. In: W. B. Walsh, K. H. Craik, & R. H. Price (Ed.), *New directions in person–environment psychology* (pp. 1–24). Hillsdale, NJ: Lawrence Erlbaum.

Kielhofner, G. W. & Burke, J. P. (1977). Occupational therapy after sixty years: An account of changing identity. *American Journal of Occupational Therapy*, 31 (10), 675–689.

Kutner, L. (1991). *Parent and Child. Getting Through To Each Other*. New York: Avon.

Markus, H. & Nurius, P. (1986). Possible selves. *American Psychologist*, 41, 954–969.

Meyer, A. (1922). The philosophy of occupation therapy. *Archives of Occupation Therapy*, 1 (1), 1–10.

Shannon, P. D. (1977). The derailment of occupational therapy. *American Journal of Occupational Therapy*, 31, 229–234.

Vygotsky, L. S. (Ed.) (1978). *Mind in society: The development of higher psychological process*. Cambridge, MA: Harvard University Press.

World Health Organization (2001). *International classification of functioning, disability, and health* (ICF). Geneva, Switzerland: Author.

PREFACE

The idea for this book started to take form about five years ago with the realization that there was a need in the occupational therapy literature for broad discussion about children's occupations and promoting their participation across home, school and community. We have drawn upon contemporary research to examine children's roles, their occupations and the skills which underpin their ability to participate in society. In the process of this undertaking it became clear that socio-environmental as well as child centred factors can either facilitate or hinder occupational mastery. Our goal is to help occupational therapists and childhood professionals develop an understanding of how to optimize the participation of children in the various environments in which they are required or choose to engage.

This book comprises two sections. The first focuses on children's roles and occupations in contemporary society at a broad level. The World Health Organization (WHO, 2001) *International classification of functioning, disability and health* (ICF) is used to frame the concept of children's occupations and societal participation. Within this context the impact of personal and environmental factors on children's activities and participation is explored. Specific chapters in this section address children's participation in society today; family influences on children's occupational roles and performance; environmental influences on children's participation, in particular at school and in the community; and children's changing occupational time use and the impact this has on health and wellbeing.

The second section focuses on childhood as a period of significant development and skill acquisition. As well as taking a developmental perspective to understand children's occupations, the concept of occupational roles, occupations and the skills required to engage in occupations (self-care, play, productivity/school, rest and relaxation) are described. This section looks specifically at the acquisition of skills needed for engagement in occupations required of children's occupational roles. Various chapters cover the importance of doing, being and becoming for children; communication and social skills for occupational engagement; supporting the role of player and developing play skills; the development and management of the self-carer role; transition into the role of school student; developing the student role and enabling participation in the classroom; the place of physical activity while at school; and supporting children's participation beyond the school grounds.

We hope that we challenge occupational therapists' and students' thinking about children's roles, the occupations in which children engage and the development of occupational and environmental mastery which supports children's participation at home, school and within their communities.

Sylvia Rodger
Jenny Ziviani

ACKNOWLEDGEMENTS

The ideas for this book could not have been realized without the stimulation and support of many individuals.

We are grateful to our colleagues and friends in the School of Health and Rehabilitation Sciences at the University of Queensland who afforded us this opportunity. This book could not have come together, however, without the commitment of exceptional contributors who are acknowledged internationally for their expertise in the fields of occupational therapy, speech pathology, social work, human movement science and educational psychology. Their adherence to timelines and acceptance of word limitations greatly facilitated the process of editing this book.

Our perspective has been maintained by the presence of our research assistant David Dickson who has always been positive, encouraging and diligently attentive to much administrative detail. Aided by the challenging discussions and critical reviews provided by colleagues and contributors we experienced a real team commitment.

Finally, we are grateful for the ongoing support provided to us by our respective husbands John Worthington and David Wadley. Also, to our children, Elise and Sam Worthington, Owen Wadley and their friends, a special thank you for providing us with rich first hand experience of what it means for children to participate in daily activities and occupations. You have taught us so much.

ABOUT THE EDITORS

Sylvia Rodger BOcc Thy, MEd St, PhD is an occupational therapist with 25 years experience in paediatric occupational therapy as a clinician, academic and researcher. She is currently Head of Division of Occupational Therapy, School of Health and Rehabilitation Sciences at the University of Queensland. She has worked with children with a range of developmental, motor and learning difficulties. She has a keen interest in curriculum development, teaches paediatric occupational therapy and supervises higher degree research students. Her research interests are primarily in the areas of developmental coordination disorder, top-down interventions, cognitive orientation for daily occupational performance, autism spectrum disorder, early intervention, family centred practice and parent education. At the time of writing she has attracted 13 major grants from competitive sources. She has over 60 national and international refereed journal publications, nine book chapters, and has given over 70 conference presentations and numerous invited presentations and workshops. She is on the editorial boards of *Occupational Therapy International* and *Physical and Occupational Therapy in Pediatrics* and reviews for many other journals.

Jenny Ziviani BApp Sc (OT), BA, MEd, PhD is Associate Professor in the Division of Occupational Therapy, School of Health and Rehabilitation Sciences at the University of Queensland. Her clinical, academic and research interests include examining functional outcomes for children who experience injury, disease and disability, the promotion of healthful participation for all children, and the study of socio-environmental factors impacting participation of children with disabilities. These activities have been supported by 24 grants from competitive sources. She has over 60 publications in national and international peer reviewed journals, presented in excess of 70 conference papers and authored or collaborated on 12 book chapters. She has been and continues to be on the editorial boards for a number of professional journals including *Occupational Therapy International* and the *Hong Kong Journal of Occupational Therapy*. She has been recognized for her contribution to occupational therapy in Australia by being awarded the Libby Lucas Fellowship for leadership in occupational therapy and the Mary Rankine Wilson Award for contribution to the profession of occupational therapy in Queensland, Australia.

CONTRIBUTORS

Rebecca Abbott, BSc(Hons), Nutrition Dip Dietetics, PhD
Human Movement Scientist and Post-doctoral Fellow, School of Human Movement Studies, the University of Queensland, Australia.

G. Ted Brown, BSc OT(Hons), MSc, MPA, PhD, OT(C), OTR, AccOT
Occupational Therapist and Senior Lecturer, Occupational Therapy Program, School of Primary Health Care, Monash University, Frankston, Victoria, Australia.

Monica Cuskelly, BA(Hons), GradDipEd, MEd St, Armidale CAE, MApp Psych, PhD
Psychologist and Senior Lecturer, School of Education, the University of Queensland, Australia.

Yvonne Darlington, BA, BSoc Wk, PGDipAdv SWPractice, PhD
Social Worker and Senior Lecturer, School of Social Work and Applied Human Sciences, the University of Queensland, Australia.

Jane A. Davis, MSc, OT Reg (Ont), OT(C), OTR
Occupational Therapist and Doctoral Candidate, Department of Occupational Therapy, University of Toronto, Ontario, Canada.

Laura Desha, BOcc Thy(Hons)
Occupational Therapist and Doctoral Candidate, Division of Occupational Therapy, the University of Queensland, Australia.

Gillian King, PhD
Thames Valley Children's Centre, London, Ontario, Canada.

Mary Law, FCA OT, OT Reg (Ont), PhD
Occupational Therapist and Dean of Rehabilitation Sciences, Faculty of Health Sciences, McMaster University, Institute for Applied Health Sciences, Hamilton, Ontario, Canada.

Doune Macdonald, BHMS(Ed)(Hons), PhD
Professor and Head of School of Human Movement Studies, the University of Queensland, Australia.

Angela Mandich, PhD, OT(C)
Occupational Therapist and Assistant Professor, School of Occupational Therapy, Faculty of Health Sciences, the University of Western Ontario, London, Ontario, Canada.

Cathy McBryde, BOcc Thy(Hons), PhD
Occupational Therapist in private practice, Jindalee, Queensland, Australia.

Mary Muhlenhaupt, OTR/L, FAOTA
Occupational Therapist in private practice, Valley Forge, Pennsylvania, United States of America.

Terry Petrenchik, PhD, OTR/L
Occupational Therapist and academic, School of Rehabilitation Science, McMaster University, IAHS, Hamilton, Ontario, Canada.

Helene J. Polatajko, PhD, OT(C), OT Reg (Ont), FCAOT
Occupational Therapist and Chair of Occupational Therapy Program, Department of Occupational Therapy, University of Toronto, Ontario, Canada.

Anne Poulsen, BOcc Thy(Hons)
Occupational Therapist and Doctoral Candidate, Division of Occupational Therapy, School of Health and Rehabilitation Sciences, University of Queensland, Australia.

Patty Rigby, OT Reg (Ont), MHSc OT
Occupational Therapist and academic, Department of Occupational Therapy, University of Toronto, Canada.

Sylvia Rodger, BOcc Thy, MEd St, PhD
Occupational Therapist and Head of Division of Occupational Therapy, School of Health and Rehabilitation Sciences, the University of Queensland, Australia.

Gail Woodyatt, BSp Thy, PhD
Speech Pathologist and Senior Lecturer, Division of Speech Pathology, School of Health and Rehabilitation Sciences, the University of Queensland, Australia.

Jenny Ziviani, BApp Sc (OT), BA, MEd, PhD
Occupational Therapist an Associate Professor, Division of Occupational Therapy, School of Health and Rehabilitation Sciences, the University of Queensland, Australia.

SECTION 1

CHILDREN'S ROLES, OCCUPATIONS AND PARTICIPATION IN CONTEMPORARY SOCIETY

CHILDREN, THEIR ENVIRONMENTS, ROLES AND OCCUPATIONS IN CONTEMPORARY SOCIETY

Sylvia Rodger and Jenny Ziviani

This chapter provides an overview of children in contemporary society. It further highlights the dynamic interaction between the developing child, the communities within which they live and the impact on the child of rapidly changing social, economic, physical, cultural and technological environments. The objectives of this chapter are to:

(1) Describe what life is like for children in contemporary post-industrial societies and to examine the impact of rapid environmental change
(2) Introduce the *International Classification of Functioning, Disability and Health* (ICF) (World Health Organization, 2001) as a means of understanding how children's health and wellbeing can be impacted by various health conditions and the interactive effect of environment and the activities in which they are engaged
(3) Describe how occupational therapists understand children's roles and how these roles shape children's occupations and their participation in contemporary society

Children in contemporary society

Talk to parents, teachers, or read the newspaper and it becomes clear that, as with every previous generation, there is currently concern about children. Yet the experience of growing up has not changed dramatically over time and still involves an interaction between individual biology and the social, economic, physical, cultural and technological environments. It is the change in these environments and the way children respond to them that results in uncertainty on the part of adults who are concerned with children's welfare. But is there a need for alarm? Surely, the first step is to understand the impact of these changes on children. It is incumbent upon occupational therapists and others concerned with children's wellbeing to come to terms with these influences, both advantageous and deleterious, and advance the most supportive environments for healthful participation.

Social environment

If we consider the social issues currently facing children we need first to examine the impact of changing family structure. In Australia single parent families represented 29% of all families in 2001 (Australian Bureau of Statistics [ABS], 2001; 2003a). Complicating these demographics is the growing number of blended families in which children might need to accommodate step-siblings as well as another parent figure. The emotional adjustment necessitated by these situations is often also accompanied by practical factors such as relocation and living between two households. Add to this the distancing from extended families that now occurs as a result of an increasingly mobile community and the lessening of community connectedness and we have a picture of fragmenting familial and social support networks.

Another demographic reality is that couples are choosing either not to have children or delaying parenting and then only having one or two children (ABS, 2003a; 2003b). This is a striking change from previous generations in which families were larger and hence provided a ready network of playmates. Both older parents and those with fewer offspring often seek more structured play and social opportunities for their children. This is manifesting in an increase in paid group activities which previously occurred informally in local parks, playgrounds and family homes. Many of these engagements appear to be targeting insecurities in parents and promoting often unrealistic expectations of the impact of early learning, play and musical exposure on children's success in schooling, sport and the creative arts. Some have even suggested that these children are so closely monitored that they are 'bubble-wrapped' (Jane Cadzow, Good Weekend, 17 January 2004). Others have gone further, remarking that we are producing the equivalent of battery-reared chickens (Hillman, 1999) who are restricted from exploring their environments and now lack the initiative and resourcefulness of their predecessors. This phenomenon appears to be largely post-industrial and urban. There is evidence that children growing up in rural environments lead a less restricted existence and that some societies (such as Germany) (Hillman, 1999) and indigenous communities (Nelson & Allison, 2000) are more supportive of independence for children.

For others the experience of childhood is in sharp contrast to that described above. Children growing up in poverty can either experience marginalization when they are in a society of 'haves' and 'have-nots' or experience a sense of solidarity when they are part of a broader community all sharing the same hardships. The type of insecurity experienced by these children relates more to basic needs such as shelter, food and familial stability. Life for children today, however, can pose challenges in both these contrasting situations.

The social and economic phenomenon of two working parents became more pronounced in the late 1990s and continues to be the norm rather than the exception in the twenty-first century (Organization for Economic Co-operation and Development [OECD], 2003). As a result, more children are now being cared for by people other than parents (such as paid carers, relatives) both at home and in childcare centres. Estimates are as high as 60% for children in their preschool years (Mackay, 1999). In order to accommodate the schedules of working parents and the needs of children, many families have developed highly structured routines as a way of juggling these multiple demands. As such, young children's routines need to conform to adult work habits and are characterized by long hours (often away from home) and structured tight schedules. The concept of the 'hurried child' advanced in 1981 by David Elkind is now a reality. Social commentators question the impact that this pressure is likely to have on children's experience of childhood, parent's experience of parenthood and the role models being provided for our next generation of parents (Mackay, 1999).

Physical environment

The physical environment in which children are growing up has changed, and continues to change. Increasingly, children have physically less play space both at home, with small or non-existent yards, and in the community, with the encroachment of housing on limited open space. Compounding this cramping is the perception held by many parents that the physical and social environment is no longer safe for unsupervised play activities and simple activities such as walking to school (Sallis et al., 1997). This fear can lead parents to limit children's activities and participation. In turn, the fear can be internalized, making children anxious and more restricted in how they engage with their environment. For example a ten-year-old child who has never been allowed to cross a road independently or access the local park with friends might not have developed the basic skills of road sense, confidence to travel independently and negotiate and problem solve play rules with friends, or have a sense of personal safety.

Cultural environment

Many post-industrial societies have become increasingly multicultural. Children are growing up interacting with children from diverse cultural backgrounds. The point of connection for children is shared activity. For some this engagement may be fostered at home through parental networks, while for others this can occur at childcare, preschool or formal schooling. People working with children need to acknowledge differing cultural attitudes towards children and childhood. These attitudes influence expectations of children, the value and the range of activities in which children participate. For example, a demographic shift in a school population can result in changing popularity of a number of extra-curricular activities. What might have been a well attended and parent supported rugby team in an Australian school may not continue to be so if the school population is more accustomed to soccer as part of their cultural background.

Technological environment

Rapid developments in communication and entertainment technology have had an unprecedented impact on how children interact, spend their time and process world events. The first consideration is that of substitution. What is watching TV or videos, playing with video games or using the Internet replacing? We already have evidence that, for children in their primary school years, this activity consumes the same amount of daily time as their engagement in physical activity (Ziviani et al., in press). We also know that childhood obesity is on the increase and that it is associated with a reduction in physical activity, as well as changing dietary patterns (Trost et al., 2001), and has long-term implications for adult health outcomes (Malina, 1996). Extended periods of screen use have been implicated in eye strain, development of myopia, headaches, neck and back pain in adults (Burgess-Limerick et al., 1999). The implications for children are only just beginning to emerge (Harris & Staker, 2000).

The second consideration relates to the often insular nature of these activities. It is both easy entertainment and 'safe' for children to be at home engaged in screen based activity. Yet, this potential insularity can change the way in which children engage with families and peers (The Royal Australasian College of Physicians [RACP], 2004). Play has become increasingly virtual, with little need to negotiate or communicate with other players. The implications for social and mental health of this shift are also being questioned. For example, the Brisbane *Sunday Mail* newspaper (29 February 2004) ran a headline 'Kids love PCs, not People', reporting that many children considered their PC as a trusted friend. For some, time at the keyboard made them happier than time with family and friends.

The third consideration is the impact on children of graphic exposure to world events. Young children repeatedly experienced 11 September 2001 in an unprecedented way. The immediate footage that appeared on television screens around the world and interrupted regular viewing schedules exposed children to a horrifying event which challenged their concept of living in a safe world. Every day children watching television confront world events such as this.

The Internet and mobile phone have also impacted on the way children learn to communicate. Messages are cryptic when sent electronically either by MSN or SMS. Reliance on virtual, rather than face to face communication, has the potential to change the way this generation interacts with one another, negotiates social contact and remains connected. All these communication technologies have the potential to decrease the need for mobility. For example, a child can access literature on the Internet instead of visiting the local library, chat to friends on email or MSN instead of visiting, and listen to downloaded music without leaving their home workstation. While these practices are increasingly becoming the norm, and some would argue for their time efficiency, they have potential influences on the way in which children interact and lead to physical inactivity. The impact on their physical and emotional health and wellbeing is yet to be determined.

While every generation struggles to come to terms with the way in which the next is growing up and the type of world in which this is happening, some of the issues highlighted above have the potential to change what it means to be a child in the twenty-first century. There are also some health issues which need to be considered. If biology or health is compromised, and even if it is not, the social, economic, cultural and technological environment in which children grow up can either facilitate or hinder their development. This view of health has been encapsulated by the World Health Organization in its *International classification of functioning, disability and health* (ICF) (WHO, 2001), which has acknowledged the multidimensional and multidirectional nature of health and wellbeing for people. It is this framework which underpins the way we will advance our understanding of children, their roles, occupations and environment in today's society.

International classification of function framework

Occupational therapists have a history of viewing their practice as an interaction of individuals, their environments and the activities in which they engage to enable occupational performance. The 1990s produced literature rich in espousing this view (Canadian Association of Occupational Therapists, 2002; Christiansen & Baum, 1997; Dunn et al., 1994; Kielhofner, 1995; Law et al., 1996;). The turn of the century has seen the core principles of individual, environment and activity/participation given an international and cross-disciplinary voice by the World Health Organization in the form of the ICF (WHO, 2001).

The ICF was proposed as a scientific framework for understanding and studying health and health related states, outcomes and determinants. Its authors also argued that if adopted broadly it would enhance communication between health care workers, researchers and the public by providing a classification system for grouping different domains for a person with a given health condition (WHO, 2001). The ICF has three important tenets:

(1) Universal application, whereby all people, not only a minority traditionally referred to as disabled, can have their experience of a health condition described
(2) An integrated approach that acknowledges the impact of individual characteristics and social factors as contributing to the way in which a health condition is experienced and how interventions can be considered
(3) An interactive structure that acknowledges the complex and multidimensional phenomenon of health and wellbeing when impacted by a medical condition

Another advance made by the ICF on earlier versions of classification systems developed by WHO is the attempt to make terminology neutral. Instead of using terms such as impairments, used in the earlier version known as the International Classification of Impairments, Disabilities and Handicaps (ICIDH) (Wood, 1980), the ICF adopts the word function (for example, mental functions instead of intellectual impairments).

ICF structure

If the universality of the ICF is to be incorporated into occupational therapy thinking and practice, the first step is to understand its structure and terminology. Figure 1.1 represents the overall structure of the ICF as a classification system. Broadly speaking it is divided into two parts. The first is *Functioning and disability*. *Functioning* and *disability* are used as two contrasting terms. The term 'functioning' relates to the successful completion of major daily activities across a broad range of life areas or expected roles. Disability is described as an inability to perform these critical life activities in ways that would be described within the normal range. Within this first part are the components of *Body functions and structures*, and *Activities and participation*. *Body functions* refer to the physiological functions of the body system including psychological and *Body structures* refer to anatomical parts of the body, organs, limbs and their components. *Activities* involve the execution of a task or action, and *participation* refers to involvement in life situations. The terms *constructs* or *qualifiers* are used to talk about how the various components can be interpreted. *Body functions and structures* can be qualified on the basis of how a health condition has changed them. *Activities and participation*, however, are qualified on the basis of performance (what an individual does in their environment) and capacity (how an individual is able to execute a task or action in a standardized environment).

The second part is contextual and includes *Environmental and personal factors*. Environment in this context is seen to relate to the physical, social and attitudinal environment in which people live and is described as pertaining to:

(1) Products and technology
(2) Natural environment and human made changes to the environment
(3) Support and relationships
(4) Attitudes
(5) Services, systems and policies (Schneidert et al., 2003)

These are seen to have either a positive or negative influence on the individual's health and functional performance. *Personal factors* are concerned with the particular background of an individual's life and living and comprise features of the individual that are not part of a health condition or health state (for example gender, age, upbringing, education). There remains some debate as to the location of some of these features, for example the ICF places 'fitness' and 'coping abilities' here, while it could be argued that these features are health states capable of modification. *Environmental factors* are qualified as facilitators or barriers/hindrances to functioning but *personal factors* are taken as given and not interpreted.

The model of the ICF depicted in Figure 1.1 looks at the parts and components alone and demonstrates the next fundamental shift in the view of health and wellbeing adopted by WHO (2001), namely, that it is multidirectional. The ICF is based on an integration of a medical model of disability which views it as a problem of the person that requires medical intervention, and a social model of disability which

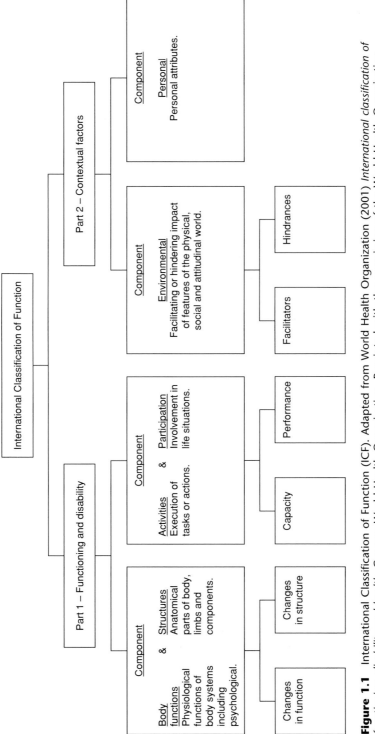

Figure 1.1 International Classification of Function (ICF). Adapted from World Health Organization (2001) *International classification of functioning, disability and health*. Geneva: World Health Organization. Reprinted with the permission of the World Health Organisation.

sees the issue mainly as a socially created problem requiring social action to enable an individual to fully participate in the community. Thus, the ICF adopts a 'biopsychosocial' approach (WHO, 2001). No longer are connections between components unidirectional, as might be assumed in the medical model, rather it is clearly acknowledged that body function does not just influence the ability to perform activities and hence enable participation, but also that *Environmental factors* can impact on the performance of activities and even modify *Body function and structures*. This is clearly a more global view of health and wellbeing and one highly consistent with occupational therapy philosophy and practice (Baum & Baptiste, 2002), particularly with its emphasis on participation (Christiansen & Baum, 2005).

The framework is not only applicable to individuals with disabilities, but also it can be applied to all people (Bickenbach et al., 1999). For example, a child born without a health condition may be exposed to lead paint in the first few years of life. The physical environment in this situation coupled with the social environment in which the dangers of this exposure are not understood, results in the child developing a health condition which in turn will impact on body function and hence activity and participation. This example highlights the multidirectional and interactive nature of this model in relation to health and wellbeing.

In another example, a child born with a club foot has alterations to the structure of their foot which can prohibit walking and hence the ability to participate with peers in a range of occupationally relevant roles. In this example, if the child is living in a country (environmental component) with advanced medical procedures, interventions would be targeted at the body structure to modify the foot to the extent that ambulation would be possible and hence participation in daily activities achievable. What, however, would happen if the child was born in a situation where medical technology was not able to offer this intervention? The child might be prohibited from involvement in activities and either marginalized or, depending on the social context, allocated a role consistent with their abilities. Alternatively, the activities and environment might be modified to accommodate the mobility restriction and hence disability might still not arise because potential barriers have been addressed.

Reactions to the ICF

Response from the clinical, research and public arena to the publication of the ICF has been largely positive. Researchers and clinicians have looked at its application for people with cognitive disorders (Arthanat et al., 2004); severe and multiple disability (Bronman, 2004); mental disorders (Kennedy, 2003); and childhood disability (Simeonsson et al., 2003). What is emerging is that the administration and interpretation of this framework has the potential to facilitate health care and promotion by being consistent and meaningful on a global and cross-cultural scale. It is a framework which can accommodate existing assessments used by health professionals and also, because of its structure, identifies where further instrumentation needs to be developed. Researchers in the area of child health (Simeonsson et al.,

2003), however, point to the need to further examine the way in which childhood disability is differentiated, the impact of developmental and environmental factors, and the purpose of assessment.

Children often present with an overlap of health condition, diagnoses and aetiological factors (often the basis of developmental difficulties is hard to specify). An illustration of where this applies with respect to receiving support services is the Individuals with Disabilities Education Act in the USA (Office of Special Education and Rehabilitation Services, 1997). Here, eligibility for special education services is determined on the basis that disability is identified as:

> '(a) children with mental retardation, hearing impairments, deafness, visual impairments including blindness, deaf-blindness, multiple disabilities, speech and language impairments, autism, traumatic brain injury, other health impairments or specific learning disabilities; and (b) who by reason thereof, need special education and related services.' (Office of Special Education and Rehabilitation Services, 1997, p. 9)

This example highlights that access to services currently encompasses aetiology, health conditions, disorders, impairments, activity limitations, as well as participation restrictions.

For children, furthermore, the mediating roles of environment and development are highly important. Children's environments change across the stages of infancy, early childhood, middle childhood and adolescence. Each of these environmental changes exposes children to new demands and experiences. The way children respond to these physical and social environmental expectations frames a developmental process which leads to the acquisition of increasingly complex skills. See Chapter 7.

Occupational therapy intervention aims to enable children (and adults) to engage in occupation to support participation in context (American Occupational Therapy Association [AOTA], 2002). Occupational therapy's focus on engagement in occupation to support participation complements the WHO perspective (WHO, 2001) articulated in the ICF. In order to understand children's activities and participation from an occupational therapy perspective, it is important to explore children's roles in contemporary society and the occupations in which they engage. The following section addresses children's roles and occupations, different types of roles and how these change during the course of childhood, the interaction between roles, socialization and learning, and how occupational therapy intervention can change role dysfunction into role competence.

Children's roles and occupations

Roles have been defined in the occupational therapy literature as 'a set of behaviours that have some socially agreed upon function and for which there is an accepted code of norms' (Christiansen & Baum, 1997, p. 56). Roles can also be defined as 'positions in society having expected responsibilities and privileges' (Christiansen & Baum, 1997, p. 56). Roles enable an individual to define themself and provide the context for occupational performance in work, play and self-care tasks (Kielhofner, 2002a; Kielhofner & Burke, 1985). Occupational role performance and, more specifically, participation in the occupations of daily life have also been proposed to have a direct and positive influence on lifestyle, health and wellbeing (Hillman & Chapparo, 1995; Laliberte-Rudman, 2002; Lambert, 1998; Law, 2002). Meaningful engagement in desired roles and occupations allows a child to participate in the daily occupations associated with these roles in their home, school and community.

Occupation refers to 'everything people do to occupy themselves, including looking after themselves . . . enjoying life . . . and contributing to the social and economic fabric of their communities' (Law et al., 1997, p. 32). It is hypothesized that occupation is positively linked to wellbeing because it fulfils a basic human need to 'do', provides a sense of purpose, provides a means to organize time and space, and is a medium for the development and expression of identity (Laliberte-Rudman, 2002). The interaction between occupation and wellbeing or quality of life is less well understood for children than it is for adults. Few studies have addressed this interaction specifically for children.

Types of roles

The concept of role is drawn from social psychology. Roles relate to positions in society which have expected responsibilities and privileges (Mead, 1934). There are many different types of roles. Matsutsuyu (1971) divided roles into three coexisting systems – familial, personal-sexual and occupational roles. *Familial roles* refer to an individual's roles within the family and extended family context (for example grandchild, sibling, niece, cousin). *Personal-sexual roles* refer to one's gender role as a male or female. *Occupational roles* refer to culturally defined roles that represent the organization of time and occupations by individuals, groups or communities (for example mother, athlete, employee, artist) (Canadian Association of Occupational Therapists, 2002). More specifically, occupational roles are composed of patterns of occupational performance that pertain to a person's occupations in the areas of work/productivity or school, play or leisure, self-care or self-maintenance, and spirituality (for example student, player, self-carer, religious participant) within specific social and cultural contexts. Occupational roles are identified both by social position (particularly formal roles such as student) and by the tasks performed within these roles. Informal roles such as family member or self-carer are often defined more by the tasks performed and expectations of role behaviour, and are influenced by family socialization, culture and norms.

Individuals may have simultaneous roles. However, at any one point in time some roles are in the foreground, while others remain in the background. Within a twenty-four hour period, the roles of an individual may change frequently in terms of which roles are pre-eminent. For example, an eight-year-old boy (Barry) lives at home with both parents and his three older brothers. He has a grandmother who lives nearby in a retirement village. He attends the local school, where he is in fourth grade. He plays baseball in summer and football in winter, training one afternoon per week and playing matches at the weekends. He also plays ball games with friends in his neighbourhood in the quiet cul-de-sac and on his PlayStation™ or computer. He learns the guitar and attends lessons once a week. He also collects and reads Phantom comics. He attends church on Sundays with his family. Barry's personal-sexual role is that of a *male*. His familial roles are those of *son* (describing his role in relationship to his parents), *brother* (his role with regard to his siblings), and *grandson* (role in relation to his grandmother). His occupational roles are *school student* (when attending to school work, either at school or homework, related to work/productivity occupations), *team member* (when training for and playing football or baseball, related to play/leisure occupations), *friend* (when hanging out with kids at school or playing with neighbours, which is related to play occupations), *hobbyist* as a comic collector (when collecting, reading, sorting out his comics and related to leisure occupations), *guitar player* (when attending guitar lessons, practising at home and related to leisure occupations), *self-carer* (when he attends to eating, dressing, toileting, grooming and hygiene, and makes himself snacks after school), and *religious participant* (when attending formal religious services in relation to spirituality occupations). During a weekday, his primary occupational role is that of student, as he spends most of his waking day at school and doing some homework, while secondary roles may include *friend* (when he plays at recess and after school in the neighbourhood), *guitar player* (when he does his daily practice), and *self-carer* (when he looks after his self-care needs). The primacy of these roles change at the weekend, when he has more discretionary time. During this time his occupational roles as friend, team member, religious participant, hobbyist and self-carer are more dominant. His personal-sexual role as a male remains constant, as do his familial roles. However, the amount of time he spends enacting familial roles may alter depending on the amount of daily contact he has with siblings, parents and grandparents.

According to Chapparo & Ranka (1997) occupational roles have three dimensions. First, *knowing* refers to having an intuitive understanding of desired or expected occupational performance roles. Second, the process of *doing* entails the physical action of people within their environment. Third, *being* addresses the interpersonal and socio-emotional aspects of role identity. *Being* refers to fulfilment or satisfaction with occupational role performance and is linked to personal meaning, which contributes to the valuing of one's occupational role. These dimensions will be discussed further in Chapter 6.

Occupational roles during childhood

Roles are dynamic, such that they are being acquired and replaced throughout life. They change within the context of a day and throughout the life cycle (Heard, 1977). Roles are regulated by age, ability, experience, circumstances and time (Hillman & Chapparo, 1995). Major life roles are associated with developmental tasks and age appropriate function. Thus, occupational role acquisition is an ongoing process that transforms and builds on previously acquired skills to enable an individual to assume the demands of new occupational roles within a developmentally appropriate sequence or within an increasingly larger role collection (Heard, 1977).

The ease with which an individual acquires new roles and occupations is dependent on the adaptive nature of the individual (Heard, 1977). Each individual manages many roles (familial, sexual and occupational) that demand different obligations, activities and responses. An example will help illustrate some of these role changes during the course of childhood. When Isabelle was three years of age, her primary occupational roles were that of *player*, while her role of *self-carer* was secondary and still developing (she could undress easily but needed assistance with dressing, was fully toilet trained, fed herself most foods, but needed assistance with grooming and bathing), and the role of *student* did not yet exist. Even when she attended a half-day kindergarten session, her main role was *player*. She was just beginning to develop the social role of *friend*. Now that she is thirteen years old, her primary occupational role is that of *student* as she spends most of her week-days at school. She also has important roles as *team member* (playing softball), *self-carer*, *friend* and *player*. She plays with friends during recess and several, who live nearby, visit her at weekends, and sometimes have a sleep-over at her house. In terms of her role as *player*, she enjoys listening to music, chatting on the Internet, reading teen novels and girls' magazines in her leisure time. During adolescence, there is a transition from the concept of play to that of recreation/leisure. Her personal-sexual role of *female*, and familial roles of *child*, *sibling*, and *niece* remain relatively constant from three to thirteen years. However, the expression of these roles changes with development, skill acquisition, and as social and cultural expectations of behaviour and performance change over time. The way individuals balance the configuration of roles at any one time and the decision about which roles are discarded and which roles are assumed, form transitions in occupational role behaviour that occur throughout the lifespan in response to environmental demands (Chapparo & Ranka, 1997). Developmental transitions are important as they involve the development of new skills (the new role of school student or friend which did not exist at three years) or the integration of previously learned skills.

Role importance

The other aspect of role that alters is the importance ascribed to various roles during childhood, both by the child themself and by significant others. Importance can often be understood by looking at the amount of time children spend enacting certain roles. However, the time spent in role enactment does not necessarily always equate with the importance of the role from the child's perspective. Undoubtedly, for most teenagers, the social role of friend is of utmost importance. They spend more time with friends than family and seek out opportunities to be with friends, whether that be at school, at weekends, or before and after school – even travelling to school on public transport becomes a social event. At this age, young people may start to view their role as friend as being more important than their roles as sibling, daughter or grandchild. Certainly, more time is spent in this pursuit. From the perspective of occupational roles, while the student role continues to be both important and time consuming in the early teen years, the amount of time and importance of the self-carer role and its associated occupations becomes paramount. The amount of time and attention some young teenage girls start to spend on occupations associated with grooming is testament to the importance of this role. Much to parents' consternation more interest can be shown in these pursuits than in homework, an occupation associated with the student role, or household chores, associated with self-maintenance.

Roles, socialization and learning

Roles affect development and personality, as successful enactment of roles leads to strong social approval, while unsuccessful role enactment and failure to meet role expectations leads to strong social disapproval. Roles are therefore mediated by the child's social and cultural environment. The socialization process is therefore about the process of learning role behaviours (Christiansen & Baum, 1997). Early in a child's life the process of communicating role expectations or socialization is largely determined by parents. However, over time teachers and peers become more influential in the socialization process. Parents provide expectations of children around becoming a family member (such as where and how to play, conforming with family routines, and responsibilities for self-care and chores). These expectations are usually more informal than role expectations that come later in life (Kielhofner, 2002a; 2002b). Role socialization involves a developmental progression from informal to more formal roles as childhood progresses. Socialization, therefore, is an ongoing process because roles change throughout life. Certain role transitions are well supported and celebrated, such as entering and exiting the student role (for example transitioning to school and leaving high school), while other transitions are forced by circumstances and hence less well prepared for (for example a biking accident causing traumatic brain injury resulting in a child being forced into the patient role). Role change is complex, involving change to identity, relationships, tasks and actions needed to be performed and organization of lifestyle (Kielhofner, 2002b). This often requires significant reorganization for both individuals and their social networks and systems.

Through this socialization process, people acquire roles that derive from a social status. Socialization involves interacting over time with explicit and implicit definitions and expectations of various roles (Kielhofner, 2002b). As a result, an individual internalizes a sense of self, which impacts on outlook and attitudes, and evokes certain behaviours. For example, children learn to interact differently with their own parents from the way they interact with other adults such as teachers, neighbours and shopkeepers. Identity can be conceptualized in terms of personal and social identity, with personal identity referring to the individual's self-perceptions and self-evaluations that are personally meaningful, and social identity referring to how a person is viewed by others (Laliberte-Rudman, 2002). Therefore identity is a dynamic process involving person–environment interaction.

The individual's sense of identity implies not only an internal view of self, but also a public recognition of one's status. Some roles, such as self-carer, are defined less by social status and more by interrelated and ongoing tasks for which an individual is responsible. These roles arise out of personal circumstances or necessity (Kielhofner, 2002a), where the term 'internalized role' is defined as the 'incorporation of a socially and/or personally defined status and a related cluster or attitudes and behaviours' (p. 22). Internalizing the role refers to taking on an identity, an outlook and actions that belong to that role. This role internalization involves gaining a sense of one's relationships with others and of expected behaviours. In the case of the role of student, the child develops a sense of how they relate to other students as well as teachers, the principal, volunteers helping at the canteen or with classroom activities such as reading. Hence, the child identifies with their student role, which means both internalizing elements of what society attributes to the role, along with one's personal interpretation of that role (Kielhofner, 2002b). Each child's identification with the student role will be individual as their personal identification with, and interpretation of, that role will be unique.

From a young age, in most cultures, children start to associate certain behaviours with being male or female through play objects, how they play and with whom they associate. This embodiment of masculine and feminine behaviour is part of the socialization process associated with personal-sexual roles, which is stereotyped in many societies. Similarly, children come to learn the behavioural expectations and pro-social behaviour associated with the role of friend, such as sharing and taking turns, saying sorry when something goes wrong, helping when someone is hurt, as well as how to manage sharing a friend with other people and managing jealousy and disappointment. The role of sports team member requires learning not only the skills requisite for the team sport (such as football or basketball), but also the skills and behaviours associated with sportsmanship (for example losing graciously, encouraging all players, accepting the referee's decisions), team cooperation, and sports etiquette.

Role dysfunction and role competence

Life roles provide a framework, which helps to define the organization and type of occupations that an individual performs. As such, roles demand that a collection of occupations is performed in a logical, timely and socially appropriate manner. Christiansen (1999) proposed a hierarchy of abilities, actions, tasks, occupations and roles. It is through the occupations associated with occupational roles that individuals are able to express themselves and their identities. Performance of tasks and occupations contributes to shaping identity and the realization of acceptable identity contributes to wellbeing (Christiansen, 1999). Occupation provides a sense of purpose and structure in daily activities and over time. Individuality can therefore be expressed by engagement in meaningful occupation and enactment of roles (Laliberte-Rudman, 2002). Competence and satisfaction with role performance is based on internal as well as external perceptions of performance.

Roles shape what children do and how they view the world. They also profoundly influence who children are, that is, their identities (Forsyth & Kielhofner, 2003). Children see themselves as students, friends, siblings and team members, because they recognize themselves as occupying a certain position or status and because they experience themselves through these roles. Roles also provide an awareness of a social identity and related obligations (Forsyth & Kielhofner, 2003). For example, the role of school student provides a child with an identity as a student of a particular school. Uniforms and dress codes reinforce this identity. Expectations by principals and teachers of children's behaviour at school also reinforce this identity (for example punctuality, codes of conduct in relation to classroom and playground behaviour) and obligations are learned in relation to homework, working in class, participation in school sports activities, etc. In summary, roles impact on children's identity, their use of time and their involvement in social groups. Roles provide structure to children's days. It is important that children have a balance in their role involvement so that they are neither over-involved in roles leading to excessive demands, role conflict and stress, or under-involved resulting in boredom and 'rolelessness'.

According to Kielhofner (2002b) roles organize action in three ways:

(1) By influencing the manner and content of actions (for example school students dress and behave differently when at school compared to playing in the local park)
(2) By carrying a range of actions that make up the role in such a way that roles shape the kinds of things individuals do (for example the student is expected to attend class, take notes, undertake assignments and exams)
(3) By partitioning daily and weekly cycles into times when certain roles are inhabited or enacted (for example for younger students the student role is mostly enacted on weekdays; however, for teenagers additional homework assignments mean that they enact student roles at weekends as well)

When a person cannot perform roles to their satisfaction, due to disease or disability, deficits in skills or abilities, the conflicting demands of multiple roles (role conflict), or unclear role expectations, dysfunction is said to be present (Christiansen, 1999). Rogers (1983) defined occupational performance dysfunction as disruption in carrying out the roles of daily living. Occupational therapists work in medical, educational and community settings with children whose occupational performance has been affected by role conflict or disruption.

The following example illustrates the potency of engaging in occupations associated with childhood roles in rehabilitation and recovery. Following a traumatic brain injury, requiring a significant period of in-patient rehabilitation, ten-year-old Jeremy's occupational therapist talked to him about the things he did before his accident. She discovered that a valued role was that of Scout. Indeed, many of his friends were in the same Scout group. His roles of friend and Scout were both disrupted during his hospitalization. The hospital environment and the extent of his injury were both contributing to this role disruption. The occupational therapist arranged for his Scout leader to visit him, along with some Scout group friends. Discussion with Jeremy and his Scout leader, enabled the occupational therapist to help Jeremy to work towards the next badge (in cooking) he wished to achieve. She used her skills in adapting and grading activities and teaching new skills to assist Jeremy to master the cooking tasks he needed to obtain his next badge. This enabled him to engage in the occupations associated with his roles of Scout and friend and to experience role competence. Viewed within the ICF framework the health condition experienced by Jeremy had restricted his participation in Scouts because he could no longer attend the meetings. Yet modification to this barrier by restructuring the requirements of the task enabled him to continue to participate. Role competence has been described as the ability to effectively meet the demands of the roles in which individuals engage (American Association of Occupational Therapy [AOTA], 2002). For clients accessing occupational therapy, the development of role competence has been described as an important outcome of intervention.

Summary

In this chapter, we have started to paint a picture of what life is like for children in contemporary post-industrial societies. In particular, the impact on children today of rapid change in family and community social structures, the economic realities for families, the perceived safety of and restricted free space in urban physical environments and the increasing use of virtual communication technologies, were highlighted.

We then turned to the ICF (WHO, 2001) as a framework for understanding the impact of health conditions on children, acknowledging that occupational therapists come into contact with children when they experience some form of health condition that affects how they function and participate in home, school and community contexts. The ICF will be used throughout this book as a framework for guiding our thinking about functioning and disability (comprised of *Body function and structures*, *Activity and participation* and *Contextual factors*, *Personal and environmental*) which influence children's health and wellbeing.

Finally, we looked at children's roles and occupations in contemporary society. We described different types of roles and how these roles change throughout childhood in terms of their primacy and importance. To a large extent roles influence what children do with their time (their occupations) and their identities. The impact of health conditions on children's roles, occupations, identity and wellbeing was also highlighted. The pivotal role of occupational therapists in grading and adapting occupations and activities, promoting skill acquisition and modifying the environment, enables children to develop competence in their social, familial and occupational roles. Through occupational engagement children are able to participate in their home, school and community contexts. Such participation promotes health and wellbeing.

References

American Occupational Therapy Association (AOTA) (2002). Occupational therapy practice framework: domain and process. *American Journal of Occupational Therapy*, 56, 609–639.

Arthanat, S., Nochajski, S. & Stone, J. (2004). The international classification of functioning, disability and health and its application to cognitive disorders. *Disability and Rehabilitation*, 26 (4), 235–245.

Australian Bureau of Statistics (ABS) (2001). *Australian social trends: family, family formation – older mothers* (Catalogue No. 4102.0). Canberra: Commonwealth Government of Australia.

Australian Bureau of Statistics (ABS) (2003a). *Australian social trends: family and community, family functioning – family and work* (Catalogue No. 4102.0). Canberra: Commonwealth Government of Australia.

Australian Bureau of Statistics (ABS) (2003b). *Family characteristics, Australia*. Canberra: Commonwealth Government of Australia.

Baum, C. & Baptiste, S. (2002). Reframing occupational therapy practice. In: M. Law, C. Baum & S. Baptiste (Eds.), *Occupation-based practice: fostering performance and participation* (pp. 3–15). Thorofare, NJ: Slack Incorporated.

Bickenbach, J. E., Chatterji, S., Badley, E. M. & Ustun, T. B. (1999). Models of disablement, universalism and the ICIDH. *Social Science and Medicine*, 48, 1173–1187.

Bronman, J. (2004). The World Health Organization's terminology and classification: application to severe disability. *Disability and Rehabilitation*, 26, 182–188.

Burgess-Limerick, R., Plooy, A., Fraser, K. & Ankrum, D. R. (1999). The influence of computer monitor height on head and neck posture. *International Journal of Industrial Ergonomics*, 23 (3), 171–179.

Canadian Association of Occupational Therapists (2002). *Enabling occupation: an occupational therapy perspective*. Ottawa, Ont: CAOT Publications ACE.

Chapparo, C. & Ranka, J. (1997). *Occupational performance model: monograph*. Unpublished manuscript, Sydney.

Christiansen, C. H. (1999). Defining lives: occupation as identity: an essay on competence, coherence and the creation of meaning. *American Journal of Occupational Therapy*, 53 (6), 547–558.

Christiansen, C. & Baum, C. (1997). Person-environment-occupational performance: a conceptual model for practice. In: C. H. Christiansen & C. Baum (Eds.), *Occupational therapy: enabling function and wellbeing* (2nd ed.) (pp. 47–70). Thorofare, NJ: Slack Incorporated.

Christiansen, C. H. & Baum, C. M. (2005). The complexity of human occupation. In: C. H. Christiansen, C. M. Baum & J. Bass-Haugen (Eds.), *Occupational therapy: Performance, participation, and wellbeing* (3rd ed.). Thorofare, NJ: Slack Incorporated.

Dunn, W., Brown, C. & McGuigan, A. (1994). The ecology of human performance: a framework for considering the effect of context. *The American Journal of Occupational Therapy*, 48 (7), 595–607.

Elkind, D. (1981). *The hurried child: growing up too fast too soon*. Sydney: Addison-Wesley.

Forsyth, K. & Kielhofner, G. (2003). Model of Human Occupation. In: P. Kramer, J. Hinojosa & C. B. Royeen (Eds.), *Perspectives in human occupation* (pp. 45–86). Baltimore, MD: Lippincott Williams & Wilkins.

Harris, C. & Staker, L. (2000). Survey of physical ergonomics issues associated with school children's use of laptop computers. *International Journal of Industrial Ergonomics, 26,* 337–346.

Heard, C. (1977). Occupational role acquisition: a perspective on the chronically disabled. *American Journal of Occupational Therapy, 31* (4), 243–251.

Hillman, A. M. & Chapparo, C. J. (1995). An investigation of occupational role performance in men over sixty years of age following a stroke. *Journal of Occupational Science, 2* (3), 88–99.

Hillman, M. (1999). *The impact of transport policy on children's development.* Retrieved 14 April 2005 from http://www.spokeseastkent.org.uk/mayer.htm

Kennedy, C. (2003). Functioning and disability associated with mental disorders: the evolution since ICIDH. *Disability and Rehabilitation, 25,* 611–619.

Kielhofner, G. & Burke, J. (1985). Components and determinants of human occupation. In: G. Kielhofner (Ed.), *A Model of Human Occupation – theory and application* (pp. 12–36). Baltimore, MD: Williams and Wilkins.

Kielhofner, G. (1995). *A Model of Human Occupation – theory and application* (2nd ed.). Baltimore, MD: Williams & Wilkins.

Kielhofner, G. (2002a). Motives, patterns and performance of occupation: basic concepts. In: G. Kielhofner (Ed.), *A Model of Human Occupation – theory and application* (3rd ed.) (pp. 13–27). Baltimore, MD: Lippincott, Williams & Wilkins.

Kielhofner, G. (2002b). Habituation: patterns of daily occupation. In: G. Keilhofner (Ed.), *A Model of Human Occupation – theory and application* (3rd ed.) (pp. 63–80). Baltimore, MD: Lippincott, Williams & Wilkins.

Laliberte-Rudman, D. (2002). Linking occupation and identity: lessons learned through qualitative exploration. *Journal of Occupational Science, 9* (1), 12–19.

Lambert, R. (1998). Occupation and lifestyle: implications for mental health practice. *British Journal of Occupational Therapy, 61* (5), 193–197.

Law, M. (2002). Participation in the occupations of everyday life. *American Journal of Occupational Therapy, 56* (6), 640–649.

Law, M., Cooper, B., Strong, S., Stewart, D., Rigby, P. & Letts, L. (1996). The person–environment–occupation model: a transactive approach to occupational performance. *Canadian Journal of Occupational Therapy, 63* (1), 9–23.

Law, M., Polatajko, H., Baptiste, W. & Townsend, E. (1997). Core concepts of occupational therapy. In: E. Townsend (Ed.), *Enabling occupation: an occupational therapy perspective* (pp. 29–56). Ottawa, Ont.: Canadian Association of Occupational Therapists.

Mackay, H. (1999). *Turning point: Australians choosing their future.* Sydney: Pan Macmillan.

Malina, R. M. (1996). Tracking of physical activity and physical fitness across the lifespan. *Research Quarterly for Exercise and Sport, 67,* 48–57.

Matsutsuyu, J. (1971). Occupational behaviour: a perspective on work and play. *American Journal of Occupational Therapy, 15* (9), 291–294.

Mead, G. H. (1934). *Mind, self, and society from the standpoint of a social behaviorist.* Chicago: University of Chicago Press.

Nelson, A. & Allison, H. (2000). Values of urban Aboriginal parents: food for thought. *Australian Occupational Therapy Journal, 47,* 28–40.

Office of Special Education and Rehabilitation Services (1997). *Individuals with Disabilities Education Act Amendments. PL105–17.* Retrieved 14 March 2005 from www.ed.gov/offices/OSERS/Policy/IDEA/the_law.html

Organisation for Economic Co-operation and Development (2003). *Society at a glance 2002.* Retrieved 14 September 2004 from http://hermia.sourceoecd.org/vl=8245604/cl=26/nw=1/rpsv/home.htm

Rogers, J. C. (1983). Clinical reasoning: the ethics, science and art. *American Journal of Occupational Therapy, 37,* 601–616.

Sallis, J. F., Johnson, M. F., Calfas, K. J., Caparosa, S. & Nichols, J. F. (1997). Assessing perceived physical environmental variables that may influence physical activity. *Research Quarterly for Exercise and Sport, 68,* 345–351.

Schneidert, M., Hurst, R., Miller, J. & Ustun, B. (2003). The role of environment in the ICF. *Disability and Rehabilitation, 25* (11–12), 588–595.

Simeonsson, R. J., Leonardi, M., Lollars, D., Bjorck-Akesson, E., Hollenweger, J. & Martinuzzi, A. (2003). Applying the international classification of functioning, disability and health (ICF) to measure childhood disability. *Disability and Rehabilitation, 25* (11–12), 602–610.

The Royal Australasian College of Physicians (RACP) (2004). *Children and the media: Advocating for the future.* Retrieved 21 May 2004 from http://www.racp.edu.au/hpu/paed/ media/Guide_parents.pdf

Trost, S. G., Kerr, L. M. & Pate, R. R. (2001). Physical activity and determinants of physical activity in obese and non-obese children. *International Journal of Obesity, 25,* 822–829.

Wood, P. H. N. (1980). Appreciating the consequences of disease: the international classification of impairments, disabilities, and handicaps. *WHO Chronicle, 34,* 376–380.

World Health Organization (WHO) (2001). *International classification of functioning, disability and health: ICF* (Short Version ed.). Geneva: World Health Organization.

Ziviani, J., Macdonald, D., Jenkins, D., Rodger, S., Batch, J. & Cerin, E. (in press). Physical activity in the lives of seven to nine-year-old Australian children. *OTJR: Occupation, Participation and Health.*

Chapter 2

FAMILIES AND CHILDREN'S OCCUPATIONAL PERFORMANCE

Yvonne Darlington and Sylvia Rodger

'It takes a whole village to raise a single child.' (African proverb)

Following on from the brief overview of families in contemporary society introduced in Chapter 1, this chapter looks in depth at how a child's family impacts on their roles, occupations and performance. We acknowledge the pivotal role of the family in supporting a child's occupational performance and the uniqueness of each family in terms of the individual mix of social, cultural, spiritual and economic factors, as well as rituals and routines that contribute to family occupations. The objectives of this chapter are to:

(1) Describe the changing nature of families, particularly in contemporary western society
(2) Explore the role of society in supporting families
(3) Describe how families impact on children's roles, occupations and occupational performance
(4) Describe working in partnership with families in a family-centred manner
(5) Highlight the role of childhood professionals in family advocacy

Families in contemporary society

Across the western world since the early 1970s, significant changes have occurred in relation to family composition and function. These are still unfolding, and will have major impacts on family life in future generations. Occupational therapists, along with other health and human services professionals, work largely within the organizations that implement government health, welfare and education policy. We can expect to see significant changes in the way services are organized and delivered, as a consequence of these changing patterns of family life.

Changes in family formation and functioning

It is difficult to talk in terms of direct cause and effect when considering changing trends in family formation and functioning. Social and economic changes do, over time, lead to changes in family patterns. The availability of the contraceptive pill from the 1960s gave women control over their fertility and made it possible for them to complete education and establish a career prior to having children. The 1970s women's movement was also a catalyst for fostering women's aspirations for a wider range of roles than wife and mother, and for greater control over decisions about partnering and parenting. The impact is partly seen in the rapid expansion of formal childcare and in delayed parenthood. Government financial support for single parents, seen as highly innovative in the 1970s, is an important plank of family income support policy.

The major demographic trend currently evident in western countries is for later family formation. The ages of first marriage and of motherhood are both increasing due to a number of factors. First, increased participation of both men and women in post-secondary education has delayed economic independence and contributed to young people staying at home longer. Between 1986 and 2001, the proportion of Australian women aged 15–24 years who were studying increased from 36% to 56%. In 2001, the number of people who had completed upper secondary or post-secondary education were 62% in USA, 73% in UK and 70% in Australia (Organization for Economic Co-operation and Development [OECD], 2003). Female participation in tertiary education has increased across the OECD, with more women than men in tertiary education in 21 out of 30 countries (OECD, 2003).

At the same time, women's participation in the labour force across the years when they are most likely to have children (that is 25–34 years) increased from 48% in 1979 to 70% in 2001 (Australian Bureau of Statistics [ABS], 2001). Again, there is likely to be some economic basis for this, with young couples choosing to work to establish themselves in careers and also to financially offset later years where one partner may be substantially engaged in childrearing.

The flow-on of these changes is a trend towards older motherhood. In 1979, almost one in four births were to women over 30 years. By 1999 this had increased to almost one in two births (ABS, 2001). In developed countries a growing proportion of women and their partners are not having children. Recent predictions suggest that, in Australia, UK and USA, at least 20% of women currently in their reproductive years will not have children (Qu et al., 2000). Average family size is also decreasing. Some childlessness is involuntary, but for those who are voluntarily childless, the decision is likely to be made in the context of work, life experiences, personal health and relationships (McAllister & Clarke, 1998).

Diversity of family types

Along with later family formation, there is greater diversity of family types than in previous generations including single parent, blended and step-families, (ABS,

2003a). However, the dual parent or nuclear family remains the most prevalent family type. In Australia in 2001, around 79% of all families with children aged less than 15 years were dual parent families, and 29% were single parent families (ABS, 2003a). Dual parent families with children are, however, forming a smaller proportion of all families – 47% of families in 2001, down from 54% in 1986 (ABS, 2003a).

In 2003, 71% of all Australian families with children under 17 years of age were intact families, where the children were the natural or adopted children of both parents. Of the remainder, 22% were single parent families, 4% were step-families, with at least one child of either parent, and 3% were blended families, with stepchildren and at least one child born to both parents (ABS, 2003b).

There have also been significant changes in workforce participation by parents. In 2001, 43% of all families with children under 15 years were dual parent families where both parents worked. Dual parent families where only one parent worked were the next most common (28%), followed by single parent families where the parent was not employed (11%), single parent families where the parent was employed (10%) and dual parent families where neither parent was employed (8%). In 2000 employment rates for mothers with at least one child were 55% for Australia, 72% for UK and 75% for USA, with mothers of younger children more likely to be in part-time employment (OECD, 2003).

The challenge of combining family and paid work responsibilities is a reality for many families. Despite increased community and employer recognition of these challenges, and some moves towards family friendly workplaces, most families struggle to achieve a balance between work and family responsibility, especially at times of family crisis and increased work pressures.

Children in families

The family life of children has also undergone significant changes. With increased participation of mothers in the paid workforce, we are seeing more children in formal childcare. In 2002, 45% of Australian children aged 0–4 years and 13% of children aged 5–11 years spent some time in formal childcare (ABS, 2004). This is in addition to informal care provided by family members, mostly grandmothers. British and Australian studies have reported that between a quarter and a half of employed women have their children looked after by a grandmother (Finch, 1989; Glezer, 1991; Millward & Matches, 1995).

The role of grandmothers in childcare is also changing. Increasing numbers of older women are participating in paid employment (34% of those aged 55 to 59 years in 1991, compared with 23% in 1971 (ABS, 1993); an age which seems also to be a peak age for grandmothers being involved in childcare. With middle genera-tion women increasingly participating in the paid workforce, assisting adult children, grandchildren and their own parents, there is considerable potential for overload (Hagestad, 1987). Even so, most grandmothers who care for grandchildren report satisfaction with this role. The impact of the current trend to older motherhood on grandmothers' childcare roles remains to be seen (Millward, 1998).

Children's lives also seem to be busier and more regulated than in previous generations. With parents' work commitments being incorporated into the family schedule, rather more out of school time is spent in structured activity, whether in after-school programmes or sporting and other activities. Perceptions of unsafe neighbourhoods and sprawling cities also mean many more children are driven to and from school. For many children, there is less unstructured, 'free time'. These concerns have been expressed in a number of parenting self-help books, (Doherty & Carlson, 2002; Rosenfeld & Wise, 2000). A national American survey found that children have lost 12 hours of free time per week since the 1970s, with a 25% drop in playing and a 50% drop in unstructured outdoor activities (Doherty & Carlson, 2002).

Many children live in families constrained by financial pressures. In 2001, 18% of Australian children under 15 years lived in a household with no employed parent, with over half (61%) of these living in single parent families. Families with no employed parent have much lower household incomes than families where one parent is employed, with considerably higher proportions of families in the lowest income brackets (ABS, 2004). The rates of single parent jobless households are 61% in UK and 34% in USA, compared with 10.7% and 5.7% respectively for dual parent families. The most important factor in child poverty is parental employment (OECD, 2003).

In addition to children living in poverty, another significant group of children with special needs are those with a disability. In 1998 there were 277 400 Australian children aged 5–17 years (8% of all children in this age group) with a disability that involved a specific restriction in one or more areas of communication, mobility, self-care, and/or schooling (ABS, 2000). The significant impact of a child with a disability on parents and siblings, family routines and activities (Rodger, 1985; 1987; Stagnitti, 2005; Turnbull & Turnbull, 1990) as well as the heterogeneity of families who have a child with a disability (for example Hanna & Rodger, 2002) has been well documented.

Since the 1970s, growing numbers of children have also experienced parental separation and divorce. While it is difficult to generalize how families manage this experience, this is a major transition for children, and the range of reported impacts include reduced economic security, loss of contact with extended family or with one parent, a sense of being 'torn' between parents and self-blame. Emergent perspectives on the impact of separation and divorce on children emphasize a range of outcomes, with some benefiting and some being harmed (Pryor & Rodgers, 2001). Nonetheless, children need to accommodate changes in parental presence, involvement, routines and living arrangements that are likely to impact on their occupational engagement.

Contact with the non-resident parent brings further complexity to children's lives. Even when children want to have regular contact with their non-resident parent, patterns of contact can interfere with children's own activities and priorities, especially as they grow older. Parents can maintain children's sporting and other routines during contact, but this is not always practicable and there is not always the will to make this happen.

A significant number of children are victims of child abuse and neglect. In 2002–2003, there were 40 412 substantiated cases of child abuse and neglect across Australia. This is a substantial increase in numbers compared with previous years. Even so, this is not necessarily due to an increase in the overall incidence of child abuse and neglect, but may be due to changes in legislation, policies and practices within jurisdictions (for example the way notifications and substantiations are counted), as well as increased community awareness and willingness to report problems (Australian Institute of Health and Welfare, 2004).

Along with specific factors that make life more difficult for some children, there are also many circumstances which may make some parents more vulnerable and potentially less able to focus on their children's needs. Times of family transition, such as separation and divorce, loss of employment or death of a family member may leave parents with depleted resources for child rearing. Parental issues such as mental illness, substance abuse and intellectual disability are all risk factors for potential harm to children, particularly chronic neglect, if adequate family support is not in place (Cleaver et al., 1999).

Role of society in supporting families

As suggested in the African proverb, no person can exist independently of others, and no one person can ever meet all an individual's needs. We all have diverse needs and require a range of resources to meet these and to function effectively. Societies are premised on the assumption that what people receive, in terms of personal resources as well as support from others, enables them in turn to contribute to the wellbeing of society, both in the present and in the nurturance of future generations. In contemporary post-industrial societies, with so much personal and political emphasis on the individual and individual advancement, this communal value (such as the importance of family and community) can seem rather blurred. By contrast, in indigenous cultures in Australia the role of the family and the community is paramount.

Family support
Most people receive some form of family and community support from people outside their household (ABS, 2004). There are two major forms of social and family support. Formal support encompasses services provided through government and non-profit organizations and may or may not incur a fee for service. Examples include income support, infant health and welfare services, childcare and neighbourhood centres, through to intensive family support and counselling services. Informal support is that provided by family members, friends and others known to the family. It is less structured and more flexible. To receive informal support, a family needs to have a social network sufficiently resourced to be able to respond when needed. Informal support also tends to be bounded by a norm of reciprocity (Cameron, 1990), with all network members involved in giving and receiving help. It is not difficult to see that some families will be excluded from such caring and protective networks, whether through high levels of mobility or homelessness, family disruption and violence, social detachment, or economic deprivation

(Healy & Darlington, 1999). For these families, formal support services are essential. We would also argue that, particularly for families who are excluded from 'natural' helping systems, formal support services need to be able to mirror some of the more flexible elements of informal services.

Family support can be further delineated according to the type of support. This is useful because we know that different types of support may be more or less useful at different times and tend to be provided by different people (Miller & Darlington, 2002). A common classification includes material, practical, information and emotional support (D'Abbs, 1991). Material support refers to receiving material goods or money. Forms of formal material support vary considerably across countries. Some examples are government family payments, family tax concessions, child disability payments, childcare assistance, health care rebates and other concessions that may be available to families, as well as emergency assistance from non-profit organizations. Informal material support may come in the form of financial assistance, gifts or loans from family or friends. Practical support is any type of support that assists the family in the completion of a task such as assistance with transport, housekeeping or household repairs, and help in caring for a sick family member.

Information support concerns the availability of and access to information. This includes information about where to find the help (for example recommending a local doctor), as well as direct information about parenting and family need (for example nutritional information). Finally, emotional support refers to the assistance families receive which helps them cope with either crisis situations or day-to-day emotional difficulties (D'Abbs, 1991).

The process of giving and receiving support is interactive. Family support needs to encompass the right help, at the right time, in the right quantity and of the right quality. There needs to be a *fit* between a family's perceived need for support and the support received. A 1993 study of 53 low-income dual parent families with young children found that the quality of support received is crucial in predicting family wellbeing and functioning (Darlington & Miller, 2000). In particular, those who viewed the support that they received as being more helpful reported more intimate and open communication, less conflict, a more democratic parenting style, as well as higher levels of family esteem, a greater sense of control over their lives and greater financial wellbeing. These findings support previous research, emphasizing the importance of the quality over the amount of support (Antonucci & Hiroko, 1987; Gibson, 1986; Maxwell & Coebergh, 1986; Wilcox, 1981).

Miller & Darlington (2002) examined who provided support to these families. Parents, followed by friends, and then siblings and other family members were the most important sources of support. Parents tended to provide material and practical support, whereas friends and siblings were important sources of emotional and information support. Friends appeared to become relatively more important as sources of information and emotional support as children reached school-age. Different sources were more influential in providing particular forms of support, at different times of the family life cycle. We suggest that, to be effective in strengthening families in the long term, formal support services targeted to marginalized families need to take on more of the shape of informal networks – flexibility, timeliness and a mix of types and sources of support – as well as putting effort into strengthening families' existing informal ties.

Family support services

While formal family support services have been provided to needy families since the late eighteenth century, the family support sector has undergone a change in focus over the past decade. Across post-industrial countries, there is a renewed interest in prevention and early intervention services, initiatives designed to enhance child and family health and wellbeing, and 'whole of community' approaches (Tomison, 2002).

Much of the current approach to family support echoes and extends early intervention programmes, such as Headstart (Zigler & Styfco, 1996), trialled in the United States over the past 30 years, and aimed at improving the cognitive and social competence of disadvantaged children (Tomison, 2002). The Australian Government's *Stronger families and communities strategy* (Department of Family and Community Services, 2004–2008) is an example of an early intervention strategy focused on enhancing family and community health and wellbeing through building resilience and community capacity.

In summary, family functioning has been influenced significantly over the past several decades by changes in family formation. As a result, family life for children has changed due to increased numbers of women in the workforce, increases in divorce rates, changing patterns of childcare and changes in children's schedules. Family support systems, both formal and informal, are needed to provide a range of support to families to enable them to undertake their responsibilities. Recent government initiatives have aimed to build community capacity through preventive and early intervention strategies for families at risk. The following section aims to describe how family composition, support networks, and family life and culture impacts on children's roles and occupations.

Impact of families on children's roles and occupations

In order to understand a family's impact on children's role performance, we need first to recognize the uniqueness of each family in terms of its composition, informal and formal support networks, culture, values and expectations. As described previously, family composition varies widely in terms of dual versus single parent families, shared care arrangements (for example after separation or divorce), extended families (for example where relatives live with a family), and children living with same gender couples.

Families' social and cultural backgrounds and religious beliefs impact significantly on their values and expectations about family life (Stagnitti, 2005), children's behaviour, activities, management and discipline. It is important for childhood professionals to be aware of these beliefs because these influence children's role engagement and ultimately their occupations and occupational performance. A case study will be used to illustrate the impact of the family on children's roles and occupations and their levels of participation. As you read the case study, try to identify the social, cultural and religious values, as well as economic factors, which influence Lien. In addition, while you are reading, consider your own social, cultural, religious and economic background and how your own beliefs and values may impact on your role as a professional working with Lien and her family, and your ability to accommodate any differences (Fitzgerald, 2004; Fitzgerald et al., 1997).

Lien

Lien is an eight-year-old girl from a Vietnamese family who migrated to Australia three years ago. She lives with her elderly grandparents and parents in a small two bedroom apartment above a Vietnamese restaurant and takeaway where her parents work, her mother as a waitress and her father as the cook. Her grandfather is ill and spends most of his time at home, while her grandmother helps in the restaurant kitchen. Lien's parents work seven nights a week. They live in a working class suburb in a largely Vietnamese community. Lien attends the local public school where she has extra lessons in English as a second language (ESL).

As an only child, Lien's *personal-sexual* role of female and her family's focus on the adult role of worker are reinforced. Her *familial* roles are that of daughter, granddaughter and cousin. Her *social* role of friend or playmate is mostly engaged in with other Vietnamese children at school, as there is little time or space in the apartment after school for play. Her pre-eminent role is that of *student*. Her parents have high expectations of her ability to succeed at school, gain a good education and attend university. They are keen for her to benefit from all education can offer, hoping that she will not have to work long hours in a kitchen as they do. At school she undertakes regular classes and ESL lessons. Three afternoons per week she attends individual tutoring in maths and English at a local tutoring centre. She plays the keyboard and has lessons on Saturday mornings. She spends every night on school homework. Her *self-maintainer* role involves chores like taking out the rubbish and making her bed. She also has to assist with the care of her elderly grandfather when her grandmother works in the restaurant kitchen. Her parents do not allow her to play sports as they are keen for her to concentrate on her schoolwork and improve her English. As a *player*, she watches TV, plays at home and sometimes visits other Vietnamese friends.

Lien's roles and occupations are predominantly shaped by her parents' desire to see her obtain a good education. This makes the *student* role critical both in and outside school. As a result, she has limited time to play with friends or engage in other activities, sports or hobbies. Unlike many other children her age, she undertakes an additional *carer* role for her grandfather. Her small apartment limits her play occupations and her neighbourhood environment restricts her play engagements to those with other Vietnamese children.

This case study illustrates the pivotal influence of family expectations, beliefs and values, as well as family composition and socio-economic factors on children's role engagement and consequently their occupations. The next section addresses how professionals work in partnership with families when children and/or parents experience occupational challenges.

Working in partnership with families

In the last two decades there has been much written about best practice when working with children and their families. Two aspects of best practice include the provision of family-centred care (that is the honouring of a family's priorities and style in designing programmes and intervening with children) and partnership (that is acknowledging that professionals and families have a mutual and reciprocal right and responsibility to involve each other in the organization and structure of services) (Dunn, 2000). It is beyond the scope of this chapter to deal with these concepts in detail. However, they will be briefly reviewed in order to make child-hood professionals aware of the need to understand parents' expectations about their involvement in intervention.

Family-centred practice

Family-centred practice (FCP) means that professionals value, encourage and commit to the meaningful involvement of families in the planning and imple-mentation of services (Salisbury & Dunst, 1997). Edwards et al. (2003) identified factors that encourage FCP in occupational therapy intervention. Recognition of family individuality is crucial. This involves viewing families as unique, deter-mining their optimum style of learning and ascertaining their preferred forms of communication and support. Support from therapists is highlighted through their accommodation of family schedules, incorporation of parents in determining goals and in therapy sessions, and establishment of effective relationships with parents. Incorporating education, communication, and sibling and care-giver participation into natural family routines was also critical. Hence, professionals need to under-stand these routines and rituals and how they are influenced by a family's customs and beliefs (Werner DeGrace, 2003).

Assumptions and principles of family-centred services

Rosenbaum et al. (1998) proposed three basic assumptions of family-centred services (FCS):

(1) Parents and other family members are the most consistent people in children's lives and the most knowledgeable about their own children
(2) Families are different and unique
(3) Optimal child functioning occurs within a supportive family and community context

Table 2.1 highlights the requirements of family-centred care and provides examples of how this care may be ensured.

Table 2.1 Family-centred service (FCS) requirements.

Family-centred service (FCS) requirements	Examples of how to ensure FCS
(1) Development of successful communication strategies	Avoiding jargon Using interpreters Using positive, non-verbal strategies such as active listening Determining the regularity and type of contact desired by families (Salisbury & Dunst, 1997)
(2) Sensitivity to the unique features of the family unit	Recognizing impact of family composition, culture, religious beliefs, values, expectations, socio-economic status, willingness to engage in therapy, acceptance of suggestions, scheduling of meetings, etc. (Werner DeGrace, 2003)
(3) Effective team collaboration	Involving parents as team members. (Dunn, 2000)
(4) A set of guiding principles	Encouraging families to decide the level of involvement they wish to have in decision making for their child Recognizing parental responsibility for the care of their children Treating family members with respect Considering the needs of all family members Supporting and encouraging involvement of all family members (Rosenbaum et al., 1998)

Effectiveness of FCS

Benefits of FCS, such as increased parent satisfaction, positive child and family outcomes, and decreased parental stress have been reported (Rosenbaum et al., 1998). In addition, children whose parents participate in intervention have more successful outcomes than those of parents who do not (Epstein, 1993). Law et al. (2003) examined factors that are important in determining parent perceptions of family-centredness of care and parent satisfaction with services using a cross-sectional survey of 494 parents and 324 service providers, from children's rehabilitation services in North America. The principal determinants of parent satisfaction with services were the family-centred culture of the organization and parent perceptions of FCS. Parent satisfaction was also influenced by the number of places where services were received and the number of health and developmental problems experienced by the child. In summary, parents are more satisfied when services are provided in a family-centred manner. Satisfaction with services has been shown to increase adherence to treatment recommendations and to decrease feelings of distress and depression, as well as improve parental wellbeing (King et al., 1999; Rosenbaum et al., 1998). FCS should be considered a 'best practice approach' to meeting the needs of children with disabilities and their families.

Finding the right *fit*

FCS recognizes the family as the consumer, respects families' priorities and decisions, and provides services and support to assist families in achieving their goals (Wehman, 1998). Support is most beneficial when it matches the need for aid and assistance as identified by the family. According to Wehman (1998), when this *fit* exists, families are empowered. When considering family participation, there is a continuum of family involvement varying in form, focus and complexity. The type of involvement families choose depends on their individual needs, values and lifestyles. We must respect family preferences for involvement and reconsider our own expectations about how families 'should' be involved.

Collaborative parent and service provider partnerships

Partnership between parents and service providers is one of the theoretical foundations of FCS. A collaborative partnership implies a balance of power. This requires mutual acceptance, respect, caring, the recognition of each other's expertise, and the opportunity for purposeful and meaningful participation (Wehman, 1998). Hanna & Rodger (2002) explored parent-therapist collaboration in occupational therapy. They proposed along with Lyons (1994) that collaboration involves a partnership entered on an equal basis, with respect for each other's skills and knowledge and a willingness to learn from each other's skills. Therapists must strive to understand parents' unique perspectives and parenting styles (resulting from differing cultural, ethnic and socio-economic backgrounds), especially when these differ significantly from their own.

Due to the increased care-giving demands on mothers when a child has a disability, Brown (2004) proposed that supporting parental roles enhances FCS. Along with Hanna & Rodger (2002), she also suggested that partnerships are based on the premise that 'two heads are better than one' and that parents and professionals together learn the best way to meet a family's needs. Professionals can be restricted by viewing themselves only as advocates for children's needs (Anderson & Hinojosa, 1984). Brown (2004) made suggestions for professionals about home therapy programmes as part of family-centred care. In particular, she emphasized the importance of helping the family become and remain a stable, happy and functional unit; creating a home environment where the child feels secure, content and able to develop their own role in the family and participate in family life; and addressing the child's needs constructively within family routines. Finally, Brown proposed that within FCS there is a continuum of participation, with parent-professional collaboration being pivotal. This continuum involves family as informant, assistant, co-worker, partner, collaborator and service director.

Family occupations

Drawing from the occupational science literature, Hanna & Rodger (2002) proposed that therapists have much to learn about the occupations of parenting, exploring the nature of parenting and family occupations and how these are

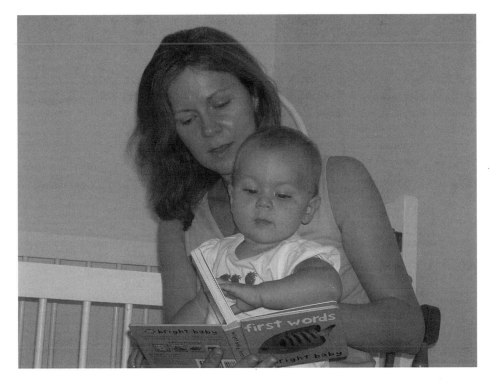

Figure 2.1 Bedtime story routines.

orchestrated in order to maintain health and wellbeing. Werner DeGrace (2003) also challenged occupational therapists to consider how each family unit constructs its meaning of family. She postulated that we need to look beyond family *doing* to *being* and *becoming*. This requires consideration of the meaning of each family's occupations. 'Being' a family implies being able to derive meaning from engaging in daily living experiences. She claimed that the crux of FCS and occupation based practice is understanding who families want to be and how they can engage in meaningful experiences together.

Family rituals and routines contribute to a common identity among family members. They preserve family meaningfulness, maintain cohesion and contact (Werner DeGrace, 2003). Rituals may include mealtime routines, weekend leisure activities, bedtime stories, goodnight kiss, the tooth fairy and birthday celebrations. See Figures 2.1 and 2.2. Segal (2004) reported that routines give life order, while rituals give it meaning. Rituals are the mechanism for constructing and affirming family identity through their symbolic and affective components. We need to consider both family *doing* and *being* goals as key aspects of occupation based family-centred interventions. Importantly, occupational therapists have a role in assisting families to *be* through promoting and facilitating engagement in rituals to enable them to create meaning. In this way we are able to address the meaningful occupations of the family unit and support individual family

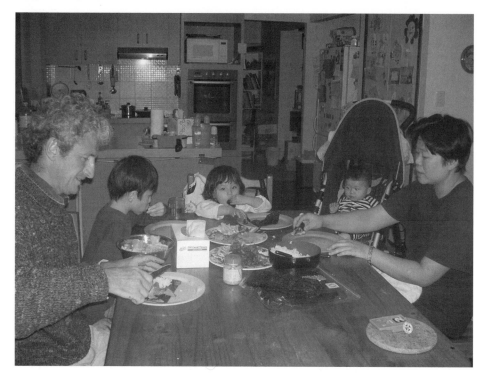

Figure 2.2 Family mealtime routines.

members in *being* a family. This in turn promotes family occupations, health and wellbeing.

The role of childhood professionals in advocacy

Finally, we turn to addressing the role of childhood professionals in advocating for families within the health, welfare and education systems. Childhood professionals primarily focus on individual children and their families. We identify the child's and family's needs and in consultation with parents develop an intervention plan based on the family's goals. We recognize that the family is very much the key to the success of the child's intervention. However, there are frequently many competing demands on families.

Many families will be highly motivated and have the financial, emotional and social resources to be able to focus on their child's needs and incorporate therapy into daily routines without undue stress. However, some families may require additional assistance and resources to be able to complete home programmes; and sometimes these needs seem quite separate to the child's issues. This is when advocacy may be an appropriate response.

Advocacy is primarily concerned with obtaining resources and helping people to overcome difficulties, as well as to secure their rights. These activities fit comfortably within the range of activities performed by health professionals (Bateman, 2000). For example, a child may be denied a disability payment, or an indigenous family may need transport assistance to attend an early intervention service.

O'Connor et al. (2003) describe advocacy as 'an effort to influence the behaviour of decision makers in relation to another or group of others' (p. 190). Advocacy is not just a role for professionals, but for anyone who sees a need to assist others who are experiencing hardship due to service gaps, or who are discriminated against or denied their legal rights. An advocacy response should be considered when a client is refused a service or benefit to which they may be entitled, when agency or government policies adversely affect people in need of services (for example cultural insensitivity of mainstream services), or when decisions are made about individuals or groups by institutions that are not aware of the totality of individual or group needs (Hepworth et al. 2002).

An example of family advocacy when parents have an intellectual disability will illustrate where advocacy may be appropriate. You are working with a preschool girl who has a global developmental delay. Both parents have a mild intellectual disability and are struggling to manage everyday home management and parenting. A home visit indicates that this family's life is chaotic. The child appears to be reasonably well cared for and is cheerful and responsive with both parents. You know that if this family had come to the attention of statutory child protection authorities, they would be receiving some extra family support to help them to develop simple household management routines. While you do not consider this to be an immediate child protection matter, you believe that support for these parents now would benefit them and the child, and potentially prevent a crisis in the future.

You contact a local family support service and discover that they take most of their clients on referral from the child protection service, as these are the most urgent cases and have a long waiting list for other families. You believe that, not only is the situation requiring immediate action, but that when a place eventually became available, the parents may not link it to the current situation and, not understanding what it is about, reject the service. You talk with the parents and they are agreeable to having someone come into the house to help them 'get organized'. Rather than have this family 'fall through the cracks', you write a detailed letter to the family support service, explaining the situation and asking that this family be treated as an urgent case.

Advocating for clients

In making decisions as to how to approach advocacy, Bateman (2000) distinguished between bounded and unbounded issues. Bounded issues are those that are circumscribed by a clear structure and procedures for seeking redress. Examples would be an appeal against a social security decision or a complaint against a health practitioner. In such situations, the procedures themselves form the basis for any action. Unbounded problems are those which lack a clearly regulated structure and are most likely to require interpersonal efforts to resolve, usually in the form of negotiation with the relevant body. Unbounded problems are more likely to result from interpersonal disputes. Whatever the situation, there are a number of ethical and procedural principles fundamental to effective advocacy. Bateman (2000) (pp. 47–63) offered some useful principles to guide advocacy efforts:

- Act in the client's best interests
- Act in accordance with the client's wishes and instructions
- Keep the client properly informed
- Carry out instructions with diligence and competence
- Act impartially and offer frank, independent advice
- Maintain rules of confidentiality

When considering an advocacy response, work within your own expertise. This is the basis upon which your credibility as an advocate rests. For example, as an occupational therapist you will be on safe ground if you link your advocacy attempt to the child's needs and the family's capacity to meet those needs. You also need to ensure that there is a realistic possibility of success. Raising false hopes, when there really is little or no possibility of success, can result in frustration and further compound an existing sense of failure.

The first step is to assemble all relevant information and to be clear about what service or redress the client is seeking. Next, find out about possible courses of action. Who are the relevant decision makers and what processes are in place for making representation to them (Bateman, 2000; O'Connor et al., 2003)? It is essential to direct your advocacy attempt to the right person – to get your message to someone with the authority to decide.

Any advocacy attempt must also be carried out in adherence with legal and administrative procedures and rules. Where legal and highly structured administrative processes are involved, enlist appropriate help, for example from a legal aid office or welfare rights service (Bateman, 2000; O'Connor et al., 2003). Another important principle is to 'adopt a position of least contest' (O'Connor et al., 2003), to use the least force necessary to achieve a result. If repeated attempts fail, then a more formal approach at a higher level may prove necessary. Remember, the object is to obtain needed supports and services for a family. In many cases you will be talking to someone with a sympathetic ear, who will do all they can to oblige. The better your working relationship with them, the better able you will be both to work together to achieve positive outcomes.

Class advocacy

So far we have been talking about advocacy on behalf of individual families, and this is most likely to be where the majority of your advocacy efforts will be. With individual advocacy, the advocate attempts to alter how an individual is dealt with in the situation. While this is an effective form of advocacy, there are some limitations. In a situation where resources are scarce, for example public housing, or places in respite care, advocacy may result in your client being placed further up the list, but someone else put down. Overall, there is no change for the group.

When a large number of people are affected by the same situation, class advocacy, which is directed at changing policy, practices and laws, may be required. While the principles are the same, the processes are likely to be more complex and require the combined efforts of a committed group of advocates.

Advocacy skills

The most fundamental skills in advocacy have much in common with everyday professional communication skills. These include the interpersonal skills of interviewing, active listening, being able to elicit full details of the issue, as well as the basis for the client's concern and what they would like to happen. Equally important is being able to explain clearly what you are able to do and to report back to the client throughout the process. For unbounded problems, skills of assertiveness and negotiation will form the basis of the advocacy action (Bateman, 2000).

The tools of advocacy include conferring with another agency or others in your agency, developing inter-agency networks, letter writing, formal appeals, oral or written submissions and providing expert evidence. For a problem that affects numbers of clients, additional tools could include documenting the problem through research, creating general or specific public awareness through education, lobbying, seminars or other publicity, organizing client groups, or legal action (O'Connor et al., 2003).

Summary

In this chapter, we have provided an overview of the changing landscape of family life in contemporary society and addressed how family composition, culture, expectations and values shape children's roles and occupations. We discussed how family-centred practice has become a cornerstone of therapy provision within early childhood intervention settings and provided an overview of principles of FCS. We focused on partnerships between parents and professionals as being critical to effective FCS provision to address children's occupational performance and family functioning.

Finally, we turned to advocacy as a method of enabling families who are unable to promote themselves in complex organizational systems, to meet their own needs. Advocacy should not be considered radical or unusual behaviour for childhood professionals. When linked to a family's needs and based upon your professional expertise, we would suggest it is an integral part of professional responsibility. Grounded in an understanding of the broader social, political and economic contexts in which families live, and the impact that these factors can have on a family's capacity to meet their children's needs, advocacy is an important means by which professionals can contribute to social justice. What is required is awareness of opportunities to effectively advocate for children and families and sufficient skills to approach it ethically and systematically.

References

Anderson, J. & Hinojosa, J. (1984). Parents and therapists in a professional partnership. *American Journal of Occupational Therapy, 38,* 453–461.

Antonucci, T. & Hiroko, A. (1987). An examination of sex differences in social support among older men and women. *Sex Roles, 17* (11–12), 737–749.

Australian Bureau of Statistics (1993). *Census characteristics of Australia, 1991 Census* (Catalogue No. 2710.0). Canberra: Commonwealth Government of Australia.

Australian Bureau of Statistics (2000). *Australian social trends: education, participation in education – disability and schooling* (Catalogue No. 4102.0). Canberra: Commonwealth Government of Australia.

Australian Bureau of Statistics (2001). *Australian social trends: older workers – family formation* (Catalogue No. 4102.0). Canberra: Commonwealth Government of Australia.

Australian Bureau of Statistics (2003a). *Australian social trends: family and community, living arrangements – changing families* (Catalogue No. 4102.0). Canberra: Commonwealth Government of Australia.

Australian Bureau of Statistics (2003b). *Family characteristics, Australia.* Canberra: Commonwealth Government of Australia.

Australian Bureau of Statistics (2004). *Australian social trends: family and community, family functioning – families with no employed parent* (Catalogue No. 4102.0). Canberra: Commonwealth Government of Australia.

Australian Institute of Health and Welfare (2004). *Child protection Australia 2002–03* (Child Welfare Series No. 34). Canberra: Australian Institute of Health and Welfare.

Bateman, N. (2000). *Advocacy skills for health and social care professionals* (2nd ed.). London: J. Kingsley.

Brown, G. (2004). Family-centred care, mothers' occupations of care-giving and home therapy programs. In: S. A. Esdaile & J. A. Olson (Eds.), *Mothering occupations: challenge, agency and participation.* Philadelphia: F. A. Davis.

Cameron, G. (1990). The potential of informal social support strategies in child welfare. In: M. Rothery & G. Cameron (Eds.), *Child maltreatment: expanding our concept of helping.* Hillsdale, NJ: L. Erlbaum and Associates.

Cleaver, H., Unell, I. & Aldgate, J. (1999). *Children's needs – parenting capacity: the impact of parental mental illness, problem alcohol and drug use, and domestic violence on children's development.* London: The Stationery Office.

D'Abbs, P. (1991). *Who helps?: Support networks and social policy in Australia.* Melbourne, Victoria: Australian Institute of Family Studies.

Darlington, Y. & Miller, R. J. (2000). Support received by families with dependent children: the importance of receiving adequate support. *Journal of Family Studies, 6* (1), 65–77.

Department of Family and Community Services, A. (2004–2008). *Stronger families and communities strategy 2004–2008.* Retrieved 19 April 2005 from http://www.facs.gov.au

Doherty, W. J. & Carlson, B. Z. (2002). *Putting family first: successful strategies for reclaiming family life in a hurry-up world.* New York: Owl Books.

Dunn, W. (2000). Best practice philosophy for community services for children and families. In: W. Dunn (Ed.), *Best practice occupational therapy in community service with children and families* (pp. 1–9). Thorofare, NJ: Slack Incorporated.

Edwards, M. A., Millard, P., Praskac, L. A. & Wisniewski, P. A. (2003). Occupational therapy and early intervention: a family-centred approach. *Occupational Therapy International, 10* (4), 239–252.

Epstein, J. (1993). Make parents your partners. *Instructor*, *19*, 119–136.

Finch, J. (1989). *Family obligations and social change*. Oxford: Polity Press.

Fitzgerald, M. (2004). A dialogue on occupational therapy, culture and families. *American Journal of Occupational Therapy*, *58*, 489–498.

Fitzgerald, M., Mullavey-O'Byrne, C. & Clemson, L. (1997). Cultural issues from practice. *Australian Occupational Therapy Journal*, *44*, 1–21.

Gibson, D. M. (1986). Interaction of wellbeing in old age: is it quantity or quality that counts? *International Journal of Aging and Human Development*, *24* (1), 29–40.

Glezer, H. (1991). Cycles of care: support and care between generations. *Family Matters*, *30*, 44–46.

Hagestad, G. (1987). Parent-child relations in later life: trends and gaps in past research. In: J. B. Lancaster, J. Altman, A. S. Rossi & L. R. Sherrod (Eds.), *Parenting across the life span: biosocial dimensions*. New York: Aldine de Gruyter.

Hanna, K. & Rodger, S. (2002). Towards family-centred practice in paediatric occupational therapy: a review of the literature on parent–therapist collaboration. *Australian Journal of Occupational Therapy*, *49*, 14–24.

Healy, K. & Darlington, Y. (1999). Family support and social inclusion: practice and policy issues in Australia. *Just Policy*, *16*, 3–10.

Hepworth, D. H., Rooney, R. H. & Larsen, J. A. (2002). *Direct social work practice: theory and skills*. Pacific Grove, CA: Brooks/Cole-Thomson Learning.

King, G., King, S., Rosenbaum, P. & Goffin, R. (1999). Family-centred care-giving and wellbeing of parents of children with disabilities: linking process with outcome. *Journal of Pediatric Psychology*, *24*, 41–53.

Law, M., Hanna, S., King, G., Hurley, P., King, S., Kertoy, M., et al. (2003). Factors affecting family-centred service delivery for children with disabilities. *Child: Care, Health and Development*, *29*, 357–366.

Lyons, M. (1994). Reflections on client–therapist relationships. *Australian Occupational Therapy Journal*, *41*, 27–30.

McAllister, F. & Clarke, L. (1998). *A study of childlessness in Britain*. London: Joseph Rowntree Foundation.

Maxwell, G. M. & Coebergh, B. (1986). Patterns of loneliness in a New Zealand population. *Community Mental Health in New Zealand*, *2* (2), 48–61.

Miller, R. J. & Darlington, Y. (2002). Who supports? The providers of social support to dual-parent families caring for young children. *Journal of Community Psychology*, *30* (5), 461–473.

Millward, C. (1998). *Family relationships and intergenerational exchange in later life* (Australian Institute of Family Studies Working Paper No. 15). Melbourne: Australian Institute of Family Studies.

Millward, C. & Matches, G. (1995). *Children's services report: childcare in nine Australian urban localities – Australian living standards study report to the Department of Health and Human Services*. Melbourne: Australian Institute of Family Studies.

O'Connor, I., Wilson, J. & Setterlund, D. (2003). *Social work and welfare practice* (4th ed.). Sydney: Pearson Education Australia.

Organization for Economic Co-operation and Development (OECD) (2003). *Society at a glance 2002*. Retrieved 14 September 2004 from http://hermia.sourceoecd.org/vl=8245604/cl=26/nw=1/rpsv/home.htm

Pryor, J. & Rodgers, B. (2001). *Children in changing families: life after parental separation*. Oxford: Blackwell Publishers.

Qu, L., Weston, R. & Kilmartin, C. (2000). Effects of changing personal relationships on decisions about having children. *Family Matters*, (57), 14–99.

Rodger, S. (1985). Siblings of handicapped children: a population at risk? *The Exceptional Child*, 33, 47–56.

Rodger, S. (1987). A comparison between parenting a normal and handicapped child across the lifespan. *British Journal of Occupational Therapy*, 50, 167–170.

Rosenbaum, P., King, S., Law, M., King, G. & Evans, J. (1998). Family-centred service: a conceptual framework and research review. *Physical and Occupational Therapy in Pediatrics*, 18, 1–20.

Rosenfeld, A. & Wise, N. (2000). *The over-scheduled child: avoiding the hyper-parenting trap*. New York: St Martin's Press.

Salisbury, C. & Dunst, C. (1997). *Homes, school and community partnerships: building inclusive teams. collaborative teams for students with severe disabilities*. Baltimore, MD: Paul H. Brookes Publishing Co.

Segal, R. (2004). Family routines and rituals: a context for occupational therapy interventions. *American Journal of Occupational Therapy*, 58, 499–508.

Stagnitti, K. (2005). The family as a unit in post-modern society: considerations for practice. In: G. Whiteford & V. Wright St-Clair (Eds.), *Occupation and practice in context*. Sydney: Elsevier.

Tomison, A. M. (2002). *Preventing child abuse: changes to family support in the twenty-first century. Issues paper no. 17*. Melbourne: Australian Institute of Family Studies: National Child Protection Clearinghouse.

Turnbull, A. P. & Turnbull, H. R. (1990). *Families, professionals and exceptionality: a special partnership* (2nd ed.). Columbus, OH: Merrill Publishing Company.

Wehman, T. (1998). Family-centred early intervention services: factors contributing to increased parent involvement and participation. *Focus on Autism and Other Developmental Disabilities*, 13, 80–86.

Werner DeGrace, B. (2003). Occupation-based and family-centred care: a challenge for current practice. *American Journal of Occupational Therapy*, 57, 347–350.

Wilcox, B. L. (1981). Social support, life stress and psychological adjustment. *American Journal of Community Psychology*, 9 (4), 371–386.

Zigler, E. F. & Styfco, S. (1996). Headstart and early childhood intervention: the changing course of social science and social policy. In: E. F. Zigler, S. L. Kogan & N. W. Hall (Eds.), *Children, families and government: preparing for the twenty-first century*. New York: Cambridge University Press.

Chapter 3

ENVIRONMENTAL INFLUENCES ON CHILDREN'S PARTICIPATION

Jenny Ziviani and Sylvia Rodger

Participating in the activities of childhood requires children to interact with the physical, social, cultural, economic and organizational aspects of their environment (Rigby & Letts, 2003). For the purpose of our discussion, *physical environment* refers to the non-human aspects of context (natural terrain, buildings, furniture, objects, tools and devices). *Social environment* refers to the availability and expectations of important persons such as family, care-givers and social groups, within the norms, expectations and routines of a child's life. *Cultural environment* refers to customs, beliefs, activity patterns, behaviours and expectations accepted by society (Dunn et al., 1994). Economic and organizational parameters influence participation through the availability of resources and the structures which mediate their distribution.

Occupational therapists view the environment as a facilitator of occupational performance, as well as a feature that can present barriers or excessive demands, which hinder performance. *Fit* is the congruence or balance of what a person brings to a transaction and the environmental demands or resources available (Rigby & Letts, 2003). As practitioners we aim to assist children in obtaining the best *fit* to enable optimal occupational performance. It is therefore incumbent on us to advocate for environments which are conducive to the health and wellbeing of all children.

Consistent with the *International classification of functioning, disability and health* (ICF) (World Health Organization [WHO], 2001), and socio-ecological paradigms (Bronfenbrenner, 1979), occupational therapists advocate that:

(1) Interventions can occur at the levels of family, neighbourhood, school, community and society
(2) Environmental factors may be more important in predicting health behaviour and outcomes than individual characteristics alone (Stewart & Law, 2003)

Those charged with the responsibility of promoting child wellbeing (Commission for Children and Young People [CCYP], 2004), have identified the provision of enriching, safe and supportive environments; connectivity across generations, families, cultures and communities; and children's participation in policy decisions, as central to this outcome. In keeping with this position, we propose that occupational therapists need to collaborate with consumers (both children and families) and professionals (in childcare, educational, recreational, health and community settings) to advocate for supportive environments for children.

The objectives of this chapter are to:

(1) Examine the role of the environment on children's activity engagement and participation
(2) Review methods of evaluating environments as they pertain to children and the contexts in which they live, play and learn
(3) Highlight collaboration with professionals in the fields of urban planning, design, architecture and children themselves as a means of promoting environments which are conducive to their participation

The nature of children's environments

The WHO (2001) has proposed an extensive range of environmental factors (for example physical, social, economic) that influence healthful participation. These factors influence what children will be able to engage in and how this will happen (Law, 2002). Most children grow up oblivious to broader political and economic environmental influences. For them the most salient environments relate to physical places and the people within these (Meucci & Schwab, 1997). The impact of these environments is important for all children, but is particularly the case for those with disabilities. For children with disabilities, physical and social support can promote positive development and adaptation (King et al., 2000).

Built environments demonstrate clear examples of how children can be deprived of participation opportunities. Despite increased awareness and legislative support of the need for accessibility, there remain numerous examples of environments where children with ambulatory difficulties cannot participate without significant human intervention (see Figure 3.1). If participation in occupational roles enhances life quality and wellbeing (Larson & Verma, 1999), then restrictions to this involvement could be conceived as occupational deprivation (Whiteford, 2000). In this context, deprivation can arise as a result of environmental barriers. Universal design has been endorsed as a way of creating both products and environments that are usable by everyone, regardless of age or ability (Ringaert, 2003). A core principle in this approach is that the design of environments (buildings, parks, streets) considers the needs of people with ranging abilities and ages. Designing spaces which are accessible to prams and wheelchairs can make them more commodious for the general public. Yet, while accessibility may be achieved by compliance with building codes and standards, universal design requires creativity to allow for broad participation (Salman, 2001). Ringaert (2003) identified occupational therapists' skill set as including knowledge of activity analysis, human functioning, human–environment fit, energy conservation, work simplification and human rights' legislation, that enables involvement in enhancing environments for all.

Another aspect of children's environment which has a profound influence on their participation is meaningful group membership (Leavitt, 1999). Group membership

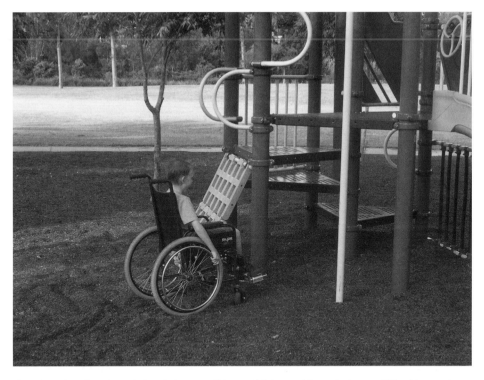

Figure 3.1 Playground that is inaccessible to children with ambulatory difficulties and wheelchair dependent children.

can provide emotional support, identity, personal security and a means of mediation between an individual and society. Furthermore, it has the potential to facilitate social problem resolution, self-help and action (Korten, 1984). These groupings can be formal, such as family, school, church and voluntary organizations, or informal, arising from networks of individuals with shared values, interests and needs (for example people who regularly catch a bus together or meet walking their dogs).

When formal and informal community structures break down, children can become vulnerable. For children, the experience of community has been impacted upon by an increasing number of parents who both work, single parent families, decreased extended families as a result of increasing mobility and fewer people accessing traditional churches. The importance of maintaining community structures for both children and families has been recognized by government programmes designed to build local community capacity. One example of this is the Stronger Families initiative in Australia (Commonwealth Department of Family and Community Services, 2002). The aim of this initiative was to help families and communities work collaboratively to prevent long-term problems and to improve the quality of family life through early intervention. Building local community capacity and engaging citizen participation in community development has been linked to improvements in neighbourhoods and communities, stronger social relationships and feelings of personal and political efficacy (Florin & Wandersman, 1990). Associated with this is the sense of empowerment, whereby individuals and groups act to gain mastery over their lives in the context of changing their social and political environments (Wallerstein & Bernstein, 1994).

Home environments

When children are physically and socially supported they are more likely to seek involvement in activity and develop confidence. Children deprived of safe play spaces may feel alienated and replace more physically active pastimes, such as exploring and socializing, with more solitary and sedentary activities, such as watching television (CCYP, 2004). An example of children growing up feeling unsafe is when they are exposed to abuse, be it physical, emotional or sexual. The manifestation of this environmental influence is particularly evident in the way children play and engage in social activities. For children who have been abused, play has been reported to be repetitive, stereotypic, disorganized and less developmentally mature than that of their peers who have not been abused (Alessandri, 1991; Cooper et al., in press).

The home is also known to be very important in the preparation of children for the important transition into school (McBryde et al., 2004). Maternal variables, including disciplinary style, affective tone or responsiveness and expectations for the child's achievement have been found to predict a child's perceived school readiness. In addition, the physical learning environment of a child's home, such as educational play materials, has also been found to support this transition (Parker et al., 1999). Discussed further in Chapter 11, the social and physical support of children in their preschool years has the potential to influence their transition into new environments.

Neighbourhood environments

A neighbourhood refers to 'a number of persons living near one another or in a particular locality' (Delbridge et al., 1997, p. 1442). For children, a neighbourhood is more than a physical setting; it defines a social universe and influences the things that they do, like to do and are able to do. Neighbourhoods affect children's play patterns and play partners (Berg & Medrich, 1980), thus enabling them to develop social relationships. Physical features, such as major streets, traffic safety conditions, local parks and playgrounds influence how far away from home children are allowed to explore independently (see Figure 3.2). The presence of other children in the neighbourhood is the strongest influence for children's desire to make contact, whereas for parents, concerns related to personal and traffic safety influence how far they allow children to venture (Berg & Medrich, 1980).

For the children in Berg & Medrich's study (1980), parks were not always accessible (due to traffic or major roads), so they tended to 'make do' with what was available. They found their own places, constructing forts and hiding spaces out of rubbish bins or fallen trees. These places were circumscribed as their play spaces in an environment built for adults. A particularly interesting finding for children

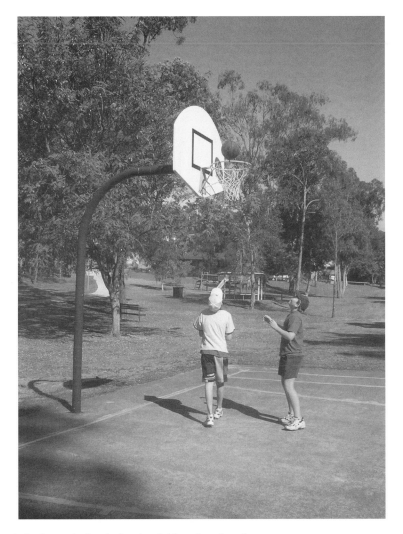

Figure 3.2 Boys playing in local neighbourhood park.

in middle childhood was the dislike of being dependent on parents for transport, instead craving opportunities to travel on their own by walking or riding bikes.

In a very different environment to urban America (cited above), children in Jordan are reported to use the street as a playground (Abu-Ghazzeh, 1998). As such, the street environment is seen as an agent of socialization. Hence, urban streets need to provide a balance between the recreational needs of children and the needs of vehicles. Abu-Ghazzeh viewed street play as a 'universal cultural phenomenon' serving an important role in children's social structures by providing a locus for peer contact close to home. All over the world, children make play opportunities from mundane features and objects such as curbs, parked cars, trees, piles of waste, stairs and patches of dirt. For children, the absence of special equipment is not

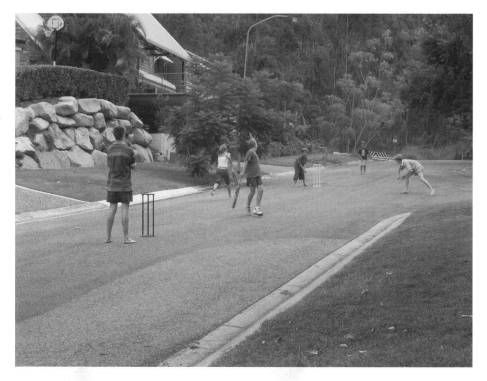

Figure 3.3 Neighbourhood children playing in quiet cul-de-sac in suburban Brisbane, Australia.

necessarily a barrier. Their play is spontaneous and casual, and is guided by features of the landscape and their imaginations.

For streets to accommodate play, they must be free from excess traffic, diverse in character, have adequate space for street games, have locations for hiding and building things, and opportunities to learn about nature. Urban innovations such as traffic calming allow safer play. For those living in high-rise apartments, play activities requiring more space, such as ball games, bike riding, skipping, running and hiding, tend to be played outside in the street or proximate park (see Figure 3.3). Schools in neighbourhoods dominated by high-rise buildings often provide indoor playgrounds as there is no outdoor space (see Figure 3.4).

There is increasing recognition that children's needs are largely unmet and unrecognized in the built environments of many cities (Blakely, 1994). With increasing urban density, there is less likelihood that children will live in houses with their own large gardens for play. Instead, it is likely that children (particularly in middle childhood) will look to the streets and facilities in their neighbourhoods as places to play. As professionals and community citizens, we need to advocate at local, state and national levels for children's play needs. Additionally, we must collaborate with urban designers and planners to ensure that children's needs for safe play spaces are met through appropriate street scape design, traffic calming, footpaths and accessible green parklands.

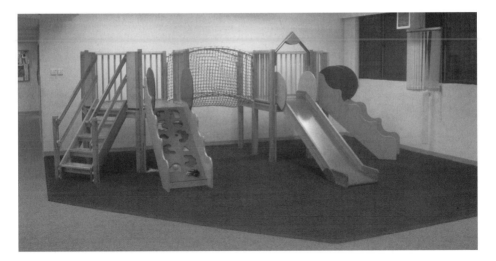

Figure 3.4 Indoor school playground, Hong Kong.

Community environments

Whereas neighbourhood has a physical dimension, community is a more social concept, defined as a 'group of any size whose members reside in a specific locality, share government and have a cultural and historical heritage' (Delbridge et al., 1997, p. 446). Communities are recognized as resources to support parents and families in their roles of nurturing children's development and journey to adulthood. Community capacity is the extent to which community members:

> '(a) demonstrate a sense of shared responsibility for the general welfare of the community and its members, and (b) demonstrate collective competence in taking advantage of opportunities for addressing community needs and confronting situations that threaten the safety and wellbeing of community members' (Bowen et al., 2000, p. 7).

Community capacity building is simply about 'helping people to discover how to better use everyone and everything to enhance their community's vitality and sustainability' (Bercuvitz & Gilman, 1992, p. 16). Concepts related to community capacity building are 'community development' and 'empowerment', which aim to increase the capabilities of people to articulate and address community health issues, and overcome barriers to achieve improved quality of life outcomes (Labonte et al., 2002). The process of community capacity building also fosters belonging, friendships, confidence and self-esteem, and encourages new networks for support.

Increasingly, human service professionals working with families are focusing their attention on the communities in which families live and work, in order to strengthen families through community based prevention and education activities (Bowen et al., 2000). This context in which families operate represents a nexus between formal and informal networks of social care. For example, a family with a child with significant disability may access formal support through a non-profit organization that provides support at home and respite services. In addition, the family may have their own informal supports such as relatives, family friends, neighbours, members of school and/or church groups. For each family, there is a unique mix of formal and informal support networks at times of need.

Recognition of the importance of informal networks was encapsulated in the Stronger Families initiative (Commonwealth Department of Family and Community Services, 2002), a government funded programme designed to build community capacity and support families in raising children. In a project funded through this initiative (Rodger, 2004), parents of children who had recently been diagnosed with autism spectrum disorder (ASD) were involved in parent education workshops designed to help them understand ASD, learn about social communication and play, community supports and experiment with management approaches at home (Rodger, in press). Parent-education group workshops were designed to:

(1) Be family-centred
(2) Based in the family's natural context
(3) Promote synchrony of interaction between parents and child (Braithwaite et al., 2003)

Parents were also supported by ten sessions of home based early intervention, focusing on parent chosen goals.

An innovative aspect of the project was the inclusion of a community session (Braithwaite et al., 2003). This involved a two-hour evening session to which parents invited anyone who had had contact with their child. For example, parents invited relatives, friends, baby-sitters, speech pathologists, childcare workers and swimming teachers. Following an informative lecture designed to help them understand the condition and various challenges it may pose there was time for questions and sharing of experiences. The incorporation of light refreshments enabled families to strengthen their formal and informal networks. These sessions also helped to build community capacity through the provision of information and enhancing support for families in their local communities.

Virtual environments

Virtual environments, created by access to electronic media, are of growing importance to children both at home and school. The extent of children's engagement with this technology has motivated some authors to refer to a 'digital childhood' (Calvert & Jordan, 2001). By virtual environments, we are referring to the activities and opportunities afforded to children through:

(1) The Internet that enables access to websites for information, to play games, chat rooms and email for social communication
(2) Console games such as PlayStation™

(3) Computer and simulation games
(4) Virtual fun parlours or arcade games

In addition, there has been a proliferation of virtual toys such as virtual pets, which represent an integration of computers into the social world of children through simulation (Subrahmanyam et al., 2001).

While virtual environments can provide potentially barrier free access for children with and without disabilities, as with other environments a number of concerns have been raised (The Royal Australasian College of Physicians [RACP], 2004). The relevance and appropriateness of the use of computers in early childhood education has been debated with respect to the quality of resources and effectiveness of learning experiences provided by software (for example Downes et al., 2001; Finegan & Austin, 2002; Freeman & Somerindyke, 2001); social interactions and collaborations (for example Roschelle et al., 2000; Scott et al., 2003); as well as the use of chat rooms to support after school learning (for example McCreary et al., 2001). However, the use of computers and the Internet at home has been less well researched, except for time use studies which have addressed the amount of time children spend engaged in screen based activities in the United States (Wright et al., 2001) and Australia (Yelland & Lloyd, 2001). American data suggests that children are on average (including weekends and holidays) engaged with various electronic media for six and a half hours per day (RACP, 2004). Such figures have caused many researchers to question the impact that this activity is having on our children.

The age and developmental maturity of children has been found to influence their reactions to media content. Children under four years have difficulty understanding that what they see on television is not real. However, the visual properties of the presentation are highly attractive regardless of content (Weddell, 2001). Another feature of exposure to media, such as television, on children is the impact that it has on their play. Beyond the displacement of play, the presence of television can distort the play transaction for children when it occurs as a background stimulus (Anderson & Evans, 2003). Engagement in television and Internet activity also exposes young children to advertising. For young children the fine line between reality and overt and covert advertising messages has been implicated in the increased consumption of high energy fast food (Robinson, 2001), the desirability of unrealistic body forms (McLellan, 2002) and 'label' driven consumerism (Turow, 2001).

The effect of children's exposure to terrorism and violence through the media also remains debated. While some point to an increase in symptoms of posttraumatic stress disorders such as fear, psycho-physiological arousal, anger and hyper-vigilance (Hayes & Casey, 1992; Parson, 1997), others argue that responses are mediated by the context and viewing partners involved (Wright et al., 2001). The use of the television as a baby-sitter has more detrimental implications than as an activity in which the family is involved and what is viewed becomes part of family discussion. These discussions are a way of socializing a child into the social and political environment in which they must function.

While moderate use of computers to play games has not been found to have a negative impact on children's friendships and family relationships, increased use of the Internet has been linked to increases in depression and loneliness, particularly in susceptible individuals (Griffiths, 1997; Subrahmanyam et al., 2001). Subrahmanyam et al. (2001) reported that social impact was complicated by the fact that most children engaged in email or chat room contact with 'strong' social ties or people with whom they already had a real life connection. The Internet did not replace face-to-face social contact but complemented it, particularly for girls, who engaged more in Internet use for social connectedness. The more concerning social impact reported was that of 'loose' social ties or those established in chat rooms where children had no previous contact with these individuals. Further concern is reported when computer/arcade game players become 'addicted', playing for 30 or more hours per week, becoming socially withdrawn and losing friends, and regarding their computers as a 'best friend' (Griffiths, 1997; Mitchell, 2000).

While parents and professionals have voiced concerns about children's use of the Internet, some authors (for example Quigley & Blashki, 2003) described these concerns as being related to adult anxieties about the crossing of boundaries between childhood and adulthood, private and public, and work and leisure. They proposed that children are active participants in virtual environments and can be empowered by appropriate information and education about how to manage themselves in these contexts. Hence, it is incumbent upon parents and professionals to not only be aware of the potential risks, but also to equip children to manage the reality of ongoing and informed engagement in virtual environments.

Children need to learn how to be discerning about their Internet usage and viewing choices, just as they must be with television viewing. However, while parents are advised to monitor their children's computer and Internet usage, they are often not as computer literate as their children. This 'digital generation gap' can make monitoring difficult (Livingstone, 2003). What is important, however, is adherence to family rules with respect to Internet access and use in relation to not providing personal information in chat rooms or via email, never allowing children to arrange personal meetings with other computer users without parental permission or supervision and appreciating that people online may not be who they seem.

Evaluating children's environments

With the increasing focus on preventive practice, we are now challenged to look at the quality of environments in which children live and how to better connect and support children within these environments. Strong and varied connections with people and organizations have been shown to provide a buffer for children at risk (Jessor et al., 1995). In this section we will look at two approaches for evaluating environments. The first focus will be at the population level and will describe how geographic information systems have the potential to inform occupational therapists and their collaborators about ways of promoting children's wellbeing by better understanding and working with the physical and social environment. The second relates to the methods currently available to enable the evaluation of specific environmental contexts.

Geographic information systems

Geographic information systems (GIS) are computer based systems for storing, maintaining, querying and analysing geographic data (Barndt, 1998). The key word in this description is 'data', and no amount of sophisticated hardware and other resources can replace the need for issue and geographic specific data. There are a number of databases available, including census, transport, facilities and services (Brownell et al., 2002). Researchers and practitioners, however, need to play an active role in acquiring data from government and non-government agencies, manipulating data, and then utilizing the findings to inform local communities and government authorities of emerging needs.

Communities that have access to information have reported increased individual participation in a range of activities and services (Barndt, 1998). For example, in a study of a community's access to its health care system (Plescia et al., 2001), researchers enlisted GIS in conjunction with survey assessment to determine community awareness of services and facilities. The findings indicated disparity between perceptions of needs and services, and demographic data on health issues and supporting resources. It also highlighted that greater access to spatial data by the community was able to facilitate change in behaviour.

Another example where this system can be applied to the health and wellbeing of children can be found in the extension of a recent project which examined the declining numbers of children walking to school (Ziviani et al., 2004). The health issue of concern was the increase in obesity and the corresponding decrease in physical activity in children. Increasing incidental physical activity for children, such as walking to school, was identified as one way to establish early healthy activity patterns which might extend into adult life. The study in question utilized a survey to ascertain the perceived barriers to children walking to school. The barriers most frequently cited were distance, traffic conditions and safety concerns. Data available from local government databases was then spatially presented as a way of informing the school community of ways in which participation could be facilitated. The available data sets accessed in this exercise included the location of parks, playgrounds and commercial areas, road systems, pavement network, pedestrian crossings, road-side parking, accident locations for the past five years, sign post locations and elevations. The way in which this data can be presented to a community is demonstrated in Figure 3.5, which maps the distribution of children attending the particular school, along with spatial data on access, crossing and transport considerations. Matching the issues raised by families in the survey with the data available through GIS is a way of involving the community in problem solving spatial as well as social barriers. Furthermore this level of information can allow communities to advocate to local authorities about bus routes, paths and safe crossing areas.

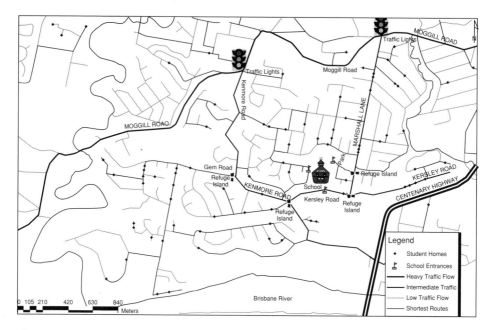

Figure 3.5 Application of GIS to support a walk to school programme in a local community. The map depicts residential locations of school children and identifies the shortest and safest walking routes to and from school. Reproduced with permission of the State of Queensland (Department of Education and the Arts).

GIS has been widely used by planners and demographers for many years to conceptualize spatial characteristics. Occupational therapists may not be the prime users of this information in everyday practice at present, but with rapid developments in technological access to this type of information it is important for therapists to be informed of its potential and to be aware of its utility.

Evaluating specific environments

Occupational therapists are often involved in evaluating children's performance within specific contexts. While there are limited assessments available that are embedded in a specific environmental context, the emergence of measures such as the School Function Assessment (SFA) (Coster et al., 1998) indicate the potential for this approach. The SFA is designed to determine the functional performance of children within their specific school context. Inherent in this approach is the distinction drawn in the ICF (WHO, 2001) between *capacity* (what a child can do) and *performance* (how well they can do it in a specific environment). A key challenge which faces occupational therapists is the development of more measures, such as the SFA, which can address the diversity of environments in which children find themselves and their impact (Mulligan, 2003). Actual measures of environments (physical and socio-cultural) in which children function (for example schools, playgrounds, home, childcare centres), however, are currently underdeveloped. The lack of such assessments has been identified by the profession (Law et al., 2001) and also by advocates of the ICF (Kuipers et al., 2003).

There has been some work undertaken on a taxonomy of physical environmental qualities and the type of engagement that they can afford children (Kytta, 2002). For example: flat, smooth surfaces can afford cycling, skating and game play; attached objects afford jumping over and jumping down from; shelter affords hiding and the opportunity for quiet reflection; mouldable materials such as sand, dirt and snow can afford opportunities for building and shaping. Connected with the physical possibilities of environmental structures, of course, is the social dimension when a number of children and/or adults are also involved. The ability to learn taking turns, role-play and cooperation may happen in part from the physical environment, but more commonly if supervisory and cooperative social structures are in place. Taxonomies such as this can provide a useful basis for the development of environment measures for playgrounds. Table 3.1 provides a summary of some of the measures currently available which focus on environment. Most of these measures were developed more than twenty years ago and though some such as the Home Observation for Measurement of the Environment (HOME) (Caldwell & Bradley, 1984) still appear in the research literature, there has been little development in these areas in recent times.

An assessment still in the early stages of development, which specifically targets the environment in which children play and is a companion to the Test of Playfulness (ToP) (Bundy, 1997) is the Test of Environmental Supportiveness (TOES) (Bundy, 1999). The TOES was designed to assess elements of a particular environment which have the potential to support play engagement. The TOES examines care-givers, playmates, objects, play space, and the sensory environment, as these elements can support or interfere with the player (Bundy, 1999). This model of teaming assessments again provides promise of a valuable direction in which assessments can be developed. The WHO (2001) identified measurement of the environment as a critical aspect of ongoing work for people with health conditions. Occupational therapists are well positioned to accept this challenge. Next we turn to how occupational therapists can impact on environmental design and engage in appropriate advocacy.

Collaborative environmental design and advocacy

There is a growing awareness of the need to:

(1) Develop policies and programmes that enhance children's sense of inclusion in their community
(2) Review urban design and planning regulations to facilitate community cohesion and provide safe environments for children (CCYP, 2004)

Table 3.1 Measures focusing on assessment of the environment.

Measure	Age range	Environment	Description	Psychometric properties
HOME Observation for measurement of the environment – revised (Caldwell & Bradley, 1984)	Birth to six years of age	Home	An observation/interview designed to sample aspects of the quantity and quality of social, emotional and cognitive support made available to children in their home environment. There is an infant, preschool and elementary school version. Scoring is binary with 1 indicating the presence of a developmentally supportive aspect of the environment and 0 its absence. Items are summed to produce an overall score.	Reliability: subtest stability over time (six months to two years) yielded alpha coefficients of .30–.70. Inter observer consistency routinely report ICC values greater than .80 (Bradley, 1994). Internal consistency alpha coefficients of .53–.93 for subtests and .93 for total score. Validity: factor analysis support subtest structure (Mundrom et al., 1993). Significant (low to moderate) correlations reported with measures of SES, intelligence and school attainment (.20–.60)
Infant/toddler environment rating scale (Harms et al., 1990)	Birth to 30 months	Childcare environment	Designed to rate the quality of centre based childcare. Uses a seven point adequacy rating scale which evaluates facilities and practices. A total score is obtained as well as subscale scores for: furnishings and display; personal care and routines; listening and talking; learning activities; interaction; programme structure; and adult needs.	Inter-rater reliability reported as .80 for total score and ranging from .58 to .89 for subscales. Test/retest reliability reported as .79 for total score ranging from .58 to .76 for subscales. Cronbach's Alpha for overall scale was .83. Criterion validity studies also undertaken (Clifford et al., 1989).

Measure	Population	Environment	Description	Psychometric properties
Environment assessment index (EAI) (Poresky, 1987)	3 to 11 years old	Home environment in rural areas	Developed as an extension of HOME, the EAI is a maternal interview and home observation procedure to determine the educational/developmental quality of a child's home. It comprises 44 items and has a 24-item short form. Scoring is dichotomous, with a score of 1 provided for a positive response/observation and 0 for a negative response.	Cronbach's Alpha for the 44-item scale was .74 and .82 for the short form. Correlation between the long and short form was .93. Test/retest reliability ranged from .66 to .96 depending on age groups and time period (Poresky, 1987).
Classroom environment scale (Moos & Trickett, 1986)	Junior and high school children and their teachers	Teacher and student perception of classroom social climate	Developed to evaluate social climate in junior and high school classrooms. Comprises nine subscales concerned with relationships (involvement, friendship, support), personal growth/goal orientation (activity completion, competition) and system maintenance and change (classroom functioning, novelty, variety). There is both a full scale (90 items) and a short form (36 items).	Normative data established on 465 students in 382 classrooms and 295 teachers located on east and west coast USA. Internal consistency ranged from .67 to .86. Test/retest reliability ranged from .90 to .98 over a six week interval. Validity studies reported.
Test of environment supportiveness (Bundy, 1999) undertaken in conjunction with the test of playfulness (Bundy, 1997).	Children (ages not specified)	Play environments	Seventeen item four-point rating scale which assesses the extent to which care-givers, playmates, objects, play space and sensory environment support or interfere with player engagement.	Preliminary results supportive of inter-rater reliability and some evidence for validity (Bronson & Bundy, 2001). Research is ongoing.

In the following discussion, we will examine how children can collaborate in the development and modification of environments and how they can review playgrounds as a dimension of space created primarily for their use.

Children as collaborators

Involving children and young people in environmental design and planning, and public health programmes, is a recognized aspect of community consultation (CCYP, 2004; ; Chawla & Heft, 2002; Francis & Lorenzo, 2002; Freeman, 1995; Meucci & Schwab, 1997; Sutton & Kemp, 2002). UNICEF has reinforced the rights and needs of children as global citizens to be involved with urban and environmental design and planning (Francis & Lorenzo, 2002), as well as planning for access to natural environments (natural open spaces, green corridors, national parks, fields or bushland) (Freeman, 1995). Experience of nature (through play, hobbies, family outings) in children's formative years is critical to their development into environmentally aware adults who are capable of safeguarding the earth's fragile ecosystem. Furthermore, natural spaces provide children with play, recreational and restorative opportunities that can harness creative potential, an environmental aspect which is not possible with designated fixed-equipment play areas.

The process of involving children in urban planning and environmental policies is relatively new, and the means by which they can be included are still underdeveloped. If given a choice, over 52% of children would prefer to go to parks and public spaces with friends after school, without adult supervision (Smith, 1995). While not always realistic, these views need to be considered with respect to how facilities and supervision are structured. An individually administered qualitative word association activity was used as part of a survey with children and youth to determine their perceptions of neighbourhood areas and residents (Polivka et al., 1998). This enabled them to identify themes around safety issues, pollution, noise and violence, which could form the basis of collaborative community initiatives to improve the neighbourhood for children. An intensive, hands-on, week long workshop, called a design 'charette', was used by Sutton & Kemp (2002). They engaged Washington children in grades 4–5 and 9–12 as active participants with designers and planners in neighbourhood place making to solve a community design problem. Benefits to children included opportunities to influence public decision making, increased social and environmental awareness, and the development of environmental competence. The 'charette' offers a methodology for bringing children and adults together to imagine landscapes that enhance social and ecological relationships and highlight children's voices.

Occupational therapists and other health professionals who understand children with and without disabilities, and who are child-centred, are in a prime position to advocate for children's roles in consultation processes. They can also assist and facilitate children's engagement in such consultations, and can play a key role in assisting children to have a voice, through preparing them for consultations, facilitating such forums where children can raise issues of concern, and developing action research and participative evaluation methods for use with community groups. Given the relative recency of children's participation in policy, decision making and design issues, the CCYP (2004) recommends the development of guidelines for good practice in how to involve children in decision making on issues that affect them.

Children's playgrounds

Planners, designers and educators alike are aware of the importance of outdoor play spaces and experiences for children. As many infants and school-age children spend much of their time indoors, outdoor playgrounds at childcare facilities and school need to afford children opportunities for quality play experiences. In addition, urban planners have become aware of the importance of designing playground spaces in neighbourhoods where children can safely play together, close to home.

A range of professionals are particularly interested in playground design, including architects and urban planners, childhood educators, public health officials and rehabilitation professionals such as occupational therapists, who have an interest in design for children with physical disabilities. It is increasingly recognized that outdoor play offers opportunities not only for physical and motor development, but also for developing and enhancing social interaction skills through sharing, cooperation and mutual goal seeking. The importance of fitness and the opportunities afforded in children's outdoor playgrounds for physical activity cannot be underestimated given the recent concerns about increasing obesity in children (Sutterby & Frost, 2002). Further, well designed playgrounds can enhance all aspects of children's development – motor, cognitive, social and emotional (see Figure 3.6). They provide opportunities for creativity, problem solving and fun (Hennger, 1993; Hudson et al., 2000).

There are four key considerations for playground safety: age or developmental appropriateness, equipment and equipment placement, supervision and maintenance (Gibbs, 2000; Wardle, 1998). From the perspective of age appropriateness, it is self-evident that toddlers and preschoolers have different play needs to those of school-age children. Specifically, size, placement and type of equipment in terms of physical demands must be considered (see Figure 3.7). Playground equipment needs to be safe and to match the developmental level of the children who use it (Taylor & Morris, 1996). In particular, children during middle childhood have additional needs for challenge and risk taking and if not provided with sufficiently challenging playground equipment (for example overhead rings, chin-up bars, ladders and overhead ropes) may misuse it and take inappropriate risks with play equipment (Wallach, 1983). Older children are also interested in having places to 'hang out' and socialize on the playground with their friends, and to become more involved in athletic pursuits such as basketball, soccer and football. There is a need, for example, for basketball courts or volleyball nets in outdoor spaces to accommodate playing in groups and for the mastering of games with rules (see Figure 3.2).

With respect to equipment and placement, the most critical safety concerns are providing adequate fall zone materials under and around all equipment; avoiding head entrapments by ensuring minimum safe openings; providing adequate guard railings to prevent falls; ensuring that there are no entanglements for catching clothes;

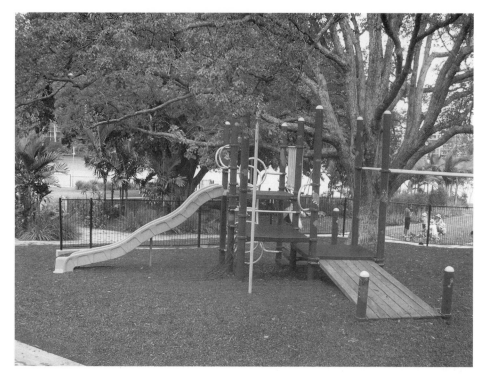

Figure 3.6 Children's playground demonstrating physical, motor and cognitive aspects.

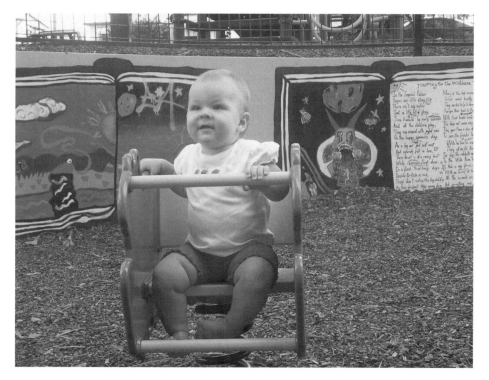

Figure 3.7 Playground for toddlers and young children.

and ensuring that equipment is away from traffic areas (Wardle, 1998). Maintenance of damaged or deteriorated equipment is critical to avoid safety hazards. Regular safety audits are important (Gibbs, 2000) and examples of playground safety checklists can be found in the literature (for example Taylor & Morris, 1996). Those working in school or early childhood settings should be aware of playground equipment safety and supervision, and like all childhood professionals they should be cognizant of and contribute to playground design and safety features, as appropriate.

Playground environments can be categorized as *defined* and *creative* (Storage & Bowers, 1983). *Defined* environments channel play activities in prescribed directions. For example, swings and slides define play according to their functions, with limited scope for experimentation. These environments tend to limit access for children with disabilities. By contrast, *creative* play environments appeal to the imagination and lend themselves to inclusion of children with disabilities. The presence of movable toys and equipment that can be returned to storage facilities provides alternative play options in school and early childhood playgrounds. These additional materials allow for creative play in outdoor spaces, lending themselves to dramatic play (for example tent, cooking stove, sleeping bags or steering wheel mounted in a wooden box) (Hennger, 1993); or obstacle courses that can be recreated and built with supervision regarding safety and with the input of children's imaginations (Griffin & Rinn, 1998). It is increasingly recognized that children, as the primary users of playgrounds, can offer invaluable insights into creating appealing and challenging play environments.

Playgrounds also have restorative potential for children. Children need play spaces and environments that allow them to select their own play themes and playthings, be free from adult rules and restrictions, and be with valued friends so that they can 'just be kids' and have fun (Talbot & Frost, 1989). Restoration involves 'renewing diminished functional resources and capabilities' (Hartig & Staats, 2003, p. 103). Attention is being paid to the socio-physical and temporal characteristics of environments that support restoration for people, as well as how unwanted demands can be reduced, such as noise, crowding and pollution. Enhanced restoration appears to be evident in natural versus urban environments (Hartig & Staats, 2003). Hence, outdoor green spaces, parks and playgrounds may be particularly important for their restorative potential for children (see Chapter 6).

Designing for difference

Occupational therapists are often consulted when schools or childcare centres need to design playgrounds for access for a child with a disability, or to find better ways of including children with limited physical abilities in the school grounds. The most obvious issues are those of physical access for children who are wheelchair dependent or who otherwise have severe mobility restrictions. Integrated playground design does not mean that every piece of equipment or every surface must be usable by every child. Ideally, accessible playgrounds offer a range of experiences, because all children are different (see Figure 3.8).

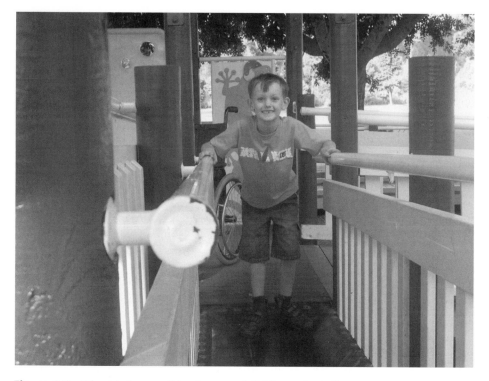

Figure 3.8 Wheelchair accessible playground, Brisbane, Australia.

To be truly inclusive, play environments must address access, activity and variability (Winter et al., 1994). Access refers to the ability to enter the desired location, while activity refers to the ability to actively take part or engage in an experience. Variability relates to the opportunity to select from a range of options to find a personally appropriate choice. Ensuring inclusion requires analysis of the activities that can be engaged in at a playground and opportunity to choose from an array of creative play opportunities. Like all children, those with disabilities need to achieve an individual balance of success and challenge. Some useful strategies for increasing inclusion include using low-cost movable pieces of equipment, increasing sensory input to playgrounds and designing around themes that foster cooperative play (Winter et al., 1994). Using a similar philosophy to universal design, playgrounds can be designed to benefit everyone. Hence, they can provide opportunities for all children, such as those with temporary mobility restrictions (for example leg plaster), in addition to those with permanent limitations (Wallach, 1983).

Another significant consideration for enhancing inclusion of children with special needs in the playground relates to teaching educational and support staff about how to facilitate friendships and to coach children during social play activities, using peer modelling of safe play and teaching peer role models how to interact with children with various physical or social disabilities (Winter et al., 1994). Given the critical role of play in the development of children, the playground provides a very important venue for social interaction, as well as for physical play. This opportunity needs to be harnessed for all children if they are to experience all that playgrounds can offer.

Summary

This chapter has provided an overview of the home, neighbourhood, community and virtual environments in which children interact. It has emphasized the complex interplay of physical, social and cultural aspects of these environments. When occupational therapists consider environmental influences on children's participation, they must understand both the context or place, and the physical, cultural and social aspects underpinning each environment. We have proposed that childhood professionals have an important advocacy role in ensuring that all children can engage in safe, appealing and child-friendly environments. Additionally, occupational therapists have a role in enabling children to collaborate with adults regarding the environments which are meaningful for them, in providing their own unique perspective which can influence future environmental design. The chapter has also highlighted the importance of the restorative capacity of environments, particularly natural spaces, in children's busy lives.

In terms of collaboration with urban planners, designers and geographers, the potential of databases such as those within GIS at a population level was identified. Occupational therapists' understanding of the human–environment fit at an individual level was also discussed and the need to address the lack of psychometrically sound and relevant measures of environment highlighted. Finally, this chapter has also identified some ways in which the physical, social and cultural environment can be harnessed or modified to enable children's participation.

References

Abu-Ghazzeh, T. M. (1998). Children's use of the street as a playground in Abu-Nuseir, Jordan. *Environment and Behavior, 30* (6), 799–831.

Alessandri, S. M. (1991). Play and social behavior in maltreated preschoolers. *Development and Psychopathology, 3*, 191–205.

Anderson, D. R. & Evans, M. K. (2003). The impact of the Internet on children: lessons from television. In: J. Turow & A. Kavanaugh (Eds.), *The Internet and the family: new views on a new world*. Evans, M. K. Cambridge: MIT Press.

Barndt, M. (1998). Public participation GIS barriers to implementation. *Cartography and Geographical Information Systems, 25* (2), 105–112.

Bercuvitz, J. & Gilman, R. (1992). Community animation. *In Context, 33*, 16–21.

Berg, M. & Medrich, E. A. (1980). Children in four neighborhoods: the physical environment and its effect on play and play patterns. *Environment and Behavior, 12* (3), 320–348.

Blakely, K. S. (1994). Parents' conceptions of social dangers to children in the urban environment. *Children's Environments, 11* (1), 16–25.

Bowen, G. L., Martin, J. A., Mancini, J. A. & Nelson, J. P. (2000). Community capacity: antecedents and consequences. *Journal of Community Practice, 8* (2), 1–21.

Bradley, R. H. (1994). The home inventory: review and reflections. *Advances in Child Development and Behavior, 25,* 241–287.

Braithwaite, M., Keen, D. & Rodger, S. (2003, 30 November–3 December). *The stronger families and ASD project*. Paper presented at the third Australian families and community strengths conference, Newcastle, Australia.

Bronfenbrenner, U. (1979). *The ecology of human development: experiments by nature and design*. Harvard, MA: Harvard University Press.

Bronson, M. J. & Bundy, A. (2001). A correlational study of a test of playfulness and a test of environmental supportiveness for play. *Occupational Therapy Journal of Research, 21,* 241–259.

Brownell, M., Mayer, T., Martens, P., Kozyrskyj, A., Fergusson, P., Bodnarchuk, J., et al. (2002). Using a population based health information system to study child health. *Canadian Journal of Public Health, 93,* S9–S14.

Bundy, A. C. (1997). *Test of playfulness (Version 3)*. Ft Collins, CO: Colorado State University.

Bundy, A. C. (1999). *Test of environmental supportiveness*. Ft Collins, CO: Colorado State University.

Caldwell, B. M. & Bradley, R. H. (1984). *Home observation for measurement of the environment (HOME): administration manual (rev. ed.)*. Little Rock: University of Arkansas.

Calvert, S. L. & Jordan, A. B. (2001). Children in the digital age. *Applied Developmental Psychology, 22,* 3–5.

Chawla, L. & Heft, H. (2002). Children's competence and the ecology of communities: a functional approach to the evaluation of participation. *Journal of Environmental Psychology, 22,* 201–216.

Clifford, R. M., Russell, S., Fleming, J., Peisner, E., Harms, T. & Cryer, D. (1989). *Infant/toddler environment rating scale: reliability and validity studies*. Chapel Hill, NC: Frank Porter Graham Child Development Center, University of North Carolina.

Commission for Children and Young People (CCYP) (2004). *A head start for Australia: an early years framework* (ISBN 0 7347 7115 0). Sydney: Commission for Children and Young People.

Commonwealth Department of Family and Community Services (2002). *Stronger families and communities strategy*. Canberra, ACT: Commonwealth Department of Family and Community Services.

Cooper, R., Ziviani, J. & Nixon, J. (in press). Playskills of preschool children who have experienced intrafamiliar child abuse and neglect. *Child Abuse and Neglect*.

Coster, W., Deeney, T., Haltiwanger, J. & Haley (1998). *School function assessment (SFA)*. San Antonio, TX: Psychological Corp.

Delbridge, A., Bernard, J. R. L., Blair, D., Butler, S., Petty, P. & Yallop, C. (Eds.) (1997). *The Macquarie dictionary* (3rd ed.). North Ryde, NSW: Macquarie Library.

Downes, T., Arthur, L. & Beecher, B. (2001). Effective learning environments for young children using digital resources: an Australian perspective. *Information Technology in Childhood Education Annual,* 139–153.

Dunn, W., Brown, C. & McGuigan, A. (1994). The ecology of human performance: a framework for considering the effect of context. *The American Journal of Occupational Therapy, 48* (7), 595–607.

Finegan, C. & Austin, N. J. (2002). Developmentally appropriate technology for young children. *Information Technology in Childhood Education Annual, 16,* 87–102.

Florin, P. & Wandersman, A. (1990). An introduction to citizen participation, voluntary organizations and community development: insights for empowerment through research. *American Journal of Community Psychology, 18* (1), 41–54.

Francis, M. & Lorenzo, R. (2002). Seven realms of children's participation. *Journal of Environmental Psychology, 22,* 157–169.

Freeman, C. (1995). Planning and play: creating greener environments. *Children's Environments, 12* (3), 381–388.

Freeman, C. & Somerindyke, J. (2001). Social play at the computer: preschoolers scaffold and support peers' computer competence. *Information Technology in Childhood Education Annual,* 203–213.

Gibbs, C. J. (2000). Elementary school playground design. *School Planning and Management, 39* (7), 54–55.

Griffin, C. & Rinn, B. (1998). Enhancing outdoor play with an obstacle course. *Young Children, 53* (3), 18–23.

Griffiths, M. (1997). Friendship and social development in children and adolescents: the impact of electronic technology. *Educational and Child Psychology, 14* (3), 25–37.

Harms, T., Cryer, D. & Clifford, R. M. (1990). *Infant/toddler environment rating Scale.* New York: Teachers College Press.

Hartig, T. & Staats, H. (2003). Guest editors' introduction: restorative environments. *Journal of Environmental Psychology, 23,* 103–107.

Hayes, D. S. & Casey, D. M. (1992). Young children and television: the retention of emotional reactions. *Child Development, 63* (6), 1423–1436.

Hennger, M. L. (1993). Enriching the outdoor play experience. *Childhood Education, 70* (2), 1–4.

Hudson, S., Thompson, D. & Mack, M. (2000). Planning playgrounds for children of all abilities. *School Planning and Management, 39* (2), 35–40.

Jessor, R., Bos, J. V., Vanderryn, J., Costa, F. M. & Turbin, M. S. (1995). Protective factors in adolescent problem behavior: moderator effects and developmental change. *Developmental Psychology, 31,* 923–933.

King, G. A., Cathers, T., Polgar, J. M. & MacKinnon, E. B. (2000). Success in life for older adolescents with cerebral palsy. *Qualitative Health Research, 10,* 734–749.

Korten, D. C. (1984). People-centred development: toward a framework. In: D.C. Korten & R. Klaus (Eds.), *People centred development: contributions toward theory and planning frameworks* (pp. 299–309). Conn.: Kumarian Press.

Kuipers, P., Foster, M. M. & Bellamy, N. (2003). Incorporation of environmental factors into outcomes research. *Expert Review of Pharmacoeconomics and Outcomes Research, 3* (2), 125–129.

Kytta, M. (2002). Affordances of children's environments in the context of cities, small towns, suburbs and rural villages in Finland and Belarus. *Journal of Environmental Psychology, 22,* 109–123.

Labonte, R., Woodard, G. B., Chad, K. & Laverack, G. (2002). Community capacity building: a parallel track for health promotion programs. *Canadian Journal of Health, 93* (3), 181–182.

Larson, R. W. & Verma, S. (1999). How children and adolescents spend time across the world: work, play and developmental opportunities. *Psychological Bulletin, 125* (6), 701–736.

Law, M. (2002). Participation in the occupations of everyday life. *American Journal of Occupational Therapy, 56* (6), 640–649.

Law, M., Baum, C. & Dunn, W. (2001). *Measuring occupational performance: supporting best practice in occupational therapy.* Thorofare, NJ: Slack Incorporated.

Leavitt, R. L. (1999). *Cross-cultural rehabilitation: an international perspective.* London: W. B. Saunders.

Livingstone, S. (2003). Children's use of the Internet: reflections on the emerging research agenda. *New Media and Society, 5* (2), 147–166.

McBryde, C., Ziviani, J. & Cuskelly, M. (2004). School readiness and factors that influence decision making. *Occupational Therapy International, 11* (4), 193–208.

McCreary, F. A., Ehrich, R. W. & Lisanti, M. (2001). Chat rooms as 'virtual hangouts' for rural elementary students. *Information Technology in Childhood Education Annual,* 105–123.

McLellan, F. (2002). Marketing and advertising: harmful to children's health. *Lancet, 360,* 1001.

Meucci, S. & Schwab, M. (1997). Children and the environment: young people's participation in social change. *Social Justice, 24* (3), 1–9.

Mitchell, P. (2000). Internet addiction: genuine diagnosis or not? *Lancet, 355,* 632.

Moos, R. H. & Trickett, E. J. (1986). *Classroom environment scale.* Palo Alto, CA: Consulting Psychologists Press.

Mulligan, S. (2003). *Occupational therapy evaluation for children: a pocket guide.* Philadelphia: Lippincott, Williams & Wilkins.

Mundrom, D. J., Bradley, R. H. & Whiteside, L. (1993). A factor analytic study of the infant-toddler and early childhood versions of the HOME inventory. *Educational and Psychological Measurement, 53* (2), 479–489.

Parker, F. L., Boak, A. Y., Griffen, K. W., Ripple, C. & Peay, L. (1999). Parent-child relationship, home learning environment and school readiness. *School Psychology Review, 28,* 413–423.

Parson, E. R. (1997). Post-traumatic child therapy (P-TCT): assessment and treatment factors in clinical work with inner-city children exposed to catastrophic community violence. *Journal of Interpersonal Violence, 12* (2), 172–195.

Plescia, M., Koontz, S. & Laurent, S. (2001). Community assessment in a vertically integrated health care system. *Journal of Public Health, 91* (5), 811–814.

Polivka, B. J., Lovell, M. & Smith, B. A. (1998). A qualitative assessment of inner-city elementary schoolchildren's perceptions of their neighborhood. *Public Health Nursing, 15* (3), 171–179.

Poresky, R. H. (1987). Environmental assessment index: reliability, stability and validity of the long and short forms. *Educational and Psychological Measurement, 47,* 969–975.

Quigley, M. & Blashki, K. (2003). Beyond the boundaries of the sacred garden: children and the Internet. *Information Technology in Childhood Education Annual,* 309–407.

Rigby, P. & Letts, L. (2003). Environment and occupational performance: theoretical considerations. In: L. Letts, P. Rigby & D. Stewart (Eds.), *Using environments to enable occupational performance* (pp. 17–32). Thorofare, NJ: Slack Incorporated.

Ringaert, L. (2003). Universal design of the built environment. In: L. Letts, P. Rigby & D. Stewart (Eds.), *Using environments to enable occupational performance* (p. 314). Thorofare, NJ: Slack Inc.

Robinson, T. (2001). Television viewing and childhood obesity. *Pediatric Clinics of North America, 48,* 1017–1025.

Rodger, S. (2004, 14–15 May). *Building stronger families with autism spectrum disorder: an innovative approach to strengths and community-based support*. Paper presented at the 2004 autism conference: 'Reach for the stars', Brisbane, Australia.

Rodger, S. (in press). Children and families: partners in education. In: K. McKenna & L. Tooth (Eds.), *Client education: a partnership approach for health practitioners*. Sydney: UNSW Press.

Roschelle, J. M., Pea, R. D., Hoadley, C. M., Gordin, D. N. & Means, B. M. (2000). Changing how and what children learn in school with computer-based technologies. *The Future of Children*, *10* (2), 76–101.

Salman, J. (2001). US accessibility codes and standards: challenges for universal design. In: W. Preiser & E. Ostroff (Eds.), *The universal design handbook*. New York: McGraw-Hill.

Scott, S. D., Mandryk, R. L. & Inkpen, K. M. (2003). Understanding children's collaborative interactions in shared environments. *Journal of Computer Assisted Learning*, *19*, 220–228.

Smith, F. (1995). Children's voices and the construction of children's spaces: the example of playcare centres in the United Kingdom. *Children's Environments*, *12* (3), 389–396.

Stewart, D. & Law, M. (2003). The environment: paradigms and practice in health, occupational therapy and inquiry. In: L. Letts, P. Rigby & D. Stewart (Eds.), *Using environments to enable occupational performance* (pp. 3–15). Thorofare, NJ: Slack Incorporated.

Storage, T. W. & Bowers, L. E. (1983). Playgrounds of the future. *Parks and Recreation*, *18* (4), 32–35.

Subrahmanyam, K., Greenfield, P., Kraut, R. & Gross, E. (2001). The impact of computer use on children's and adolescents' development. *Applied Developmental Psychology*, *22*, 7–30.

Sutterby, J. A. & Frost, J. L. (2002). Making playgrounds fit for children and children fit for playgrounds. *Young Children*, *57* (3), 36–41.

Sutton, S. E. & Kemp, S. P. (2002). Children as partners in neighborhood placemaking: lessons from intergenerational design charrettes. *Journal of Environmental Psychology*, *22*, 171–189.

Talbot, J. & Frost, J. L. (1989). Magical playscapes. *Childhood Education*, *66* (1), 11–19.

Taylor, S. I. & Morris, V. G. (1996). Outdoor play in early childhood education settings: is it safe and healthy for children? *Early Childhood Education Journal*, *23* (3), 153–158.

The Royal Australasian College of Physicians (RACP) (2004). *Children and the media: advocating for the future*. Sydney: The Royal Australasian College of Physicians.

Turow, J. (2001). Family boundaries, commercialism, and the Internet. A framework for research. *Journal of Applied Developmental Psychology*, *22*, 73–86.

Wallach, F. (1983). Play in the age of technology. *Parks and Recreation*, April, 36–38.

Wallerstein, N. & Bernstein, E. (1994). Introduction to community empowerment, participatory education and health. *Health Education Quarterly*, *21* (2), 141–148.

Wardle, F. (1998). Playgrounds for schoolage after-school programs. *Child-care Information Exchange*, *121*, 5–30.

Weddell, C. (2001). Media-savvy young children: understanding their view. *Every Child*, *7*, 4–5.

Whiteford, G. (2000). Occupational deprivation: global challenges in the new millennium. *British Journal of Occupational Therapy*, *63* (5), 200–204.

Winter, S. M., Bell, M. J. & Dempsey, J. D. (1994). Creating play environments for children with special needs. *Childhood Education, 71* (1), 28–32.

World Health Organization (WHO) (2001). *International classification of functioning, disability and health: ICF* (Short version ed.). Geneva: World Health Organization.

Wright, J. C., Huston, A. C., Vandewater, E. A., Bickham, D. S., Scantlin, R. M., Kotler, J. A., et al. (2001). American children's use of electronic media in 1997: a national survey. *Applied Developmental Psychology, 22,* 31–47.

Yelland, N. & Lloyd, M. (2001). Virtual kids of the twenty-first century: understanding the children in schools today. *Information Technology in Childhood Education Annual, 13,* 175–192.

Ziviani, J., Scott, J. & Wadley, D. (2004). Walking to school: incidental physical activity in the daily occupations of Australian children. *Occupational Therapy International, 51,* 69–79.

Chapter 4

PARTICIPATION OF CHILDREN IN SCHOOL AND COMMUNITY

Mary Law, Terry Petrenchik,
Jenny Ziviani and Gillian King

Participation in childhood occupations in school and community is essential for children and youth to grow and develop. Through participation, children develop skills, engage in collaborative activities with others, learn to express themselves, find meaning and promote health (King et al., 2003). Participation is the means by which children interact with other people and their environment. Yet our study and understanding of participation and the factors that influence participation in childhood occupations is still unfolding. While there is a growing body of literature about childhood participation for children and youth, there is much less information about the experience of participation in the context of developmental difficulties, disability, social marginalization and poverty.

The objectives of this chapter are to:

(1) Explore the concept of participation by way of definition and classification
(2) Examine the relationship of childhood participation to health, wellbeing and occupation
(3) Describe how physical, socio-cultural, political and economic environments affect the experience of childhood participation in school and in the community
(4) Identify how occupational therapists contribute to participation for children and youth

Participation

How is participation defined? The word participation is derived from the Latin word *participatus*, the past participle of *participare*. In turn, this word derives from *pars*, meaning 'part', plus *capere*, meaning 'to take' (Merriam-Webster online dictionary, 2004). Thus, the literal definition of participation is to 'take part' in something. Current definitions of participation also emphasize the active element of the meaning, expanding the literal definition to include participation as sharing, being involved with, being active, or experiencing something (The free dictionary, 2004).

Conceptually, participation is both a process and an outcome. As a process, participation is conceptualized as the act of engaging in everyday activities within physical, socio-cultural, economic and institutional environments. Implicit in this conceptualization is the assumption that participation has temporal and spatial qualities, as well as personally ascribed meaning. A thorough understanding of the meaning of participation requires therapists to consider dimensions of participation such as *with whom* and *where* activities take place, as well as children's activity enjoyment and preferences (Law, 2002).

Participation is the stated goal of occupational therapy intervention (American Occupational Therapy Association [AOTA], 2002; Canadian Association of Occupational Therapists [CAOT], 1997; Law, 2002). The outcome of participation is also a frequently used indicator of child health, wellbeing and development (Canadian Council on Social Development [CCSD], 2001; Federal Interagency Forum on Child and Family Statistics, 2003; Waters et al., 2002; World Health Organization, 2001).

While participation has a general meaning for all persons, it has been introduced into health care by the World Health Organization (WHO) within classification schemes of functioning and disability (2001). In a revision of the International Classification of Disability, the concepts of both participation and environment became central to understanding the relationship between people, their participation and the environments in which they live. The International Classification of Functioning, Disability and Health (ICF) identifies participation as the ultimate outcome for people who have disabling conditions. In this classification, participation is defined as involvement within a life situation (WHO, 2001). Participation can only be understood in the context of people in the environment in which they live, work and play. As defined in the ICF, participation is of central interest to occupational therapists, whose focus is to facilitate and promote the participation of children and youth with and without disabilities in childhood occupations.

Classification of participation

Since participation is a complex concept, classification schemes or typologies have been developed to aid our understanding of its meaning and factors influencing outcomes. We will now briefly review several of these classification schemes.

In the ICF (WHO, 2001), participation and activity are considered synonymously. The categories of participation in the ICF include *Learning and applying knowledge*, *General tasks and demands*, *Communication*, *Movement*, *Self-care*, *Domestic life areas*, *Interpersonal interactions*, *Major life areas*, and *Community, social and civic life*. In the past, there have been criticisms of the revised ICF and its perceived applicability to children and youth. For example, Simeonsson et al. (2000) comment that it has few items covering the childhood areas of learning, behaviour and school/community function. Recently, a version of the ICF for children and youth has been developed and is available on the WHO website (WHO, 2004). Specific details regarding the proposed subcategories of participation within the children's version are listed in Table 4.1.

Table 4.1 Proposed children's version of the international classification of functioning, disability and health.

Participation category	Subcategories
Learning and applying knowledge	Purposeful sensory experiences Basic learning Applying knowledge Learning and applying knowledge, other specified Learning and applying knowledge, unspecified
General tasks and demands	Undertaking a single task Undertaking a complex task Undertaking a single task independently Undertaking a single task in a group Undertaking single tasks, other specified Undertaking single tasks, unspecified
Communication	Communicating – receiving Communicating – producing Conversation and use of communication devices and techniques Communication, other specified Communication, unspecified
Mobility	Changing and maintaining body position Carrying, moving and handling objects Walking and moving Moving around using transportation Mobility, other specified Mobility, unspecified
Self-care	Washing oneself Caring for body parts Toileting Dressing Eating Drinking Avoiding potentially dangerous situations and harm to self Looking after one's health Self-care, other specified Self-care, unspecified
Domestic life	Acquisition of necessities Household tasks Caring for household objects and assisting others Domestic life, other specified Domestic life, unspecified
Interpersonal interactions and relationships	General interpersonal interactions Particular interpersonal relationships Interpersonal interactions and relationships, other specified Interpersonal interactions and relationships, unspecified
Major life areas	Education Economic life Major life areas, other specified Major life areas, unspecified

(Continued)

Table 4.1 (cont'd)

Participation category	Subcategories
Community, social and civic life	Community life School life and related activities Recreation and leisure Religion and spirituality Community, social and civic life, other specified Community, social and civic life, unspecified

Source: World Health Organization (2004) *International classification of functioning, disability and health: children and youth version*. Available online at www3.who.int/icf/icftemplate.cfm. Reproduced with permission.

Studies conducted around the world concerned with how children and youth spend their time have used activity categories to classify children's participation. Typically, time budget studies focus on categories very similar to those used by occupational therapists, that is, personal maintenance or self-care, work and leisure (Larson & Verma, 1999). Research measuring children's participation has expanded the leisure category to include recreation, active physical activities, social activities, skill based activities, and self-improvement activities (King et al., 2004).

Recreational and leisure participation have been further classified according to formality (King et al., 2004; Sloper et al., 1990). Formal activities involve structure and organization, and are usually carried out with other people. Examples of formal activities for children include sports teams, lessons, drama clubs and community groups such as Scouts. In contrast, informal activities are more spontaneous in nature, completed alone or with others, and require less planning. Examples of informal activities include playing with puzzles, talking to a friend, drawing or reading. Making the distinction between formal and informal activities is important for developing an understanding of the specific and unique benefits attributable to these two classes of activities (Beauvais, 2001).

Participation: relationship to health, wellbeing and development

Participation in day-to-day activities is an important aspect of children's health, wellbeing and development (see Figure 4.1). Participation, being a performer rather than an onlooker, contributes to children's physical and psychosocial development (Beauvais, 2001; CCSD, 2001; Waters et al., 2002). The health benefits of recreation and physical activity are well documented and include reduced obesity, improved cardiovascular health and fitness, and the facilitation of motor skill development. Psychosocial benefits include an improved sense of wellbeing, decreased incidence of depression, improved self-esteem and self-image, and greater life satisfaction (Beauvais, 2001; CCSD, 2001; Waters et al., 2002).

Through sustained participation in increasingly complex activities, children acquire the basic skills and competencies necessary for a successful transition into adulthood (Bronfenbrenner, 1999; Corsaro, 1997). Furthermore, participation in

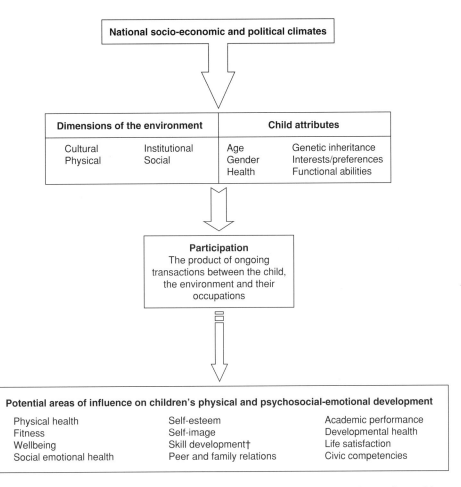

Figure 4.1 Elements of participation. † Skills: motor, social, communicative and cognition.

structured activities has been shown to decrease the incidence of behavioural and emotional problems among children in high-risk environments (Sandler et al., 2004; Werner, 1993). Additional benefits of participation in structured activities include improved school engagement, peer relations and educational outcomes (Masten & Coatsworth, 1998) and reductions in school drop out and delinquency (Mahoney & Cairns, 1997). Participation in structured activities reputedly also buffers the effects of living with a parent with mental health problems (Rutter, 1990).

While considerable evidence shows that participation in formal and informal activities benefits children's health, wellbeing and development, it is important to keep in mind that participation in more activities is not necessarily better (Forsyth & Jarvis, 2002; Henry, 1998). For example, a child might choose to participate in few recreational or leisure activities but may have intense involvement in these activities. Another child might be involved in several activities, but may participate in them very infrequently. The important consideration is whether children are able to participate in activities in which they need or would like to be involved.

Participation: relationship to occupation and occupational performance

Participation, as implemented within the ICF, is part of a conceptual classification scheme used by health practitioners to develop a common understanding of the process of disablement and the complex relationships between people and their environment. Occupational therapy, as a profession, is unique in its consideration of occupation as the central focus of human life. Occupation has been defined as:

> *'groups of activities and tasks of everyday life, named, organized and given value and meaning by individuals and a culture. Occupation is everything people do to occupy themselves, including looking after themselves (self-care), enjoying life (leisure), and contributing to the social and economic fabric of their communities (productivity)'* (CAOT, 1997, p. 34).

Occupational performance is considered to be the act of *doing* an occupation (Christiansen & Baum, 1997). Occupational therapists understand occupational performance to be the point at which the person, environment and occupation intersect to support the tasks, activities and roles that define that person as an individual (Christiansen & Baum, 1997). Thus, occupational therapists think of participation as a person's experience of participating in occupations that are personally meaningful and important. The outcome of participation would therefore be very similar to the outcome that occupational therapists measure as occupational performance.

There is little information in the occupational therapy literature examining the relationship between occupational therapy models of practice and the concept of participation as delineated within the ICF (WHO, 2001). Townsend et al. (1990) explored the relationship between the Canadian model of occupational performance and the predecessor to the ICF, the International Classification of Impairments, Disability and Handicap (ICIDH) (WHO, 1980). They proposed a mirror categorization between the Handicap dimension of the ICIDH and the three areas of occupational performance: self-care, productivity and leisure. Similarly, in the new ICF framework, the outcome of participation encompasses the three areas of occupational performance within the Canadian model of occupational performance and other conceptual models of occupational therapy.

Participation in school

School is a major influence on children and, outside their families, is a primary contributor to social, economic and psychological outcomes. When considering schools with respect to child and youth participation, we need to appreciate the cultural context in which school is embedded, the political agenda driving participation, and the physical and social environments of educational institutions.

Political agenda

While considered to be one of the most significant influences on social and economic outcomes, participation in education, be it in the physical environment of a school building or in a home setting, is not the experience of all children. It has been estimated (UNICEF-EAPRO, 2000) that 113 million children around the globe do not have access to education and that having a disability reduces an individual's chance of involvement even further. These figures may seem alarming to those in post-industrial nations, where there has been a well established political agenda of 'Education for all', and for the inclusion of children with disabilities in the least restrictive educational environment (Price, 2001). We will now present two examples where political structures are used to promote the participation of children in school. These will illustrate how a distinction can be drawn between political efforts being efficient versus effective.

Iyanar (2001) reported on the situation of education for children in India. The state government of Tamil Nadu, in south-eastern India, has a scheme of compulsory elementary school education for both boys and girls. Special emphasis is given to female education, particularly girls from lower socio-economic classes whose parents are not educated. Any girl admitted into first grade is given 500 rupees per year as a scholarship, which rises to 1000 rupees when she reaches the eighth grade[1]. In the case of working children, parents are provided with government subsidized housing if their children are sent to school. The government also increased the (educational) budget fivefold for children with disabilities, thus encouraging the inclusion of children with disability within ordinary schools. These measures can be considered effective as many children who would not have attended school are now able to do so. However, are they efficient?

If we examine the situation in a country such as Australia, which is similar to that in many post-industrial countries, then we see a stark political contrast to that in the example above. First, it is legally mandated that all children attend school (formal, distance or home). For children with disabilities, while segregated special education facilities still exist, the adoption of the least restrictive educational environment is advocated (Queensland Department of Education, 2000). In practice this means that children can experience 'mainstreaming', in which they receive some instruction in a special segregated unit but are also included in regular classes. The other model involves 'inclusion', in which the support services (modified curriculum, therapy support and environmental modification) for an individual child are provided in the classroom, thereby enabling the child to participate in the regular educational programme. In this situation it could be argued that practice is both effective (that is, all children are required to participate in education) and efficient, in that adequate support and structures are in place for those children with special needs.

---

[1] At the time of writing this book, 1000 Indian rupees was equal to approximately $22 USD, $28 CAD, €18 and $30 AUD.

Physical environment

The physical structure of schools and their facilities can be instrumental in enabling the participation of children in education. Access to school is the first physical feature which needs to be examined. As many as 50% of children in post-industrial countries access school via private transport (National Center for Chronic Disease Prevention and Health Promotion, 2002; Ziviani et al., 2004). While distance from school is often cited as the reason for use of motorized transport, there are also factors related to family routine and safety which influence this decision. The growing tendency for children not to walk to school reduces the amount of physical activity which can otherwise be obtained and also opportunities for social connectedness among children within a geographical area. There are now a number of communities (in Australia, Canada and the USA) involved in trying to make schools more accessible by non-motorized means (National Center for Chronic Disease Prevention and Health Promotion, 2002; Pedestrian Council of Australia, 2003). This has involved parents, teachers and local authorities collaborating to examine physical and social barriers to walking, as well as encouraging participation in 'walk to school' days as a way of establishing walking as a daily activity (see Figure 4.2).

Once at school the nature of the physical environment and the facilities available can impact upon the way in which children engage in the educational and social aspects of school. Schools that lack ventilation can make children drowsy or cause behavioural changes. Open classrooms with noise and visual distractions can interfere with the delivery of classroom material. Drab interiors, poor lighting and the lack of pleasant social gathering spots can also make schools a less than inviting place to be for both children and staff (Sanoff, 2000). Children have identified ideal classrooms as comfortable places with interesting activities (Sanoff, 2000). They also prefer not to spend all day at a desk and still look for places where they

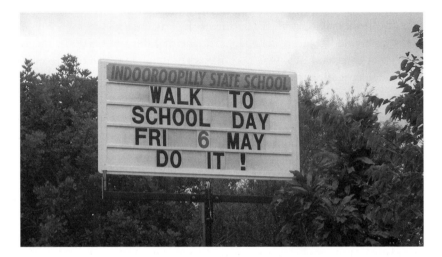

Figure 4.2 Sign promoting walk to school day, Brisbane, Queensland.

can be alone. These insights from children in regular classrooms have largely informed the design of new school buildings. For children with disabilities, however, there may be additional parameters which need attention.

When a child's occupational performance is impaired by physical, developmental, sensory, attention and/or learning challenges, occupational therapists try to match the student's skills and abilities with environmental expectations. This process may involve physical modifications to enable non-ambulatory access to rooms, task modification to facilitate performance, or the provision of assistive technology to enhance performance (Hanft & Place, 1996). These interventions are aimed primarily at the physical or structural school, which remains an important part of their contribution to the educational team.

Social environment

Resiliency has been defined as a dynamic process encompassing positive adaptation within the context of significant adversity. While it is widely accepted that resiliency has an individual and family component, schools have also been acknowledged as playing an important role in fostering in children a sense of being able to overcome obstacles (Borman et al., 2002). Schools which foster caring relationships among students and between students and staff, have high expectations with respect to behaviour and effort, and promote a sense of belonging, which will nurture resilience (Bernard, 1995).

Participation in community

Children's activities take place in diverse physical, socio-cultural and economic environments that play a powerful role in shaping children's participation in neighbourhoods and communities. This section will provide an overview of environmental, physical, socio-cultural and economic factors that occupational therapists consider when designing interventions to foster children's participation in the community.

Physical environment

Physical environments which are external to the child include natural and built surroundings. The natural environment includes land, air, water, plants and animals, whereas the built environment includes human built structures such as buildings, roads, parks and other infrastructure. In the natural environment, the season of the year affects children's participation in activities such as television viewing, outdoor play and sports (McHale et al., 2001; Sallis & Oweb, 2002). Likewise, the characteristics and quality of the physical environment influence children's participation. For example, in combination with child and family preferences, the geography and accessibility of physical environment influences whether, on a hot summer day, a child splashes in the waters of a clean lake, plays along the banks of a muddy river, or swims in a pool.

Around the globe, urban populations are typically thought to have advantages over rural populations, having better access to goods and services, secondary schools, childcare, hospitals, health related services, parks, playgrounds and recreational facilities (Beauvais, 2001; Satterthwaite, 2001). Research also suggests urban and rural differences in children's levels of participation in physical activities. In Canada, children living in rural communities with fewer than 1000 residents appear to be less physically active than their counterparts living in larger communities (Beauvais, 2001). Similar disparities have been found among urban and rural families in Australia (Bennet, 1999), with rural families participating in less recreational physical activities than their urban counterparts. In the USA, a comprehensive review of correlates of youth physical activity described the effects of milieu (rural/urban settings) as indeterminate (Sallis et al., 2000), though less access to structured recreation has been found in small rural communities (Beauvais, 2001).

Environmental characteristics, such as neighbourhood safety, public transportation, land use patterns and urban design, are known to influence children's activity patterns. In the USA, parent's perceptions of poor neighbourhood safety have been associated with physical inactivity among children and youth (Centers for Disease Control and Prevention [CDCP], 1999; 2003; Sallis et al., 1997). Sallis et al. (1997) argued that parental concerns about children's safety in the community are likely to increase reliance on organized activities. If accurate, this prediction poses challenges for low-income families who cite transportation, expense, and neighbourhood safety as barriers to their children's recreational and leisure participation in the community (Beauvais, 2001; CCSD, 2001; CDCP, 1999; CDCP 2003).

It has been observed that spatial and temporal structures of neighbourhoods (for example flow of daytime and night-time visitors) directly influence the situations and opportunities available to children and youth (Sampson, 2001). Sampson observed that: 'The ecological placement of bars, liquor stores, strip-mall shopping outlets, subway stops, and unsupervised play spaces play a direct role in the distribution of high-risk situations for children' (p. 11). Mixed-use neighbourhoods (commercial-residential land use) offer greater opportunities for youth crime and increased opportunities for children to congregate with peers in unsupervised community meeting places (Booth & Crouter, 2001; McHale et al., 2001).

Conversely, the availability of play spaces, parks, playgrounds and recreational facilities which are perceived as safe is associated with higher rates of children participating in formal sports and physical activities (Beauvais, 2001; CDCP, 2003; Offord et al., 1998; Sallis et al., 2000), and to a lesser extent participation in the arts and informal sports (Offord et al., 1998). Similarly, children, particularly low-income children in post-industrial societies, benefit when high quality, local, after school programmes are accessible (Larner et al., 1999).

Social and cultural environment

Social environment is an umbrella term that encompasses the people and institutions with whom a child interacts. Social environment is often described as an interconnected web of relationships at home, in the community and within larger social systems (Bronfenbrenner, 1979; Garbarino, 1992). Layers of the social environment include family, peers, neighbourhood, community (including schools, churches), as well as local, regional and national culture. These layers are comprised of individual and group relationships that form the proximal (for example family) and distal (for example historical and societal level of influences) social contexts in which children live, play and learn. Social environments are dynamic, changing over time as children grow and develop. Adding to this complexity are the operating cultural and social customs, beliefs and norms.

The cultural context and pressures within societies and families define, modify and influence children's participation in the community (Coll & Magnuson, 1999; Göncü, 1999; Super & Harkness, 1999). Parental preferences, values, religiosity and beliefs about how children develop are examples of cultural forces operating within a child's social environment. Parental beliefs about the nature of the world are cultural frameworks that form the basis of judgements about what is good and bad, safe and dangerous, important and irrelevant (McLoyd, 1999). These beliefs lead to very specific opportunities for (or limitations on) children's activities. For younger children especially, parental beliefs are strong determinates of where, when, with whom and how children participate in activities.

The activities available to children vary depending upon parental and societal beliefs about what constitutes valuable childhood experiences (Garbarino, 1992; Göncü, 1999; Holloway & Valentine, 2000). For example, in urban Bangladesh, many families live in homes without running water and indoor plumbing. Here, it is customary for children to collect family drinking water from communal wells. On average, children are required to make two thirty-minute water trips per day. Not only do obligatory water trips shape children's daily routines, but carrying heavy loads of water long distances may drain children's energy for other activities. In some instances, the time required for daily water trips also prevents regular school attendance (Bartlett, 1999). In this example, family needs and customs, which may or may not reflect a child's activity preferences, strongly influence how children participate in community life.

How children spend their time is strongly influenced by local customs and family culture. Family culture includes beliefs, customs, values, preferences, needs and norms. Gaskins' (1999) longitudinal study of children's activities in a traditional Mayan village demonstrates how children's activity patterns are culturally constructed. In these villages, children's activities typically revolve around adult work activities. Because adult work centres on meeting the essential needs of the household, little consideration is given to children's interests and activity preferences. Similarly, Mayan parents believe their children's development unfolds naturally. Consequently, they see no need to create additional opportunities for children to participate in activities intended to foster a child's interests and development.

How are these socio-cultural forces evident in the activity patterns of young Mayan children? First, it is important to note that western classification schemes are not useful for characterizing how Mayan children engage in their communities. That is, the western concepts of recreation, organized sports and self-improvement

activities have little cultural relevance. Rather, Gaskins (1999) found the categories of maintenance activities (self-care), social orientation, play and work best
describe Mayan children's activities. With this framework in mind, we will see how
the socio-cultural environment shapes the activity patterns of Mayan children.

In terms of maintenance activities (self-care), by age five, Mayan children take
full responsibility for their own self-care. Gaskins (1999) noted the customary degree
of freedom afforded young Mayan children may appear neglectful from a western
perspective. Yet, this level of independence is a valued cultural norm in traditional
Mayan cultures.

From infancy, children living in traditional Mayan villages are socialized to
be keen, silent, non-participatory observers of family and village life. This abiding
awareness of village activity is a cultural goal modelled by parents and siblings.
In these villages, it is customary for young Mayan children to spend between
25–30% of their time as non-participant observers. Typically, silent observations
of community and family activities, even distressing ones, do not include action
or a response from the child (Gaskins, 1999).

Within traditional Mayan societies, 'play is not culturally supported as an activity – at best it is tolerated and it is often discouraged' (Gaskins, 1999, p. 49).
Therefore, recreation and play, particularly symbolic play, are not primary forms
of activity. The opposite pattern is seen in western societies in which play and recreation are culturally encouraged and supported activities. Viewing Mayan children's
level of involvement in play activities from a western perspective may lead to mis-
interpretations about the diversity and quality of these children's participation. In
reality, these children spend their time engaged in activities which are culturally
meaningful and valued in their society.

These scenarios exemplify the effects of socio-cultural environments on children's
activity patterns. Understanding children's participation in the community
requires that we attend to specific aspects of the social context and culture in which
activities take place.

Economic environment

In this section we focus on a single aspect of the economic environment – how the
distribution of family and neighbourhood wealth influences children's participation. Family income and local economies affect the availability and accessibility of
recreational and community facilities. The economic structure of children's environments also influences the social organization of children's neighbourhoods and
schools.

Studies conducted in North America illustrate how children's participation in
organized and informal sports, clubs, lessons and artistic activities is linked to
family income. Greater family income is associated with more diverse and regular
participation in formal and community based activities. The opposite pattern is true
– participation in structured physical activity, recreation and artistic activities is
low and irregular among children in low-income families (Beauvais, 2001; CCSD,
2001; Lugalia, 2003; Offord et al., 1998; Ross & Poberts, 1999). In general,

children in low-income families spend more time in unstructured and informal activities than children from middle and high-income families (Medrich et al., 1982; Posner & Vandell, 1999). These children participate in fewer family outings (Lugalia, 2003), read less, watch more television, and spend more time in informal outdoor recreational activities such as bike riding (McHale et al., 2001; Medrich et al., 1982; Posner & Vandell, 1999). Conversely, participation in activities like dance, gymnastics, art, drama, music lessons and camps has been shown to increase as family income levels rise (CCSD, 2001).

The number of parent and youth reported barriers to child and youth participation in physical activities and structured recreation also rises and falls according to family income, with lower income families reporting the greatest number of barriers (Beauvais, 2001; CDCP, 2003). The most commonly cited barriers include transportation problems, expense, lack of opportunities available in the immediate community, parental time constraints, and concerns about neighbourhood safety (CDCP, 1999; Offord et al., 1998).

A family's lack of disposable income and material resources is not the only economic factor affecting children's participation. Often, low-income families live in impoverished communities and neighbourhoods with poor resources. Children in these neighbourhoods are typically exposed to higher rates of crime and violence, attend poorer quality schools, and have access to fewer community institutions, resources and role models that foster and support their participation in positive community activities (Brooks-Gunn et al., 1997; Sampson, 2001).

In sum, the political, physical, socio-cultural and economic structure of children's daily environments profoundly influence the nature, scope and quality of children's participation in school and the community. As we have illustrated, children's participation in these areas varies by geographic location, family culture and norms, social class and income. These are just a few of the many child, family and environmental variables that may influence the educational, recreational and leisure participation of children around the globe. Given the complex nature of participation, efforts to promote and support participation must be based on an understanding of the dynamic interplay between children, their environments and occupations.

Occupational therapists and participation

Enabling participation is the stated objective (or *raison d'être*) of occupational therapy (AOTA, 2002; CAOT, 1997; Law, 2002). Fulfilling our role as enablers of participation requires us to deepen and broaden our knowledge of children's activities and person–environment–occupation relations. Developing comprehensive knowledge of children's activities demands that we reach beyond an understanding of the age appropriateness of a given object or activity. Likewise, understanding children's activity patterns requires more than decontextualized lists of children's daily activities and pie graphs of children's time use. Certainly, understanding how children spend their time contributes significantly to our understanding of children's engagement in the world. However, in our efforts to analyse and promote participation, it is important to remember that children's time use is but a single chapter in a larger story. To understand variations in children's participation, we must understand not only *what* children do, we must also understand child and family activity preferences as well as how, where and with whom children participate. In sum, fulfilling our role as enablers of children's participation requires us to study both the process and outcome of participation within the environmental and cultural contexts in which children's activities occur.

An ecological approach to facilitating children's participation

A sizeable literature in the health and social sciences emphasizes the powerful association between child and youth outcomes and the characteristics of home, school and community environments. There is emerging consensus that health related research and interventions should be based on ecological models (Smedley & Syme, 2000; WHO, 2001). Ecological models are concerned with the inter-relationships between individuals and their socio-physical environments. Because participation is a product of the dynamic interplay between children, their occupations and environments, ecological frameworks are particularly useful for understanding the complexity of children's participation.

From an ecological perspective, children's physical, social, cultural and institutional environments are not merely backdrops to participation – they are essential but variable elements. Children's environments vary in terms of the nature and extent of participation they enable or permit. Children vary in their abilities to shape, adapt and make use of their everyday environments. Attention to the *fit* between children, their activities and environments is important for ensuring that children who need them will have the social and environmental supports necessary to participate in desired or requisite activities.

Environments are not static, nor are they inherently supportive or constraining. The degree to which the immediate environment is perceived as supportive depends in large measure upon factors within the child and the demands of the desired activity. In this way physical and social environments can serve as both barriers and facilitators to participation. Environmental factors that are beneficial in one circumstance may be a hindrance in another. However, certain features of a child's socio-economic environment can and often do limit children's participation in the community. When the structure, organization, or arrangement of physical, social, economic, or institutional environments results in barriers to children's participation, these barriers are said to be structural or systemic.

A model by Donnelly & Harvey (as cited in Beauvais, 2001) is useful for understanding the range of systemic barriers that are most likely to constrain child and youth participation in structured recreation. In this model, environmental factors are organized into three categories:

(1) Infrastructural barriers
(2) Superstructural barriers
(3) Procedural barriers (see Table 4.2)

Table 4.2 Typology of barriers limiting child and youth participation in structured recreation.

Infrastructural barriers	⟶	Limits emerging from costs, lack of transportation and time, location and availability of resources
Superstructural barriers	⟶	Limits emerging from the nature of activities, cultural ideas and prejudices
Procedural barriers	⟶	Limits emerging from a lack of social support, organizational structure and management arrangements

Source: adapted from Donnelly & Harvey (as cited in Beauvais, 2001).

Keep in mind that this model of structural factors is only one piece of a puzzle of factors important for understanding children's participation in school and community. We include this model to demonstrate the range of environmental factors that occupational therapists consider when designing interventions to foster children's participation in school and community.

While environments have a profound effect on children's activities, it would be an exaggeration to suggest that environments are the sole determinates of children's participation, discounting the influence of genetic inheritance and individual characteristics (Rutter, 2002). If environments were sole determinates of children's participation, activities such as play would be privileged occupations enjoyed by a select number of children in families fortunate enough to have adequate financial and social resources. Yet we know that play is a universal experience shared by children of all ages, cultures and countries (Göncü, 1999; Holloway & Valentine, 2000).

However, while children are remarkably resilient, they are not invulnerable (Garbarino, 1995), and the place is important for children's participation. As a world community we share a stake in the outcomes of children around the globe. Enabling children's participation in school and community is a way to support healthy outcomes in children. With this in mind, let us take a closer look at how we might enable and support the participation of children and youth around the world.

Enabling participation: a multi-method, multi-level approach

Our ultimate goal in enabling children's participation is to provide children and youth with opportunities to participate in desired or requisite activities in ways that are enjoyable, personally relevant and/or satisfying. We propose the most effective interventions will be multi-method and multi-level, involving a combination of direct practice, community building and research. These approaches will be strengths based, focused on maximizing the fit between children, occupations and environments, and they will target modifiable factors within the person–environment–occupation (PEO) relationship.

Adopting a strengths based approach

A strengths based perspective operates on the premise that every child, family and environment possesses identifiable strengths, capacities and resources that are stepping-stones to school and community participation (Maton et al., 2004; Saleebey, 2002). Strengths based practice and research focuses on abilities and positive potential rather than pathology and dysfunction. In this view, life circumstances, environments and genetic endowments are not destiny. Saleebey (2002) suggested: 'We do not know the upper limits of the capacity for growth in individuals, families and communities' (p. 15). As a profession, the time is right to make a significant investment in understanding the confluence of child, family and environmental factors that facilitate, support and strengthen the participation of children and youth.

Advocacy and community building

Enabling child and youth participation thorough advocacy and community building will include the following:

- Building community partnerships with schools, businesses, local government, parks and recreation, and family organizations and service providers
- Collaborating with community partners to identify, leverage and mobilize underutilized community resources and strengths
- Enhancing social support networks and social capital by facilitating community partnerships
- Empowering children and families through knowledge transfer and by facilitating access to and utilization of community resources and services
- Raising public awareness about the importance and benefits of child and youth participation
- Bridging the gap between research and practice through knowledge dissemination and education

Maximizing person–environment–occupation fit

Person–environment practice encompasses work with individuals, families, groups and neighbourhoods within two distinct levels of practice. *Micro-level practice* focuses on individuals in the immediate environment while *macro-level practice* encompasses community organizing, involvement in social policy and planning, and social action (Kemp et al., 1997). Historically, occupational therapists have engaged in micro-level practice with a predominate focus on individuals and, to a lesser extent, their physical and social environments.

Enabling childhood participation requires a shift from individual, performance component centred practice to person–environment practice which focuses on the relationship or fit between children, their occupations and environments. A goal of occupational therapy intervention is reconfiguring PEO fit to enable participation in both the immediate and broader environment. Dunn (2000) observed:

'We need to think about the gifts of occupational therapy that we withhold from families when all we do is focus on improving a person's skills. We need to start giving the gift of making things available to people the day they want to do them. We need to be willing to do whatever it takes to support performance' (p. 136).

Matthew

We will consider a specific example of how this approach to intervention would work. Matthew is an eight-year-old boy who has cerebral palsy. He walks independently, but at a slower pace than other 'typically developing' eight-year-olds. Currently, Matthew lives in a small, rural community in Canada, with his mother and older brother. The family income is low, below $30 000 per year in Canadian dollars[2]. He is being seen by an occupational therapist at the request of his mother, who is concerned that he is unhappy and spends most of his time outside school hours at home.

The occupational therapist begins by focusing assessment on Matthew's current participation in activities outside school. Using the Children's Assessment of Participation and Enjoyment (CAPE) and Preference of Activities in Children (PAC) (King et al., 2004), she gathers information from Matthew and his mother about how he spends his time. As detailed in Table 4.3, Matthew participates in a few recreational or active physical activities, and his frequency participation is very low. These activities outside school take place primarily in the home and with his family or other adults. As shown in Table 4.4, this pattern of participation is in direct contrast to Matthew's preferences as measured using the PAC. The PAC

Table 4.3 Matthew's CAPE scores.

CAPE activity types	Participation (activities/ total possible)	Frequency (1–7)	Enjoyment (1–5)	Primary location	With whom
Recreation	2/12	1	4	Home	Family
Active physical	1/13	1	5	Home	Other adult
Social	1/10	1	1	Home	Family
Skill-based	2/10	2	1	Home	Other adult
Self-improvement	3/10	5	1	School	Other adult

Frequency: 1 = once in past 4 months; 3 = once per month; 7 = once a day or more; Enjoyment: 1 = not at all; 3 = pretty much; 5 = love it.

---

[2] At the time of writing this book, $30 000 Canadian dollars was equivalent to approximately $24 000 USD, €18 000 or $32 000 AUD.

Table 4.4 Matthew's PAC scores.

PAC scale	Preference score (maximum 3)
Recreation	3
Active physical	3
Social	2
Skill-based	1
Self-improvement	1

Preference: 1 = would not like to do at all; 2 = would sort of like to do; 3 = would really like to do.

assessment clearly indicates that Matthew prefers recreational and/or active physical activities.

An occupational therapist then completes the Canadian Occupational Performance Measure (Law et al., 1998) with Matthew, specifically focusing the interview on determining the recreational and active physical activities that he wishes to perform. Matthew identifies basketball and playing board or card games with other children.

In collaboration with Matthew and his mother, the therapist investigated opportunities within the local community for these activities. A recreational basketball team did exist and the coach was very willing to include Matthew. There was an economic barrier to participation for Matthew as the cost of equipment and registration fees were high. However, a local group had recently been formed to support the participation of low-income children in community based sports activities. Matthew was able to receive funds from this group to purchase equipment and clothing and pay his registration fees. Once registered, the occupational therapist attended one team practice session to work with his coach on adaptation suggestions to maximize Matthew's involvement in basketball practice and games.

For board or card games, the therapist asked Matthew and his mother to identify several games Matthew knew or might wish to learn. The therapist analysed the requirements for these activities (cognitive, physical, social, sensory) and suggested 2–3 games that best fitted Matthew's current skills and abilities. The therapist also suggested strategies for Matthew to use to invite other children to play these games with him. Once he had learned these games, Matthew invited a child he knew from school to come over to his house to play.

As illustrated in Figures 4.3 and 4.4, this occupational therapy intervention has the potential to move Matthew along the participation continuum. The focus for intervention is primarily on changing or removing the environmental factors that are limiting current participation, while building on Matthew's strengths and interests.

Research

Enabling participation in everyday occupations is occupational therapy's unique contribution to society (Law, 2002). Therefore, our research efforts should focus

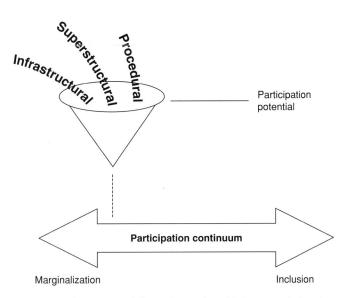

Figure 4.3 Pre-intervention: constraining effects of multiple systemic barriers on child participation.

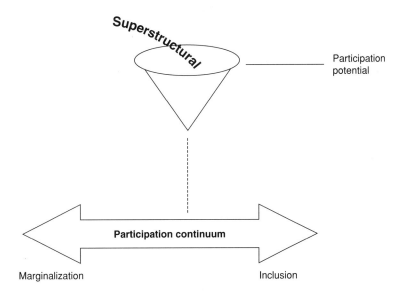

Figure 4.4 Post-intervention: facilitating effects of reduced systemic barriers on child participation.

on generating a deeper understanding of children's activity patterns and the factors that influence patterns of participation at home, school and in the community. This work demands a broader and deeper knowledge of person–environment–occupation relations.

Current occupational therapy literature contains relatively little information about children's school and community participation. A concerted effort is needed to describe the activity patterns of children and youth with and without physical disabilities. In addition, there is a need to understand the relationship between social inequities and childhood participation. This information is needed at local, regional and national levels in order to develop and support programmes aimed at promoting child and youth participation. It is important that we study facilitators and facilitating mechanisms of participation, not just barriers. Discovering the pathways and processes underlying participation and non-participation among children with developmental difficulties, disabilities and those living in impoverished environments, is essential for developing public policies aimed at overcoming the marginalization of entire groups of children and youth.

Our demands for knowledge about children's participation are great. Cross-cultural studies are needed to deepen our understanding of how children's activities are culturally constructed and supported. Currently, the bulk of our existing measurement tools are standardized and validated in white middle-class populations or representative samples (Coll & Magnuson, 1999). These are often not appropriate for studies involving different cultures, races and ethnic groups. Consequently, there is a pressing need to develop culturally and developmentally sensitive tools that will enable us to capture the effects of social and physical environments on the participation of ethnically, racially and economically diverse groups of children.

Little information exists on the causal pathways through which child, family and environmental factors influence children's participation in educational and extra-curricular activities. Longitudinal studies are needed for understanding and describing these causal pathways. In the past, health science research, irrespective of study design, has typically failed to distinguish between structured and unstructured activities (Beauvais, 2001). Oversights such as these limit our understanding of the predictors and benefits associated with specific types of activities. Going forward, studying a range of children's structured and unstructured activities will allow us to develop a more complete understanding of the nuances of children's participation in school and community.

Summary

This chapter has examined the concept of participation as detailed in the ICF and explored the reasons for this being a salient way of viewing health outcomes for children. It has further explored participation in the context of occupation and occupational performance presenting a rationale for occupational therapists to look more broadly at the ways they support children in their participation in school and community environments. The authors present an approach to enabling participation which is both multi-method and multi-level, adopting a strengths perspective, community building philosophy and optimizing the best fit between a child and their environment. The example presented provides a means whereby occupational therapists can move children along a participation continuum by influencing a range of external factors as well as attending to individual child needs. Finally, a strong case is made for occupational therapists to focus research energy on generating a deeper understanding of children's activity participation patterns and the factors which can both hinder or facilitate optimal participation.

References

American Occupational Therapy Association [AOTA] (2002). Occupational therapy practice framework: domain and process. *American Journal of Occupational Therapy, 56,* 609–639.

Bartlett, S. (1999). Children's experience of the physical environment in poor urban settlements and the implications for policy, planning and practice. *Environment and Urbanization, 11* (2), 63–73.

Beauvais, C. (2001). *Literature review on learning through recreation.* Ottawa: Canadian Policy Research Networks.

Bennet, T., Emmison, M. & Frow, J. (1999). *Accounting for tastes: Australian everyday cultures.* Cambridge: Cambridge University Press.

Bernard, S. (1995). *Fostering resilience in children.* ERIC Document No. 386 327.

Booth, A. & Crouter, A. C. (Eds.) (2001). *Does it take a village?* Mahwah, NJ: Lawrence Erlbaum Associates.

Borman, G. D., Hewes, G. M., Overman, L. T. & Brown, S. (2002). *Comprehensive school reform and student achievement: a meta-analysis.* Baltimore, MD: Centre for Research on the Education of Students Placed at Risk (CESPAR), The John Hopkins University.

Bronfenbrenner, U. (1979). *The ecology of human development: experiments by nature and design.* Harvard, Mass.: Harvard University Press.

Bronfenbrenner, U. (1999). Environments in developmental perspective: theoretical and operational models. In: S. L. Friedman & T. D. Wachs (Eds.), *Measuring environment across the lifespan: emerging methods and concepts* (pp. 3–30). Washington, DC: American Psychological Association.

Brooks-Gunn, J., Duncan, G. J. & Aber, J. L. (Eds.) (1997). *Neighborhood poverty. Volume 1: context and consequences for children.* New York: Russell-Sage Foundation.

Canadian Association of Occupational Therapists [CAOT] (1997). *Enabling occupation: an occupational therapy perspective.* Ottawa, Ont.: CAOT Publications.

Canadian Council on Social Development [CCSD] (2001). *Recreation and children and youth living in poverty: barriers, benefits and success stories.* Ottawa: Canadian Council on Social Development.

Centers for Disease Control and Prevention (CDCP) (1999). Neighborhood safety and the prevalence of physical inactivity – selected states, 1996. *Morbidity and Mortality Weekly Report, 48* (7), 143–146.

Centers for Disease Control and Prevention (CDCP) (2003). Physical activity levels among children aged 9–13 years: United States 2002. *Morbidity and Mortality Weekly Report, 52* (33), 785–788.

Christiansen, C. & Baum, C. (1997). Person–environment–occupational performance: a conceptual model for practice. In: C. H. Christiansen & C. Baum (Eds.), *Occupational therapy: enabling function and wellbeing* (2nd ed.) (pp. 47–70). Thorofare, NJ: Slack Incorporated.

Coll, C. G. & Magnuson, K. (1999). Cultural influences on child development: are we ready for a paradigm shift? In: A. S. Masten (Ed.), *Cultural processes in child development: the*

Minnesota symposia on child psychology (pp. 1–24). Mahwah, NJ: Lawrence Erlbaum Associates.

Corsaro, W. A. (1997). *The sociology of childhood*. Thousand Oaks, Calif.: Pine Forge Press.

Dunn, W. (2000). Overview of theoretical models. In: P. A. Crist, C. B. Royeen & J. K. Schkade (Eds.), *Infusing occupation into practice* (2nd ed.), (pp. 106–148). Bethseda, MD: American Occupational Therapy Association.

Federal Interagency Forum on Child and Family Statistics (2003). *America's children: key national indicators of wellbeing*. Washington, DC: Government Printing Office.

Forsyth, R. & Jarvis, S. (2002). Participation in childhood. *Child: care, health and development*, 28 (4), 277–279.

Garbarino, J. (1992). *Children and families in the social environment*. New York: Aldine de Gruyter.

Garbarino, J. (1995). *Raising children in a socially toxic environment*. San Francisco, Calif.: Jossey-Bass.

Gaskins, S. (1999). Children's daily lives in a Mayan village: a case study of culturally constructed roles and activities. In: A. Göncü (Ed.), *Children's engagement in the world: socio-cultural perspectives* (pp. 25–61). New York: Cambridge University Press.

Göncü, A. (Ed.) (1999). *Children's engagement in the world: Socio-cultural perspectives*. New York: Cambridge University Press.

Hanft, B. & Place, P. (1996). *The consulting therapist: a guide for OTs and PTs in schools*. Antonio, Tex.: Therapy Skills Builders.

Henry, A. D. (1998). Development of a measure of adolescent leisure interests. *American Journal of Occupational Therapy*, 52, 531–539.

Holloway, S. L. & Valentine, G. (2000). *Children's geographies: playing, living, learning*. London: Routledge.

Iyanar, J. (2001). Listening to different voices – inclusion and exclusion of people with disabilities in education. *Asia Pacific Disability Rehabilitation Journal*, 12 (2), 155–159.

Kemp, S. P., Whittaker, J. K. & Tracy, E. M. (1997). *Person–environment practice: the social ecology of interpersonal helping*. New York: Aldine de Gruyter.

King, G., Law, M., King, S., Rosenbaum, P., Kertoy, M. K. & Young, N. L. (2003). A conceptual model of the factors affecting the recreation and leisure participation of children with disabilities. *Physical and Occupational Therapy in Pediatrics*, 23 (1), 63–90.

King, G., Law, M., King, S., Hurley, P., Hanna, S., Kertoy, M., et al. (2004). *Children's assessment of participation and enjoyment (CAPE) and preferences activities in children (PAC)*. San Antonio, TX: Harcourt Assessment, Inc.

Larner, M. B., Zippiroli, L. & Behrman, R. E. (1999). When school is out: analysis and recommendations. *The Future of Children*, 9 (2), 4–20.

Larson, R. W. & Verma, S. (1999). How children and adolescents spend time across the world: work, play and developmental opportunities. *Psychological Bulletin*, 125 (6), 701–736.

Law, M. (2002). Participation in the occupations of everyday life. *American Journal of Occupational Therapy*, 56 (6), 640–649.

Law, M., Baptiste, S., Carswell, A., McColl, M., Polatajko, H. & Pollock, N. (1998). *Canadian occupational performance measure* (3rd ed.). Ottawa: Canadian Association of Occupational Therapists.

Lugalia, T. (2003). *A child's day: home, school, and play (selected indicators of child wellbeing), August 2003*. Washington, DC: U.S. Census Bureau.

McHale, S. M., Crouter, A. C. & Tucker, C. J. (2001). Free-time activities in middle childhood: links with adjustment in early adolescence. *Child Development*, 72 (6), 1764–1778.

McLoyd, V. C. (1999). Cultural influences in a multi-cultural society: conceptual and methodological issues. In: A. S. Masten (Ed.), *Cultural processes in child development: the Minnesota symposia on child psychology* (pp. 123–135). Mahwah, NJ: Lawrence Erlbaum Associates.

Mahoney, J. L. & Cairns, R. B. (1997). Do extra-curricular activities protect against early school drop out? *Developmental Psychology, 33* (2), 241–253.

Masten, A. S. & Coatsworth, J. D. (1998). The development of competence in favorable and unfavorable environments. *American Psychologist, 53* (2), 205–220.

Maton, K. I., Schellenbach, C. J., Leadbeater, B. J. & Solarz, A. L. (Eds.) (2004). *Investing in children, youth, families and communities: strengths based research and policy.* Washington, DC: American Psychological Association.

Medrich, E. A., Roizen, J. A., Rubin, V. & Buckey, S. (1982). *The serious business of growing up: a study of children's lives outside of school.* Berkeley, Calif.: University of California Press.

Merriam-Webster Online Dictionary (2004). Retrieved 5 July 2004 from http://www.m-w.com/

National Center for Chronic Disease Prevention and Health Promotion (2002). *Kids walk to school: a guide to promote walking to school.* Atlanta: National Center for Chronic Disease Prevention and Health Promotion.

Offord, D., Lipman, E. & Duku, E. (1998). *Which children don't participate in sports, the arts and community programs?* Ottawa: Human Resources Development Canada.

Pedestrian Council of Australia (2003). *Walk safely to school day.* Retrieved 1 September 2004 from www.walk.com.au

Posner, J. K. & Vandell, D. L. (1999). After-school activities and the development of low-income urban children: a longitudinal study. *Developmental Psychology, 35* (3), 868–879.

Price, P. (2001). Ethics and inclusion: diversity and equity. *Asia Pacific Disability Rehabilitation Journal, 12* (1), 34–43.

Queensland Department of Education (2000). *Priorities in practice – a manual for occupational and physiotherapists.* Brisbane, Queensland: Education Queensland.

Ross, D. P. & Poberts, P. (1999). *Income and child wellbeing: a new perspective on the poverty debate.* Ottawa: Canadian Council on Social Development.

Rutter, M. (1990). Psychosocial resilience and protective mechanisms. In: J. Rolf, A. Masten, D. Cicchetti, K. Nuechterlein & S. Weintraub (Eds.), *Risk and protective factors in the development of psychopathology* (pp. 181–214). Cambridge: Cambridge University Press.

Rutter, M. (2002). Nature, nurture and development: from evangelism through science toward policy and practice. *Child Development, 73* (1), 1–21.

Saleebey, D. (Ed.) (2002). *The strengths perspective in social work practice.* Boston, Mass.: Allyn and Bacon.

Sallis, J. F., Johnson, M. F., Calfas, K. J., Caparosa, S. & Nichols, J. F. (1997). Assessing perceived physical environmental variables that may influence physical activity. *Research Quarterly for Exercise and Sport, 68,* 345–351.

Sallis, J. F., Prochaska, J. J. & Taylor, W. C. (2000). A review of correlates of physical activity of children and adolescents. *Medicine and Science in Sports and Exercise, 32,* 963–975.

Sallis, J. F. & Oweb, N. (2002). Ecological models of health behavior. In: K. Glanz, B. K. Rimer & F. M. Lewis (Eds.), *Health behavior and health education.* San Francisco: Jossey-Bass.

Sampson, R. J. (2001). How do communities undergrid or undermine human development? In: A. Booth & A. C. Crouter (Eds.), *Does it take a village? Community effects on children, adolescents, and families* (pp. 3–30). Mahwah, NJ: Lawrence Erlbaum Associates.

Sandler, I. N., Ayers, T. S., Suter, J. C., Schultz, A. & Twohey-Jacobs, J. (2004). Adversities, strengths, and public policy. In: K. I. Maton, C. J. Schellenbach, B. J. Leadbeater & A. L. Solarz (Eds.), *Investing in children, youth, families, and communities: strengths-based research and policy* (pp. 31–49). Washington, DC: American Psychological Association.

Sanoff, H. (2000). Participation in educational facilities. In: H. Sanoff (Ed.), *Community participation methods in design and planning*. New York: John Wiley & Sons.

Satterthwaite, D. (2001). *The ten and a half myths that may distort urban policies among governments and international agencies.* Retrieved 9 February 2005 from http://www.ucl.ac.uk/dpu-projects/drivers_urb_change/urb_infrastructure/pdf_city_planning/IIED_Satterthwaite_Myths_complete.pdf

Simeonsson, R. J., Lollar, D., Hollowell, J. & Adams, M. (2000). Revision of the international classification of impairments, disabilities and handicaps: developmental issues. *Journal of Clinical Epidemiology, 53* (2), 113–124.

Sloper, P., Turner, S., Knussen, C. & Cunningham, C. (1990). Social life of school children with Down's syndrome. *Child: Care, Health and Development, 16* (4), 235–251.

Smedley, B. D. & Syme, S. L. (Eds.) (2000). *Promoting health: intervention strategies from social and behavioral research*. Washington, DC: National Academy Press.

Super, C. M. & Harkness, S. (1999). The environment as culture in developmental research. In: S. L. Friedman & T. D. Wachs (Eds.), *Measuring environment across the lifespan: emerging methods and concepts* (pp. 279–323). Washington, DC: American Psychological Association.

The Free Dictionary (2004). Retrieved 5 July 2004 from http://www.thefreedictionary.com/

Townsend, E., Ryan, B. & Law, M. (1990). Using the World Health Organization's international classification of impairments, disabilities, and handicaps in occupational therapy. *Canadian Journal of Occupational Therapy, 57*, 16–25.

UNICEF-EAPRO (2000) *Special roundtable: 'Inclusive education: a process, a challenge'*. Paper presented at the Asian Pacific Conference on Education for All 2000 Assessment, 17–20 January Bangkok, Thailand.

Waters, E., Goldfeld, S. & Hopkins, S. (2002). *Indicators for child health, development and wellbeing*. Melbourne, Australia: Centre for Community Child Health, Royal Children's Hospital.

Werner, E. E. (1993). Risk, resilience and recovery: perspectives from the Kauai longitudinal study. *Development and Psychopathology, 5*, 503–515.

World Health Organization (1980). *International classification of impairments, disabilities and handicaps*. Geneva: World Health Organization.

World Health Organization [WHO] (2001). *International classification of functioning, disability and health*. Geneva: World Health Organization.

World Health Organization [WHO] (2004). *International classification of functioning, disability and health: children and youth version*. Retrieved 9 February 2005 from http://www3.who.int/icf/icftemplate.cfm

Ziviani, J., Scott, J. & Wadley, D. (2004). Walking to school: incidental physical activity in the daily occupations of Australian children. *Occupational Therapy International, 51*, 69–79.

Chapter 5

CHILDREN'S OCCUPATIONAL TIME USE

Jenny Ziviani, Laura Desha and Sylvia Rodger

Adolph Meyer first posited the organization of daily activity as having the potential to impact on wellbeing (Meyer, 1977). In the emerging discipline of occupational science, researchers continue to question what constitutes a healthful balance of work, rest and leisure (Clark et al., 1991). To date, most of this work has been undertaken with adults. The current attention directed to children with respect to the increasing amount of time devoted to screen based activities, and reduced time in physical activity, has alerted all involved in children's welfare to review what constitutes a healthful distribution of time.

Unlike adults, children have much less control about how their time is structured. The family/social milieu in which children grow up and their immediate physical environment are largely under adult influence. Furthermore, because they are developing beings, time use for children has important developmental implications. Children require adequate sleep for growth, physical activity for health and the development of motor skills, and social contact to support communication and skill development. In this chapter we explore children's occupational time use, with the aim of establishing what we currently understand to be a healthful balance. The objectives of the chapter are to:

(1) Highlight the developmental significance of occupational time use patterns for children
(2) Describe factors influencing children's time use and look at the impact of culture on its distribution
(3) Discuss the impact of time use patterns on physical, cognitive and psychosocial wellbeing
(4) Explore the concept of occupational balance and discuss challenges of maintaining healthy balance in the face of disability, rapid societal change and technological advances
(5) Describe the role of occupational therapists in striving for occupational balance

The division of time

In the occupational therapy literature, the division of time was first addressed by Adolf Meyer, who identified four categories of occupation – work, play, rest and sleep (Meyer, 1977). Various authors (for example Canadian Association of Occupational Therapists, 1986; Hagedorn, 1992; Mosey, 1986; Reed, 1984) have since re-categorized occupation, with most retaining the global categories of work/productivity and play/leisure, but omitting overt reference to sleep or rest, and including activities of daily living or self-maintenance as an additional category. Christiansen (1994) criticized the lack of explicit criteria to guide classification of activities under these headings, suggesting that their ambiguity limits their value for the study of occupation.

In the wider literature on time use drawn from psychology, sociology, vocational and leisure studies, a primary distinction is made between activities of a discretionary versus non-discretionary nature. Discretionary activities are those that involve an element of freedom of choice and volition. Such activities make up much of 'free time' outside school hours, and primarily involve 'leisure' occupations (Meeks & Mauldin, 1990). Within the context of leisure, activities are further categorized into those that are structured and unstructured. Structured activities are characterized by being organized by adults, and having clear and specific social or behavioural goals. Structured activities are typically linked to school (for example band, student council or sporting teams), based in the community (for example youth groups, scouting, volunteering) or privately arranged (for example music lessons) (Fletcher et al., 2003; Meeks & Mauldin, 1990). In contrast, unstructured activities are initiated by children and tend to involve spontaneous, unorganized leisure pursuits. Unstructured activities may include time spent interacting socially with friends, an impromptu outdoor game, or more *passive* leisure such as watching television, listening to music (Huston et al., 1999). A distinction between *passive* and *active* engagement is frequently made, and refers at times to both the mental and physical demands of an activity.

The quantitative division of time into the number or percentage of hours per week spent in various activities provides a picture of engagement. Collation of these data facilitates investigation of personal and contextual influences which shape patterns of time use. In a large study of American children (0–12 years) Hofferth & Sandberg (2001) performed analysis of twenty-four-hour time recall budget diary information, finding that in 1997 children spent on average 55% of their week engaging in ADL activities (activities of daily living, for example sleeping, eating, personal care), 15% in work activities (school or day care), and the remaining 30% in discretionary activities. While many of the discretionary activities resemble leisure, the two terms cannot be simply equated. As time use in this age group is often influenced, if not dictated, by parents or other adults, the freedom of choice, intrinsic rewards, meaning and sense of pleasure that are characteristic of leisure experiences may not always be present (Suto, 1998). This highlights the categorization difficulties inherent in discussions of time use.

Activities of daily living

Time allocated to basic and instrumental ADL activities varies across different age and cultural groups. The considerable time that young children spend eating and having their personal care needs tended to (Hofferth & Sandberg, 2001; Robinson & Bianchi, 1997) diminishes as their independence in these tasks increases. For example, the amount of time children spend sharing meals with parents or siblings tends to decline as children move toward adolescence. In accordance with cultural pressures that encourage attention to physical appearances, adolescent girls in post-industrial nations are likely to spend more time bathing, dressing and grooming than their younger sisters. This is in contrast to adolescent boys who spend less time on such tasks than younger boys (Larson & Verma, 1999; Robinson & Bianchi, 1997). Larson & Verma proposed that while younger children sleep more than adolescents (Hofferth & Sandberg, 2001; Robinson & Bianchi, 1997) the average amount of time spent sleeping varies little across populations and averages 8–9 hours per day.

Accompanying parents who are performing instrumental ADL activities (for example shopping) or who are visiting friends is a frequent activity for children, particularly prior to commencing school, and accounts for 5–10 hours per week of time. It is further suggested that time spent in transit between activities consumes five hours per week of preschoolers' time, and this increases by 1–2 hours per week during the school years (Hofferth & Sandberg, 2001; Robinson & Bianchi, 1997).

Work

In post-industrial societies compulsory schooling and technological advances have eliminated the need for children to perform large amounts of household work, and well enforced child labour laws restrict income generating work to adolescents (Larson & Verma, 1999). Children's work activities therefore encompass school, homework, household chores and some labour market work for older children. Robinson & Bianchi (1997) found that in America time spent in school and on homework averages 22 hours per week during the early school years and increases to 29 hours per week in adolescence. Furthermore, 40% of children (aged 3–11) had completed close to an hour of housework during the diary day recorded.

Leisure

While the amount of discretionary time available to children from 0–11 years of age remains fairly constant, free play declines steadily from 30 hours per week in infancy to 19 hours in the early school years (Robinson & Bianchi, 1997), then dwindles to less than nine hours per week among older elementary school children (Hofferth & Sandberg, 2001). As free play diminishes, children are increasingly recruited to structured activities and also start to engage more in socializing and visiting (Robinson & Bianchi, 1997). Structured activities in the after school hours may be active (for example competitive sport) or passive in nature. Passive leisure activities frequently involve interacting with media and consume large amounts of time. Indeed, research suggests that on average American children are exposed to over six hours of media per day (Jordan, 2004). When hours devoted to television are looked at in isolation, research indicates that 5–11-year-olds watch up to 14 hours of television per week, a figure which increases by 4–6 hours for 12–17-year-olds. This is in stark contrast to the typical single hour of time spent reading (or being read to) per week, which varies little across age groups (Hofferth & Sandberg, 2001; Robinson & Bianchi, 1997).

The personal and contextual factors impacting on time use

It is clear that time use in all areas of occupational performance is heavily influenced by age and developmental level. These, however, are just two key 'personal characteristics' that contribute to the formation of time use patterns. Other personal factors as well as contextual factors will now be reviewed.

Personal factors

As has been highlighted, *age* and *developmental level* are key determinants of children's time use. As children mature, time spent performing ADL such as eating and sleeping declines, the amount of play reduces, and leisure time is increasingly occupied by structured activities (Robinson & Bianchi, 1997). With the advent of kindergarten and school the student role develops and extends to fill substantial amounts of time, potentially displacing other activities (for example leisure pursuits). Compared to adolescents, younger children tend to have less control over their time use, as adults direct activity participation out of practical necessity (for example provision of transportation) and also for more complex reasons such as a desire for a child to participate in 'team work', or develop particular skills. *Personality* and *temperament* influence how children spend their time, and parents who are attuned to their children's strengths and weaknesses may seek activities accordingly.

Significant *gender* differences in time use emerge primarily with the onset of adolescence, with boys spending more time than girls in sporting activities (Carpenter et al., 1989; Hofferth & Sandberg, 2001; Posner & Vandell, 1999), outdoor games and watching television (Bianchi & Robinson, 1997), and girls spending more time than boys reading, engaging in other academic activities (Medrich et al., 1982; Posner & Vandell, 1999), conversation and socializing (Meeks & Mauldin, 1990; Robinson & Bianchi, 1997). *Ethnicity* may impact on time use patterns due to cultural differences in the value placed on activities. Household chores, for example, are valued in many western cultures for teaching self-sufficiency and individual responsibility. However, in Japan and China, where there is greater emphasis on academic success, chores are less frequently assigned for fear that they may divert children from homework activities (Larson & Verma, 1999; Stevenson & Lee, 1990). Cultural variation in how time is experienced also exists, as demonstrated by the concept of time held in some Australian indigenous communities, where daily activities are less regimented by clock time than by social and communal obligations (Yalmambirra, 2000).

Contextual factors

The ICF (World Health Organization, 2001) delineates between environmental and attitudinal factors which impact upon activity participation. For a child, the most immediate environment consists of the home and family. Children function as part of their family unit, and their patterns of time use are woven closely with those of parents and siblings. Social coordination of a family's schedule is a complex task which depends on the flexibility of routines, and the extent of competing desires, needs and obligations (Larson & Zemke, 2003).

Parents' occupations, particularly *maternal employment* influence children's patterns of time use. However, debate continues as to the possible negative effects on longer term outcomes. When compared with children of unemployed mothers, the children of working mothers spend more time in all forms of day care (Hofferth & Sandberg, 2001). Time spent working has the potential to displace family, personal and discretionary activities (for example church attendance), and work commitments may necessitate tight scheduling which favours children's participation in structured activities (Hofferth & Sandberg, 2001). Robinson & Bianchi (1997) found that children of working mothers spend equivalent amounts of time on schoolwork and housework, to children of non-employed mothers.

Family composition, including parental factors (whether the family is headed by one or two parents, either biological or step-parents) and sibship (number and sex of siblings, as well as their relative ages and birth order) (Steelman et al., 2002) have varied implications for time use. Some research suggests that, compared to their peers, young children from single parent families tend to receive less monitoring and supervision, spend less time playing and sleeping and more time watching television (Posner & Vandell, 1999; Timmer et al., 1985). In contrast, Robinson & Bianchi (1997) found no significant differences between single or dual parent families in the amount of time spent watching television, reading, doing schoolwork or household chores. Whether they have one or two parents, children of large families may benefit from having ready access to siblings as playmates (Downey & Condron, 2004). Surprisingly, investigations into the impact of sibship have largely focused on academic outcomes, with researchers concluding that as family size increases, resources become diluted, leading to poorer academic outcomes (Steelman et al., 2002). In congruence with the resource dilution model, financial strain may curtail the time use of children from larger families by limiting participating in costly activities (for example extra-curricular music lessons) (Bianchi & Robinson, 1997; Hofferth & Sandberg, 2001).

The level of *parental education* is a reflection of parents' values and knowledge and is an indicator of socio-economic status. Higher educational attainment is typically positively associated with children engaging in activities of an educational nature and negatively related to time spent watching television (Bianchi & Robinson, 1997; Hofferth & Sandberg, 2001; Robinson & Bianchi, 1997).

Outside the realm of a child's direct family, there are many societal and environmental factors which influence time use. Funding decisions and resource allocation (both in schools and at the neighbourhood level) may determine the nature of time use in a tangible manner (for example construction of a skating rink may lead to more physical activity) or by less visible mechanisms such as policy targeting neighbourhood safety (for example reduced crime rate and improved traffic conditions may lead to less restrictions on outdoor play). Environmental conditions, including seasonal changes and daily weather variation necessarily lead to variation in children's time use patterns.

The effect of time use on wellbeing

According to ecological systems theory, the context in which time is spent is important in determining children's opportunities for development, learning and skill acquisition (Bronfenbrenner, 1979; Larson & Verma, 1999; Silbereisen et al., 1986). While the quantity of time distributed across various activity contexts may serve as an estimate of the degree to which children have been exposed to or participated in developmental experiences, caution must be exercised in interpreting this, as not all activities or contexts are *equal* in their effects on wellbeing. For example, while spending more time in school logically results in extended learning opportunities and may lead to better educational outcomes, aspects of the experience, such as high pressure, may have an overall negative impact on a child's psychological wellbeing.

The idea that there may be a curvilinear relationship between some types of activity participation and wellbeing has been explored by Marsh & Kleitman (2002), who specifically investigated extra-curricular school activities. They present five theoretical models to explain the effects of extra-curricular activity involvement (see Table 5.1) and have found evidence supporting a threshold model of participation, where moderate amounts of extra-curricular activities have benefits to students, but above an optimal level the effects were considered detrimental.

Research which goes beyond simple associations to further investigate causal relationships and mediators that influence a child's trajectory to positive or negative health and wellbeing is critical to the successful planning and implementation of health promotion programmes. Longitudinal studies are particularly valuable in establishing causal pathways. The recent commitment of substantial funding to research undertakings such as 'Growing up in Australia', a longitudinal study of Australian children which includes time use details, demonstrates heightened government recognition of a need for evidence to support social policy debate and determine appropriate intervention and prevention strategies for health and wellbeing (Sanson et al., 2002).

Wellbeing

Wellbeing is a complex, multidimensional construct which encompasses psychological, social, cognitive, physical and economic domains (Pollard & Lee, 2003). Subjective wellbeing refers to a child's assessment of their quality of life across these domains, and consists of both affective components (happiness) and

Table 5.1 Models explaining extra-curricular activity, adopted from Marsh & Kleitman (2002).

Model	Key references	Key posits of the model	Comments on the model by Marsh (1991; 1992)
Zero-sum model	(Coleman, 1961)	The quantity of time devoted to academic, social and academic pursuits are in competition with each other. Participation in extra-curricular activities may therefore detract from time spent on academic pursuits.	Marsh suggests that the *degree* of commitment (rather than *time* per se) to various pursuits may be the critical variable in determining whether they detract from time spent on academic activities.
Developmental model	(Holland & Andre, 1987)	Extra-curricular activities provide experiences which further the total development of students, aiding them in skill acquisition in non-academic areas, leading to greater maturity and social competency as well as building character.	The focus is on non-academic benefits. These are not seen as detracting from academic outcomes.
Identification commitment model	(Finn, 1989; Marsh, 1992)	Extra-curricular activities may enhance commitment to and identification with a school, as well as increasing involvement/participation. This enhances academic as well as non-academic outcomes.	Some extra-curricular activities (such as part-time employment) may undermine identification/commitment to a school.
Threshold model	(Marsh & Kleitman, 2002)	While moderate amounts of extra-curricular activities have beneficial effects, beyond an optimal point they may have diminishing returns (producing a 'non-linear' effect).	This model provides support for the concept of 'overwhelmed children' who are engaged in many extra-curricular activities.
Social inequality/gap reduction model	(Marsh & Kleitman, 2002)	This model predicts that extra-curricular activities are more beneficial for children from lower socio-economic groups and that their involvement reduces the size of the gap in academic achievement between children of low and high SES.	The differential effects of extra-curricular activity may be mediated by identification with a school. Participation may provide children of lower SES with a way to form identification with a school, whereas children of higher SES are likely to already identify with their school and be committed to its values.

cognitive–judgemental components (life satisfaction) (Bender, 1997). It is often measured by using multiple separate assessments that are presumed to be negative or positive indicators of wellbeing, such as depression or self-esteem scales (Pollard & Lee, 2003). To gain an overall picture of a child's wellbeing, indicators of wellbeing are frequently drawn from more than one domain (that is psychosocial, cognitive, physical). However, specific tests of wellbeing have also been devised. These purport to measure constructs such as global life satisfaction, for example, Student's life satisfaction scale (Huebner, 1991), general life satisfaction (where overall life satisfaction is conceptualized as the sum of responses across multiple life domains such as family, friends and school), such as Perceived life satisfaction scale (Adelman et al., 1989) and quality of life, for example PedsQL (Varni et al., 2001).

Work

The number of days a child attends school (considering the proportion of this time spent 'on task'), and the amount of time dedicated to homework are related to academic achievement and have clear benefits in terms of economic productivity. While engagement in schoolwork implies participation in activities which expand knowledge and provide opportunities for social skill development, international studies have also associated it with high rates of boredom and negative affect, and low intrinsic motivation (Larson & Verma, 1999). Spending long periods of time in such negative psychological states may have consequences, such as diminished feelings of academic competence and lessened enjoyment of learning, leading to poorer academic performance, and placing a student at risk of psychopathology.

While in some western societies chores are valued for teaching self-sufficiency and individual responsibility, empirical studies have suggested that although specific skills may be attained during completion of housework in post-industrial societies, the activities typically offer low challenge and have limited developmental benefits (for example Carr et al., 1996).

Leisure

In stark contrast to work activities, positive psychological states and high intrinsic motivation have been repeatedly associated with time spent in leisure activities (Larson & Verma, 1999). Leisure time contexts have been extensively researched, with a substantial amount of literature linking involvement in structured extra-curricular activities with psychosocial wellbeing. Structured leisure activities are thought to benefit children and adolescents by teaching positive skills and social competence, helping to develop supportive networks of peers and adults, providing a forum for the development of initiative, and preventing involvement in antisocial or risky activities (Carnegie Corporation of New York, 1992; Larson, 1994; McHale et al., 2001). Participation in structured activities also facilitates investment of time in specific skill development, which may also help children to recognize their unique abilities and thereby foster identity development (Kleiber, 1999). Alternatively, when children spend their free time in unstructured often unsupervised activities (for example hanging out with friends) there may be more opportunities for risky behaviour (Osgood et al., 1996).

Table 5.2 Typologies of why children engage in different activities.

Typology	Examples of activities	Characteristics of the activity	Links with mental health
Achievement leisure	Sports Music lessons Dancing	Provide challenge Demanding Require commitment	Enhances self-efficacy and competence Positively linked with *self-esteem*
Social leisure	Talking Visiting Eating with friends Going out	Engaged in for the primary purpose of being with others	Enhance competence (particularly in relationships and social acceptance) Positively linked with *self-esteem*
Time out leisure	Watching television Reflecting Reading Listening to music	Relaxing Socially isolating Low demand Often passive	Did not support development of competence or *self-esteem*

Farnworth (2000); Passmore & French (2000, 2001).

Unstructured activities are frequently passive in nature and have not been found to offer equivalent opportunities for development as structured activities. In a large study of Australian adolescents, Passmore (2003) identified significant positive relationships between selected forms of leisure and perceptions of self-efficacy, competence and global self-worth, supporting earlier research in which three distinct typologies of leisure had been identified. These typologies categorize activities on the basis of underlying reasons why young people engage in leisure, and include achievement, social and time-out leisure. Characteristics of the typologies and their potential relationships with mental health are outlined in Table 5.2.

Rest

Poor quality and reduced duration of sleep is known to have significant effects on mood, cognition and motor performance in adults (Pilcher & Huffcutt, 1996). Likewise, recent paediatric studies have clearly linked 'not feeling rested while at school' with reduced school functioning, and 'difficulty getting up in the morning' with lessened achievement motivation (Meijer et al., 2000). While the causal relationships are yet to be established empirically, childhood sleep disturbances have also been linked with depression and anxiety (Glaze et al., 2002).

Physical activity

The main way in which physical activity manifests in the time use of children is in structured sport, physical education components of the school curriculum and outdoor play. Physical activity during childhood and adolescence is important for maintaining normal growth and development (Parizkova, 1996). However, despite the documented benefits of regular physical activity, evidence suggests that a sizeable percentage of school-aged children fail to meet recommended daily activity guidelines of half to one hour (Trost & Pate, 1999). Trost et al. (2002) recently evaluated age and gender differences in objectively measured physical activity in a population based sample of American students in grades 1 to 12. Daily physical activity exhibited a significant inverse relationship with grade level with the largest declines occurring between grades 1–3 and 4–6. Across all grade levels, boys were more active than girls.

Is there occupational balance?

Occupational therapy philosophy is underpinned by the notion that health and wellbeing are inextricably linked with achieving a *balance* of work, leisure, self-maintenance and rest occupations. A firm belief in the value of occupational balance has since been advanced by many prominent authors (Christiansen, 1996; Kielhofner, 1977; Wilcock et al., 1997) and is frequently supported by the popular media through recommendations on how to achieve 'balanced lifestyles'. Despite the widespread assumption that an ideal *balance* exists, researchers have struggled to define this in either quantitative or qualitative terms.

One view of balance as potentially deriving from the synchrony of internal chrono-biological rhythms with patterns of activity is supported by research into the physical and mental health sequelae for adults of rhythm changes brought about intentionally (for example through shift work), or through life events such as the birth of a child (Christiansen, 1996). It has been postulated that life events which cause disruptions to social rhythms may then perturb both circadian rhythms and sleep–wake cycles, leading to psychopathology (Frank et al., 2000).

An alternate view is that balance arises through devotion of roughly equivalent amounts of time to productive, recreational and rest activities. Christiansen (1996) challenged this by arguing that 'the meaning, impact, or benefit of an activity is not always proportionate to the amount of time spent on it' (p. 435). The concept of balance may therefore be better understood by looking beyond the amount of time dedicated to an activity to investigate how these activities vary according to their individual and cumulative, positive or negative influences on psychosocial and physical health and wellbeing. Quantifying the benefits of activities is complicated by the challenge to researchers of categorization.

We propose that balance may relate to participation across a number of parameters. For example, once we account for adequate rest, it might be that for children there are optimal levels of involvement in structured, physical and social activity which are associated with general wellbeing. In Figure 5.1 we have attempted to represent this concept in a very preliminary way. Research is needed to demonstrate if particular profiles of activity engagement are indeed associated with at-risk children.

There is a dearth of knowledge regarding children's perceptions of their occupational engagement and their understanding of balance. The act of *balancing*

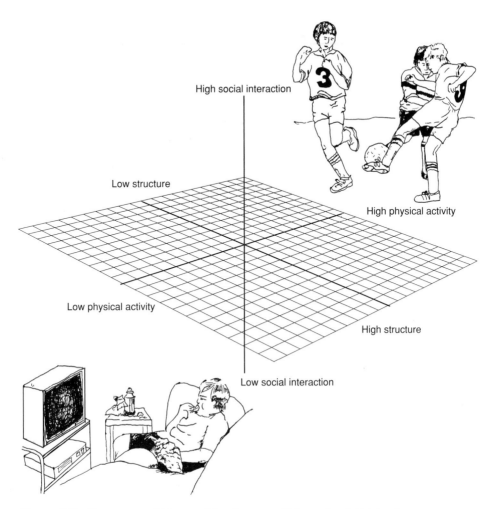

Figure 5.1 Time use could be considered as a multidimensional construct.

occupations may not be one that children consciously undertake, and children's activity profiles may indeed more closely reflect parental beliefs and social and environmental factors than their own choices and preferences. The common media representation of children growing up in an increasingly time pressured manner, where parental circumstances necessitate tightly scheduled, structured and hurried activity engagement, begs the question of how adults themselves perceive balance (Elkind, 1992).

Limited research has been conducted in this field. However, Wilcock et al. (1997) conducted a pilot study of teenagers and adults in which *ideal* and *current* balance were quantified by asking respondents to rate their ideal and current intensity of involvement in physical, mental, social and rest occupations. The most frequently chosen pattern of ideal balance comprised *moderate* involvement in all categories of occupation. In this study, heightened congruency between perceptions of ideal balance and actual time distribution was related to better self-reported health status. Rather than searching for an elusive definition of *ideal* occupational balance, it may be more pertinent to examine the considerable societal, economic and technological changes currently occurring in post-industrial societies and to investigate their impact upon temporal patterns and thus the *occupational balance* of any given individual.

How is occupational balance affected by family and societal change?

Children's participation in a range of activities is affected by their parents' ability to invest time and financial resources. Notable demographic changes which may affect both the availability of time and finances include altered family composition and changing maternal labour force participation. Furthermore, community perceptions of, or actual threats to, personal safety have led to the curtailing of freedoms previously afforded in childhood.

Families and maternal employment

Over recent decades there have been drastic changes to the structure and form of families. High divorce rates and the subsequent development of blended or step-families, cohabitation and the increasing occurrence of extramarital childbirth have contributed to this change. Family composition has also been affected by declining fertility, leading to children having fewer siblings.

It is often assumed that single parenthood results in less time spent with parents. Bianchi (2000), however, argued that maternal employment has not necessarily led to mothers spending less time with their children, and that there is inconclusive evidence to suggest that the effects of increased market work are positive or negative (Bianchi & Robinson, 1997). Although the total quantity of shared parent–child time may have changed little, Bryant & Zick (1996) found that the activities that parents engage in with their children change with maternal employment patterns. Their study showed that as mothers spent more time in the workforce, the amount of direct childcare decreased, but the amount of leisure time and housework shared by mothers and children actually increased. Bianchi & Robinson's (1997) research indicated that children's own patterns of time use are little affected by the employment status of their mothers, except that children of mothers employed part time watch less television than children whose mothers do not work outside the home. Just as the potential effects of family changes on child development are increasingly being recognized, the impact of broader societal changes is also receiving attention.

Threatening society?

Crime rates have escalated in many cities and rural areas, leading to heightened actual and perceived risk in leaving the home. Neighbourhoods differ considerably in their physical and social order, and parents report curtailing their children's free play due to concerns regarding dangers such as traffic, contact with strangers and exposure to drugs (O'Brien & Smith, 2002). Residing in an unsafe neighbourhood has been linked with reduced physical activity (Molnar et al., 2004), which has clear negative implications for children's health and wellbeing.

Opportunities for sporting activity and participation in organized extra-curricular clubs are also increasingly being jeopardized by spiralling insurance costs. Cases of personal litigation are threatening the viability of many clubs frequently led by volunteers. These trends are worrying given evidence which suggests that participation in extra-curricular activities such as Scouts, provides opportunities to develop numerous competencies (for example social skills, physical fitness) (Fletcher et al., 2003). Highly public cases of abuse within various church and youth groups have also brought some clubs into disrepute and led to withdrawal of children from such organizations. Where such circumstances are limiting opportunities, children's potential to achieve a healthful balance of occupations may be compromised.

How is occupational balance affected by technological change?

Rapid technological advances and relatively low-cost access to media, including television, video games, music, computers, the Internet and mobile phones are impacting on the experience of growing up in modern times. Media exposure has a pervasive influence on all spheres of life. However, little is known regarding its ultimate impact on children's development.

Displacement theory

A primary concern is that time spent engaging with media is displacing alternative, potentially more developmentally beneficial activities. Television watching remains a dominant pastime, occupying more of children's time than any other single activity apart from sleep (Huston & Wright, 1997). It appears, however, that burgeoning access to additional technologies (for example home computers) has not led to vastly reduced time devoted to television, but rather an increase in the total aggregate of time devoted to screen based, sedentary activities (Subrahmanyam et al., 2000).

Physical effects

Attewell and colleagues (2003) observed links between heavy home computer use (more than eight hours per week) and greater body mass in children. Similarly, a study of excessive television watching (five or more hours per day) has shown that this type of behaviour is closely linked with increased risk of obesity (Gortmaker et al., 1996). While this is possibly due to the power of screen based activities to displace physical activity, other causes might include the secondary activity of food consumption and the effects of television marketing on food choice (Jordan, 2004). Additional physical health concerns of increasing technology exposure relate to the risks of computer and video game use identified in studies of adult users, such as eye, back and wrist problems as well as repetitive strain injuries (Palmer, 1993). The potential exists for children to spend extended periods at workstations which are not appropriately adjusted to their size and needs. Hence, children may be exposed to prolonged poor postures during developmental periods of critical skeletal growth (Harris & Straker, 2000).

Cognitive effects

The impact of increased technology exposure on cognition has proven more difficult to elucidate. Media exposure may be of benefit to cognitive development when it is not displacing or precluding participation in more enriching activities. Moderate home computer use and selective television viewing has been linked with better academic performance (Attewell et al., 2003; Li & Atkins, 2004; Rochelau, 1995; The Royal Australasian College of Physicians, 2004; Subrahmanyam et al., 2000). It has also been suggested that playing computer games may contribute to computer literacy by enhancing specific visual skills (Subrahmanyam et al., 2000).

Social effects

Heightened participation in technological pursuits has diverse ramifications for social development. The type of activity, the physical and social context in which it is undertaken and the intensity of engagement determine the social impact of technology (Subrahmanyam et al., 2000). Both pro- and antisocial behaviours have been linked with media exposure (Jordan, 2004). Television viewing has been the primary focus of research, and numerous authors extrapolate those findings to suggest how exposure to violence may impact on social development. However, further research is needed to determine the specific effects of newly evolving *interactive* media such as video and computer games.

Television delivers powerful messages to children. Many studies have found links between television viewing and violent or aggressive behaviour. However, the existence of a causal relationship is disputed (Jordan, 2004). Television may also foster prosocial behaviour, and programmes designed to teach about such topics as acceptance of diversity have been found to be effective in young children (Mares & Woodard, 2001). Jordan (2004) proposed that the context of media use is of critical importance in determining its impact on prosocial behaviour, and that children may require an adult to assist them to process the information received.

Television, computer and video games are frequently enjoyed in the company of peers or family members. However, as media are often located in children's bedrooms (Jordan, 2004) this may result in children using the media in an isolated manner. Physical isolation of a computer workstation may not, however, equate with social isolation, due to the substantial potential for communication via the Internet. Research into online communication is limited. However, some studies suggest that using the Internet causes a decline in social wellbeing (Kraut et al., 1998). Greater use was associated with reduced communication with household members, a shrinking social circle and increased depression and loneliness. Researchers are yet to investigate whether intense online or mobile phone interaction may hinder or substitute for 'real life' interactions in the development of social skills.

How is occupational balance affected by disability?

In the language of the ICF (WHO, 2001) disability may impose both activity and participation restrictions on a child. The presence and severity of specific physical, cognitive or social difficulties may form barriers which limit a child's capacity to perform particular occupations. A child's access to supports which compensate for these barriers, or facilitate adaptive performance despite restrictions, has implications for their ability to achieve a healthful balance of time use.

Comparative studies between children with and without disability suggest that time use for children with disability is characterized by a slower tempo, more dependence on adults, less diversity, less involvement in activities outside the home or in education, and less involvement with friends (Brown & Wayne, 1987; Margalit, 1981; 1984). In a time use study of 239 children with disabilities and 519 children without disabilities (aged 6–19 years) Brown & Wayne (1987) found that some similarities existed in activity performance with increasing age (for example older children slept less). However, notable differences over time included greater time spent watching television and only modest increases in educational activities among disabled children, compared to the non-disabled control group. These findings are corroborated by more recent studies in which people with disabilities have been found to spend less time in productive occupations, to dedicate more time to self-care tasks and to have more free time, which is typically less active than that of non-disabled peers (Pentland et al., 1998). In a qualitative study of the perceptions of play and leisure among children with juvenile idiopathic arthritis, Hackett (2003) found that physical problems (pain, stiffness and fatigue), environmental issues (for example poor wheelchair access and the impact of climate on symptoms), overprotection and limits set by others (parents, relatives, friends and school personnel), and self-imposed constraints, all affected participation. Hackett suggested that some of these constraints may have stemmed from an inaccurate understanding of the disease process, potentially leading to needless play restrictions and social isolation. In endeavouring to facilitate physical and mental wellbeing through balanced occupational involvement, occupational therapists must campaign at the individual, familial and societal level to ameliorate barriers to activity participation.

The occupational therapist's role in the quest for balance

Occupational therapists are attuned to the 'orchestration of occupations in time and space' (Yerxa, 1997, p. 365), and espouse the value to health and wellbeing of establishing balanced involvement across occupational performance areas. Like other groups of health professionals, we are increasingly moving towards health promoting models of intervention to achieve this. In the quest for balanced and healthful lifestyles, there is a frequent focus on building competencies, personal resources and connectivity, ultimately enhancing the resilience of individuals, their families and the greater community (Passmore & French, 2000; Wilcock & Whiteford, 2003).

Historically, occupational therapists have focused on service provision to individuals and families, rather than intervening at the community level or entering political debate (Wilcock & Whiteford, 2003). Hence, the profession's potential contribution in health promotion is not always recognized by other groups with longstanding experience. Wilcock & Whiteford (2003) suggest that therapists remain conscious of their skills in promoting and enhancing health through engagement in meaningful and balanced occupation. They also emphasize the value of becoming involved with health promotion, public health and community development teams, and interacting with politicians, social planners, researchers and the media. They suggested that conducting research about occupation and incorporating a greater focus on health promotion in education and training, may also pave the way for occupational therapists to become more involved in supporting full and balanced participation.

Intervention at the individual level

While occupational therapists recognize that children function as part of a complex family unit, children can be targeted directly for individual assessment and intervention to facilitate occupational balance. An assessment of the child which identifies a lack of wellbeing could be suggestive of occupational imbalance. Clarifying children's perspectives of their individual balance between physical, social, mental and rest occupations may highlight specific areas of concern and provide a forum for education regarding the potentially harmful effects of long-term imbalance on wellbeing. In addition to education, therapeutic interventions could target the child, the environment or specific activities to facilitate participation in a well balanced range of occupations which meet developmental needs. To illustrate, a teenager with disinhibition, memory and concentration difficulties following a traumatic brain injury may require social skills training (personal intervention) and the use of a diary (environmental intervention) to ensure appropriate interactions and punctual attendance at Girl Guide events. Residual lack of coordination may necessitate intervention to reduce physical barriers to participation (environmental intervention). Liaison with the Girl Guide leader regarding grading of activities and strategies to maintain concentration might also facilitate involvement (occupation-specific intervention). Where interventions are focused on an individual, it is important to remain cognizant of the many factors which mediate the relationship between engaging in an occupation and the effect of that engagement on health (for example level of perceived control, amount of intrinsic motivation, degree to which the task challenges match skills) (Law et al., 1998).

Intervention at the family level

The support of parents and family is critical to the success of attempts to change a child's patterns of occupation. Where a child or therapist has identified that greater or reduced involvement in certain activities might be beneficial, collaboration with the family is vital. It is imperative that the impact of intervention on established routines and schedules does not undermine family cohesiveness and functioning. Where families are already burdened by the extra care needs of a child with a disability, this process requires sensitivity and compromise. Primeau (1998) suggested, for example, that where play is limited, therapists could learn about parent's daily routines and then assist parents to embed play into household work. Where parents lack understanding regarding other developmental requirements, such as a need for rest, relaxation and sleep, a therapist's role might incorporate providing education regarding the effects of sleep deprivation and supporting parent's efforts to integrate rest time and sleep into daily routines. When a child has a disability, the process of parents coming to understand and actively strive for their child's balanced occupational involvement helps them to enable performance rather than fostering dependence. By remaining informed regarding community resources, therapists are able to further encourage participation in meaningful activities and link parents with support groups. This, in turn, extends children's occupational repertoires and builds a network of community connections.

Intervention at the community and political level

Through raising awareness of the relationship between occupation and wellbeing and setting a need for children's occupational balance on the political agenda, therapists have the potential to shape public policy (Law et al., 1998). Occupational therapists have a role in advocating for equitable access to occupational opportunities and resources to enable children to fulfil their diverse needs. This is of particular importance where families and children live in impoverished circumstances, and are alienated or marginalized. Wilcock & Whiteford (2003) challenged occupational therapists to accept the 'mandate to promote health through occupation for all individuals and communities' and to then, 'in partnership with public policy makers and those they seek to assist, take a proactive stand toward the attainment of occupationally healthy social, political and economic environments' (p. 68).

Summary

The aim of this chapter was to highlight the importance of time use within the context of children's development and wellbeing. The ways in which time has been categorized were reviewed and the difficulties in developing time use taxonomies explored. The personal and contextual factors which influence the distribution of time use in children were detailed and evidence presented for the importance of understanding educational pursuits, leisure involvement, the extent of physical activity and rest for both the physical and psychological wellbeing of children. The perplexing issue of occupational balance was addressed within the context of changing family composition, societal and environmental influences. Finally, the way in which occupational therapists can support children to attain a healthful range of activity engagement was examined by looking at how therapists can influence change at individual, family, community and political levels.

References

Adelman, H. S., Taylor, L. & Nelson, P. (1989). Minors' dissatisfaction with their life circumstances. *Child Psychiatry and Human Development*, 20, 135–147.

Attewell, P., Suazo-Garcia, B. & Battle, J. (2003). Computers and young children: social benefit or social problem? *Social Forces*, 82 (1), 277–296.

Bender, T. A. (1997). Assessment of subjective wellbeing during childhood and adolescence. In: G. D. Phye (Ed.), *Handbook of classroom assessment. Learning, achievement and adjustment*. (Vol. 7, pp. 199–225). San Diego, CA: Academic Press.

Bianchi, S. M. (2000). Maternal employment and time with children: dramatic change or surprising continuity? *Demography*, 37 (4), 401–414.

Bianchi, S. M. & Robinson, J. (1997). What did you do today? Children's use of time, family composition, and the acquisition of social capital. *Journal of Marriage and the Family*, 59 (2), 332–344.

Bronfenbrenner, U. (1979). *The ecology of human development: experiments by nature and design*. Cambridge, MA: Harvard University Press.

Brown, M. & Wayne, A. G. (1987). Impact of impairment on activity patterns of children. *Archives of Physical Medicine and Rehabilitation*, 68, 828–832.

Bryant, K. W. & Zick, C. D. (1996). An examination of parent–child shared time. *Journal of Marriage and the Family*, 58 (1), 227–237.

Canadian Association of Occupational Therapists (1986). *Intervention guidelines for the client-centred practice of occupational therapy*. Ottawa: Ministry of National Health and Welfare.

Carnegie Corporation of New York (1992). Young adolescents: risk and opportunity. In: *A matter of time. Risk and opportunity in the non-school hours* (pp. 25–35). New York: Carnegie Corporation of New York.

Carpenter, C. J., Huston, A. C. & Spera, L. (1989). Children's use of time in their every-day activities during middle childhood. In: M. N. Bloch & A. D. Pellegrini (Eds.), *The ecological context of children's play* (Vol. 9, pp. 165–190). Norwood NJ: Ablex Pub. Corp.

Carr, R. V., Wright, J. D. & Brody, C. J. (1996). Effects of high school work experience a decade later: evidence from the National Longitudinal Survey. *Sociology of Education*, 69, 66–81.

Christiansen, C. (1994). Classification and study in occupation: a review and discussion of taxonomies. *Journal of Occupational Science*, 1 (3), 3–21.

Christiansen, C. H. (1996). Three perspectives on balance in occupation. In: R. Zemke & F. Clark (Eds.), *Occupational science: the evolving discipline* (pp. 431–451). Washington, DC: F. A. Davis.

Clark, F., Parham, D., Carlson, M. E., Frank, G., Jackson, J., Pierce, D., et al. (1991). Occupational science: academic innovation in the service of occupational therapy's future. *American Journal of Occupational Therapy*, 45, 303–314.

Coleman, J. S. (1961). *The adolescent society*. New York: Free Press of Glencoe.

Downey, D. B. & Condron, D. J. (2004). Playing well with others in kindergarten: the benefit of siblings at home. *Journal of Marriage and the Family*, 66, 333–350.

Elkind, D. (1992). *The hurried child: growing up too fast too soon*. Reading: Addison-Wesley Publishing Company.

Farnworth, L. (2000). Time use and leisure occupations of young offenders. *American Journal of Occupational Therapy*, 54 (3), 315–325.

Finn, J. D. (1989). Withdrawing from school. *Review of Educational Research*, 59, 117–142.

Fletcher, A. C., Nickerson, P. & Wright, K. L. (2003). Structured leisure activities in middle childhood: links to wellbeing. *Journal of Community Psychology, 31* (6), 641–659.

Frank, E., Swartz, H. A. & Kupfer, D. J. (2000). Interpersonal and social rhythm therapy: managing the chaos of bipolar disorder. *Biological Psychiatry, 48* (6), 593–606.

Glaze, D. G., Rosen, C. L. & Owens, J. A. (2002). Toward a practical definition of pediatric insomnia. *Current Therapeutic Research, 63* (Supplement B), B4–B17.

Gortmaker, S. L., Must, A., Sobol, A. M., Peterson, K., Colditz, G. A. & Dietz, W. H. (1996). Television viewing as a cause of increasing obesity among children in the United States, 1986–1990. *Archives of Pediatrics and Adolescent Medicine, 150,* 356–362.

Hackett, J. (2003). Perceptions of play and leisure in junior schoolaged children with juvenile idiopathic arthritis: what are the implications for occupational therapy? *British Journal of Occupational Therapy, 66* (7), 303–310.

Hagedorn, R. (1992). *Occupational therapy: foundations for practice.* Edinburgh: Churchill Livingstone.

Harris, C. & Straker, L. (2000). Survey of physical ergonomics issues associated with schoolchildren's use of laptop computers. *International Journal of Industrial Ergonomics, 26,* 337–346.

Hofferth, S. L. & Sandberg, J. F. (2001). How American children spend their time. *Journal of Marriage and the Family, 63* (2), 295–308.

Holland, A. & Andre, T. (1987). Participation in extra-curricular activities in secondary school: what is known, what needs to be known? *Review of Educational Research, 57,* 437–466.

Huebner, E. S. (1991). Initial development of the Students' life satisfaction scale. *School Psychology International, 12,* 231–240.

Huston, A. C. & Wright, J. C. (1997). Mass media and children's development. In: W. Damon, I. Sigel & A. Renninger (Eds.), *Handbook of child psychology* (5th ed., Vol. 4, pp. 999–1058). New York: Wiley.

Huston, A. C., Wright, J. C., Marquis, J. & Green, S. B. (1999). How young children spend their time: television and other activities. *Developmental Psychology, 35* (4), 912–925.

Jordan, A. (2004). The role of media in children's development: an ecological perspective. *Developmental and Behavioral Pediatrics, 25* (3), 196–206.

Kielhofner, G. (1977). Temporal adaptation: a conceptual framework for occupational therapy. *American Journal of Occupational Therapy, 31,* 235–242.

Kleiber, D. (1999). *Leisure in human experience: a dialectical interpretation.* Boulder, CO: Westview.

Kraut, R., Patterson, M., Lundmark, V., Kiesler, S., Mukopadhyay, T. & Scherlis, W. (1998). Internet paradox. A social technology that reduces social involvement and psychological wellbeing? *American Psychologist, 53* (9), 1017–1031.

Larson, R. (1994). Youth organizations, hobbies and sports as developmental contexts. In: R. K. Silbereisen & E. Todt (Eds.), *Adolescence in context. The interplay of family, school, peers and work in adjustment* (Vol. 3, pp. 46–65). New York: Springer-Verlag.

Larson, R. & Verma, S. (1999). How children and adolescents spend time across the world: work, play and developmental opportunities. *Psychological Bulletin, 125* (6), 701–736.

Larson, R. & Zemke, R. (2003). Shaping the temporal patterns of our lives: the social coordination of occupation. *Journal of Occupational Science, 10* (2), 80–89.

Law, M., Steinwender, S. & Leclair, L. (1998). Occupation, health and wellbeing. *Canadian Journal of Occupational Therapy, 65* (2), 81–91.

Li, X. & Atkins, M. S. (2004). Early childhood computer experience and cognitive and motor development. *Pediatrics, 113* (6), 1715–1722.

McHale, S. M., Crouter, A. C. & Tucker, C. J. (2001). Free-time activities in middle childhood: links with adjustment in early adolescence. *Child Development*, 72 (6), 1764–1778.

Mares, M. L. & Woodard, E. H. (2001). Pro-social effects on children's interactions. In: D. Singer & J. Singer (Eds.), *Handbook of children and the media* (pp. 183–206). Thousand Oaks, CA: Sage.

Margalit, M. (1981). Leisure activities of cerebral palsied children. *Israel Journal of Psychiatry and Related Sciences*, 18 (3), 209–214.

Margalit, M. (1984). Leisure activities of learning disabled children as a reflection of their passive lifestyle and prolonged dependency. *Child Psychiatry and Human Development*, 15 (2), 133–141.

Marsh, H. W. (1991). Employment during high school: character building or a subversion of academic goals? *Sociology of Education*, 64, 172–189.

Marsh, H. W. (1992). Extra-curricular activities: beneficial extension of the traditional curriculum or subversion of academic goals? *Journal of Educational Psychology*, 84 (4), 533–562.

Marsh, H. W. & Kleitman, S. (2002). Extra-curricular activities: the good, the bad, and the non-linear. *Harvard Educational Review*, 72 (4), 464–511.

Medrich, E. A., Roizen, J. A., Rubin, V. & Buckley, S. (1982). *The serious business of growing up: a study of children's lives outside school*. Berkeley, CA: University of California Press.

Meeks, C. B. & Mauldin, T. (1990). Children's time in structured and unstructured leisure activities. *Lifestyles: Family and Economic Issues*, 11 (3), 257–281.

Meijer, A. M., Habekothe, H. T. & Van den Wittenboer, G. L. H. (2000). Time in bed, quality of sleep and school functioning of children. *Journal of Sleep Research*, 9, 145–153.

Meyer, A. (1977). The philosophy of occupational therapy. *American Journal of Occupational Therapy*, 31, 639–642.

Molnar, B. E., Gortmaker, S. L., Bull, F. C. & Buka, S. L. (2004). Unsafe to play? Neighbourhood disorder and lack of safety predict reduced physical activity among urban children and adolescents. *American Journal of Health Promotion*, 18 (5), 378–386.

Mosey, A. C. (1986). *The psychological components of occupational therapy*. New York: Raven Press.

O'Brien, J. & Smith, J. (2002). Childhood transformed? Risk perceptions and the decline of free play. *British Journal of Occupational Therapy*, 65 (3), 123–128.

Osgood, D. W., Wilson, J. K., O'Malley, P. M., Bachman, J. G. & Johnston, L. D. (1996). Routine activities and individual deviant behavior. *American Sociological Review*, 61 (4), 635–655.

Palmer, S. (1993). Does computer use put children's vision at risk? *Journal of Research and Development in Education*, 26, 59–65.

Parizkova, J. (1996). *Nutrition, physical activity and health early in life*. Boca Raton: CRC Press.

Passmore, A. (2003). The occupation of leisure: three typologies and their influence on mental health in adolescence. *The Occupational Therapy Journal of Research*, 23 (2), 76–83.

Passmore, A. & French, D. (2000). A model of leisure and mental health in Australian adolescents. *Behaviour Change*, 17 (3), 208–220.

Passmore, A. & French, D. (2001). Development and administration of a measure to assess adolescents' participation in leisure activities. *Adolescence*, 36 (141), 67–75.

Pentland, W., Harvey, A. S. & Walker, J. (1998). The relationships between time use and health and wellbeing in men with spinal cord injury. *Journal of Occupational Science, 5* (1), 14–25.

Pilcher, J. J. & Huffcutt, A. I. (1996). Effects of sleep deprivation on performance: a meta-analysis. *Sleep, 19*, 318–326.

Pollard, E. L. & Lee, P. D. (2003). Child wellbeing: a systematic review of the literature. *Social Indicators Research, 61*, 59–78.

Posner, J. K. & Vandell, D. L. (1999). After school activities and the development of low-income urban children: a longitudinal study. *Developmental Psychology, 35* (3), 868–879.

Primeau, L. A. (1998). Orchestration of work and play within families. *The American Journal of Occupational Therapy, 52* (3), 118–195.

Reed, K. L. (1984). *Models of practice in occupational therapy.* Baltimore: Williams & Wilkins.

Robinson, J. P. & Bianchi, S. (1997). The children's hours. *American Demographics, 19* (2), 20–23.

Rochelau, B. (1995). Computer use by school-age children: trends, patterns, and predictors. *Journal of Educational Computing Research, 12* (1), 1–17.

Sanson, A., Nicholson, J., Ungerer, J., Zubrick, S., Wilson, K., Ainley, J., et al. (2002). *Introducing the longitudinal study of Australian children. LSAC discussion paper number 1.* Melbourne: Australian Institute of Family Studies.

Silbereisen, R. K., Noack, P. & Eyferth, K. (1986). Place for development: adolescents, leisure settings and developmental tasks. In: R. K. Silbereisen, K. Eyferth & G. Rudinger (Eds.), *Development as action in context* (pp. 87–107). Heidelberg, Germany: Springer-Verlag.

Steelman, L. C., Powell, B., Werum, R. & Carter, S. (2002). Reconsidering the effects of sibling configuration: recent advances and challenges. *Annual Review of Sociology, 28*, 243–269.

Stevenson, H. W. & Lee, S. (1990). Context of achievement. *Monographs of the Society for Research in Child Development, 55* (1–2, Serial No. 221), 33–49.

Subrahmanyam, K., Kraut, R. E., Greenfield, P. M. & Gross, E. F. (2000). The impact of home computer use on children's activities and development. *The Future of Children, 10* (2), 123–144.

Suto, M. (1998). Leisure in occupational therapy. *Canadian Journal of Occupational Therapy, 65* (5), 271–278.

The Royal Australasian College of Physicians (2004). *Children and the media: advocating for the future.* Sydney: The Royal Australasian College of Physicians.

Timmer, S. G., Eccles, J. & O'Brien, K. (1985). How children use time. In: F. T. Juster & F. P. Stafford (Eds.), *Time, goods and wellbeing* (Vol. 14, pp. 353–382). Ann Arbor, Mich.: Survey Research Center, University of Michigan.

Trost, S. G. & Pate, R. R. (1999). Physical activity in children and youth. In: J. M. Rippe (Ed.), *Lifestyle Medicine.* Malden: Blackwell Science.

Trost, S., Pate, R., Sallis, J., Freedson, P., Taylor, W., Dowda, M., et al. (2002). Age and gender differences in objectively measured physical activity in youth. *Medicine and Science in Sports and Exercise, 34* (2), 350–355.

Varni, J. W., Seid, M. & Kurtin, P. S. (2001). PedsQL[TM] 4.0: reliability and validity of the pediatric quality of life inventory[TM] version 4.0 generic core scales in healthy and patient populations. *Medical Care, 39* (8), 800–812.

Wilcock, A. A., Chelin, M., Hall, M., Hamley, N., Morrison, B., Scrivener, L., et al. (1997). The relationship between occupational balance and health: a pilot study. *Occupational Therapy International, 4* (1), 17–30.

Wilcock, A. & Whiteford, G. (2003). Occupation, health promotion and the environment. In: L. Letts, Rigby, P. & Stewart, D. (Ed.), *Using environments to enable occupational performance* (Vol. 4, pp. 55–70). Thorofare, NJ: Slack Incorporated.

World Health Organization (2001). *International classification of functioning, disability and health: ICF* (Short Version ed.). Geneva: World Health Organization.

Yalmambirra (2000). Black time . . . white time: my time . . . your time. *Journal of Occupational Science*, 7 (3), 133–137.

Yerxa, E. (1997). Occupation: the keystone of a curriculum for a self-defined profession. *The American Journal of Occupational Therapy*, 52 (5), 365–372.

SECTION 2

MASTERING OCCUPATIONS, ROLES AND ENABLING CHILDREN'S PARTICIPATION

DOING, BEING AND BECOMING: THEIR IMPORTANCE FOR CHILDREN

Angela Mandich and Sylvia Rodger

'. . . the way to improve quality of life is not through thinking, but through doing.'
(Csikszentmihalyi, 1993, p. 38)

Participation in everyday childhood occupations is fundamental to the healthy development of all children, regardless of ability or disability (Polatajko & Mandich, 2004). The occupational roles of childhood require children to develop personal independence, become productive and participate in play or leisure pursuits. Through *doing*, or participation in everyday occupations, children learn and master new skills. Engaging in new experiences and occupations enables children to develop positive self-esteem and become contributing members of society. Through *doing* with friends and family children develop a sense of belonging and social engagement, both of which contribute to health and wellbeing. Occupational therapists aim to facilitate and promote children's engagement in activities of daily living. Failure to participate in everyday *doing* can lead to marginalization and can have a profound negative impact on children (Mandich et al., 2003; Segal et al., 2002). This chapter draws on the work of Wilcock (1998) to elucidate the important role that participation in occupation holds for children. Wilcock (1998) conceptualized occupation as 'a synthesis of doing, being and becoming' (p. 249), and argued that engagement in occupation leads to health and wellbeing. She encouraged health practitioners to move beyond traditional intervention planning and focus on understanding the importance of *doing* or engaging in meaningful occupation. In this chapter we will:

(1) Address the importance of *doing* in terms of physical, cognitive, affective and social development
(2) Illustrate how successful occupational engagement leads to the development of self-esteem and self-efficacy, and how the lack of activity engagement or *doing* impacts negatively on children

(3) Address an occupational therapy approach that enables acquisition of a range of skills and hence children's ability to engage in daily occupations or *doing*

(4) Highlight the importance of *being* for all children in terms of restoration and relaxation, and in particular for those with significant disabilities and terminal conditions

The importance of doing, being and becoming

Wilcock (1998) drew on the work of Fidler & Fidler (1978) and others to provide a conceptualization of occupation as a combination of *doing*, *being* and *becoming*. Fidler & Fidler (1978) defined 'doing' as 'a process of investigating, trying out and gaining evidence of one's capacity for experiencing, responding, managing, creating and controlling' (p. 306). Wilcock believed that *doing* provides a means of social interaction and connection with the community. *Doing* furthermore, enables the acquisition and development of physical, cognitive, affective and social skills. She claimed that *doing* leads to *being*, that is the 'contemplation and enjoyment of the inner life' (Maslow, 1968, p. 214), where the individual experiences an inner sense of peace.

Further, Wilcock (1998) conceptualized *becoming* as the person whom one strives to be, as they are best fitted to be, and as they hope to be. The occupations engaged in by humans, define their *being*, and are necessary in helping people achieve whom they wish to *become*. *Becoming* or undergoing developmental change (Merriam-Webster, 2005) emphasizes the notion of growth and change that emerges from *doing* and participating in daily activities. Wilson (1990) pondered about the process of living, and considered that everything that happens to us is integral to our *becoming*. Fidler & Fidler (1978) emphasized the complexity of *becoming* by highlighting three dimensions of: *becoming I*, *becoming competent*, and *becoming a social being*. *Becoming* occurs through growth and experience and leads to the development of a sense of self-confidence and social connection.

The theoretical work of Piaget (1972), Erikson (1963), Reilly (1960) and others described in Chapter 7, highlight the contribution of *doing* to occupational development. *Doing* and positive occupational participation enables the development of self-esteem and competence that enhances *becoming*. Humans have an innate drive to explore and master their environment, which motivates them to become competent beings (Fidler & Fidler, 1978). Wilcock (1998) suggested that 'a dynamic balance between "doing" and "being" is central to healthy living and "becoming" whatever a person is best fitted to become is dependent on both' (p. 251).

Health practitioners contribute to the child's physical, cognitive, affective and social development by engaging them in *doing* activities. Wilcock (1998) stated 'occupational therapists are in the business of helping people transform their lives by facilitating talents and abilities not yet in full use . . . we are part of their process of becoming' (p. 251). Further, she proposed that occupational therapists are employed to assist people in *doing*, *being* and *becoming* by facilitating their talents and abilities through the performance of meaningful occupations. We propose that the sequence of *doing*, *being* and *becoming* is neither sequential nor linear, but rather fluid with movement through these three processes being continuous and occurring in varying order.

Virgin & Mandich (2001) interviewed children (aged from 10 to 16 years) with varying physical abilities to explore their experiences of occupational engagement, and provided further evidence for Wilcock's conceptualization of occupation as an amalgamation of *doing*, *being* and *becoming*. Their study suggested that occupational engagement is integral to child development. The children shared their views on the importance of *doing* in terms of developing self-efficacy and appreciating their accomplishments. One ten-year-old discussed how much he enjoyed playing soccer:

'It's important to me because it makes you feel good about yourself and it helps you to occupy your time and get to know other people. It sort of builds up your self-esteem, it makes you feel good, like something you can be proud of, accomplishments you can look back at.' (unpublished manuscript)

Clark (1993) claimed that engaging in childhood occupations is related to adult character building or 'becoming' who one is as a person. The children in the Virgin & Mandich (2001) study supported Clark's notion and discussed their awareness that participation in school activities leads to 'becoming':

'It is important to go to university, get a good job, you know. My marks are important, it's important to get good marks so I can become what I want and keep my options open because I don't really know what I wanna be when I grow up'. (unpublished manuscript)

This study demonstrated that children, irrespective of developmental level or physical ability, viewed occupation as important.

Outcomes of occupational engagement

Baum & Law (1998) argued that through occupational engagement people develop and maintain health. Indeed, occupations develop across the lifespan. Infants and young children begin with a small number of occupations. As they engage in *doing* with family, friends and others they build a repertoire of occupations that allow them to further develop their roles as child, student, player and friend. (Davis & Polatajko, 2004). As individual children are unique their occupational repertoire is unique in its development. Participation in the activities and occupations of childhood, contributes to children's physical, cognitive, social and affective development. These will be discussed in turn.

Research has shown that children's competence in motor based activity throughout early childhood is an important predictor of academic success (Macnab, 2003). *Physical development* involves the attainment of various motor skills through *doing* a variety of typical childhood activities. As young children engage in motor activities, they develop physical strength, coordination, motor control, as well as an awareness of their environment. Children move through various stages of physical growth and development as they participate in *doing* childhood activities, beginning with limited control of movement and progressing to more complex, voluntary movements such as walking, jumping, ball catching and cursive writing. Gross and fine motor development continues and becomes refined as the child participates in activities such as music lessons or organized sports.

Additionally, *doing* assists the child in the development of *cognitive skills*. Piaget (1972) identified four developmental stages and the processes by which children progress through them. The first stage is the sensorimotor stage that lasts from birth until about two years old. At this stage the child uses their senses and motor abilities to understand the world. From two until about seven years the child enters the next stage, namely pre-operational thought. At this stage the child has mental representations and is able to engage in pretend and creative play. The concrete operations stage occurs from about the age of seven to eleven years. During this stage the child thinks logically and concretely, and their thinking processes develop largely through hands-on experiences or *doing*. The final stage of formal operations is where the child can think logically and abstractly. Piaget emphasized the important role of experiential learning for cognitive development, as well as the role that cognition plays in the acquisition of new skills at each of these stages.

Doing also leads to *socialization and development of social skills*, which will be addressed further in Chapter 8. Learning to get along with others is accomplished through practice and engagement in daily occupations. Young children's experience of playing in the playground and taking turns assists in their social development. Bandura's social learning theory highlighted the importance of observing and modelling behaviours and *doing*. Bandura (1977) stated:

> '*Learning would be exceedingly laborious, not to mention hazardous, if people had to rely solely on the effects of their own actions to inform them what to do. Fortunately, most human behaviour is learned observationally through modelling: from observing others one forms an idea of how new behaviours are performed, and on later occasions this coded information serves as a guide for action.*' (p. 22)

Doing or engaging in activities with other children is one of the most powerful mechanisms of socialization. In a recent qualitative study by Zilberbrandt & Mandich (2004), parents and children (aged from eight to sixteen) of varying ability, were asked about children's everyday occupations. In-depth interviews were conducted with nine parents and ten children regarding the reasons why children engaged in various activities. One common theme was the importance of *doing* activities with friends. One child stated, '. . . "being" with my friends, that's high on the priority list, that's what makes life fun, it makes you enjoy it . . .'

With respect to *affective development*, Christiansen (1999) discussed the importance of occupation in defining personal identity, and that 'one of the most compelling needs that every human being has is to be able to express their unique identity in a manner that gives meaning to life' (p. 547). Each child is born with

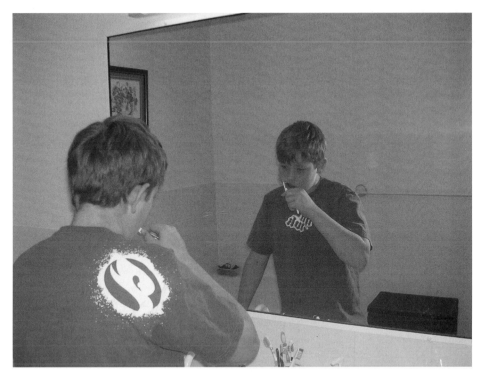

Figure 6.1   Brushing teeth is an important self-care activity mastered during childhood.

the potential to *become* and it is through children's life roles, *doing* and *being,* that this potential emerges. Our identity is formed through successful engagement in activities and occupations that are inherent in our life roles. For example, a child develops their identity as a sibling, a self-carer, a friend, a member of a basketball team, or a school student. Mastering the activities prescribed by these occupational and social roles leads to positive self-identity. A self-carer needs to be able to brush their teeth, get dressed independently, complete household chores, while a basketball player needs to dribble, shoot hoops and catch a ball on the run (See Figures 6.1 and 6.2). Through *doing* these activities most children develop and refine their skills and view themselves as successful, leading to positive self-esteem and self-efficacy, and positive self-attributions of success.

Consequences of not being able to do

Many children, for a range of physical, cognitive, social, or emotional reasons, do not have the same opportunities to engage successfully in meaningful occupations. While the consequences of physical/motor skill difficulties, cognitive impairment and emotional disturbance are frequently seen by occupational therapists, the impact of socio-economic factors may be less obvious. Some children experience occupational deprivation due to lack of social or financial capital/resources preventing them from accessing experiences that can enhance their self-identity, for

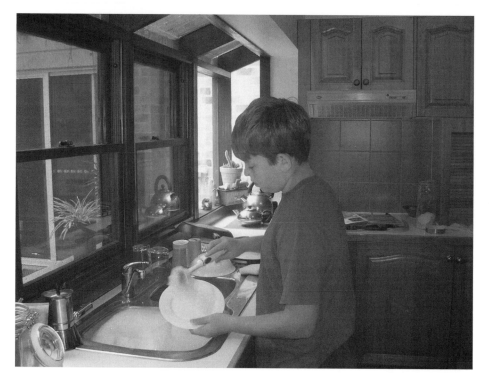

Figure 6.2 Doing chores such as washing dishes helps children learn how to contribute to the household.

example children experiencing poverty, abuse, natural disasters, terror or war. When children are unable to do the typical activities of childhood there are many negative consequences. A child who is not *doing* may not have a healthy sense of who they are (that is self-identity). In turn, this may negatively impact on who they *become* by limiting their sense of their ability to *become*. Occupation provides a sense of purpose in a person's life and meaning to one's existence (Rebeiro & Cook, 1999). Without occupation, a breakdown of habits can lead to reduced occupational performance competence or a loss of personal identity. As occupational therapists, we enable clients to do in order to fulfil their human need for occupation and allow them to *become*, hence achieving their occupational potential.

Inability to participate in typical childhood occupations can lead to marginalization and social isolation. Failing to master simple activities such as tying shoes, doing up buttons, riding a bike or learning to write can have profound negative effects (Segal et al., 2002). (See Figure 6.3.) Mandich et al. (2003) interviewed 12 parents of children with developmental coordination disorder (DCD). They reported that failure to master these everyday childhood skills was devastating for their children. Parents discussed the importance of succeeding in these everyday activities. Paul's mother was keenly aware of the marginalizing effect that her son's

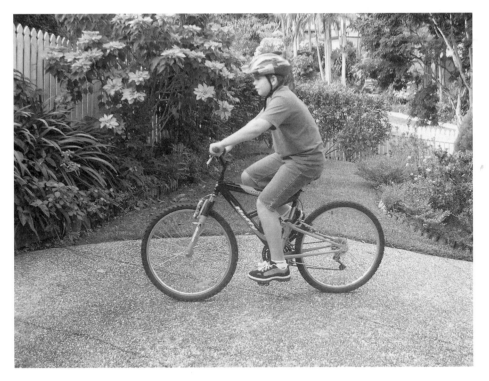

Figure 6.3 Riding a bike enables children freedom to explore their environment, become independent in travel and have adventures with friends.

inability to master bike riding and rollerblading had on his participation in extra-curricular activities. She said:

> 'Well, at Cubs they did a bike rodeo. And we were outside setting up the cones and of course you could either ride a bike or rollerblades, which excluded him from both things. (He could do neither.) He felt excluded and I know that he felt that because most of the kids turned up with bikes and I knew he felt he had a bike at home and he could not ride it and he had gotten too big for the one we had.' (Mandich et al., 2003, p. 591)

Mounting research evidence clearly illustrates that children need opportunities to engage in occupation and to have fun, for their personal health, to be accepted by peers, to make friends, to be good at something and to acquire new skills. Humans need to have meaningful occupation for their wellbeing and to become competent functioning members of society. *Doing* enables the child to develop an occupational repertoire that contributes to healthy development. By contrast Elkind (2001) highlighted the problems associated with children *doing* too much too fast. He discussed the negative consequences of high expectations on children's academic, social, or emotional development. This will be discussed further in the section of this chapter on occupational balance.

Approaches to enabling doing

Historically, intervention approaches for children with performance problems have focused on remediation of performance component deficits rather than looking more broadly at the functional difficulties with *doing* or participating in daily life (Gentile, 1992; Mandich et al., 2001). These bottom-up approaches consider foundational factors, such as performance components, first to obtain an understanding of a person's strengths and deficits (Weinstock-Zlotnick & Hinojosa, 2004). Hence, the emphasis is on components such as strength, balance, range of motion, visual perception and vestibular functioning. These are believed to be prerequisites to successful occupational performance. The inherent assumption is that acquisition of the underlying performance sensorimotor, cognitive, and psychosocial component skills and abilities will lead to successful occupational performance (Gentile, 1992). Although many of these bottom-up approaches have been used for a long time, little evidence has accrued to support them and many remain untested. Even where there is measurable improvement in general motor performance, ensuing improvements in the specific motor skills that the child wants to, needs to, or is expected to perform have not been found (Mandich et al., 2001; Sigmundsson et al., 1998).

Currently, there is a movement away from traditional approaches to intervention to enabling *doing* using contemporary or top-down approaches in which assessment focuses first on issues of role competency and meaningfulness, as well as self-care, rest, play and school occupations. The foundational factors (performance skills, patterns, context, activity demands and client factors) are considered if needed later (Weinstock-Zlotnick & Hinojosa, 2004). These approaches have been drawn from contemporary principles about motor learning and control, evidence based practice, client centred practice and the shift from a focus on disease to health (WHO, 2001). Each of these underpinning principles will be addressed in turn.

Motor learning approaches

Motor learning approaches, drawn from human movement science, work from the assumption that skill acquisition emerges from the interaction of the child, the task and the environment. The child must engage in *doing* the activity to improve performance (Thelen et al., 1987; Turvey, 1990). From this top-down perspective, performance emerges, is self-organized and arises from a heterarchical, dynamic interaction of multiple subsystems including the person's sensory, motor, perceptual and anatomical systems and environmental factors (Thelen, 1995). Current theories of skill acquisition emphasize the importance of contextual over neuro-maturational factors. Gentile (1992) argued that if the goal is to facilitate skill acquisition in children, it may be fruitful to pursue interventions based on functional activities, rather than focusing on underlying components. Contemporary treatment approaches include, the problem solving approach (Bouffard & Wall, 1990), the cognitive motor approach (Henderson & Sugden, 1992), task specific approach (Revie

& Larkin, 1993) and cognitive orientation to daily occupational performance approach (CO-OP) (Polatajko & Mandich, 2004).

Evidence based practice

In addition to current shifts in motor performance theories, health and education systems are demanding greater accountability. This shift to evidence based practice, demands interventions that are cost effective and efficient (Driever, 2002). Law & Baum (1998) reported that 'clients expect interventions that are effective, provided by competent therapists, and appropriate to their needs and preferences' (p. 132). Childhood professionals must be aware of current research, incorporate this research into practice, and measure and document intervention outcomes (Wood, 1998). Clinical research must be based on outcomes that are specific, measurable, attainable, time limited and enable the client to do the activities that are important to them.

Client centred practice

Client centred practice is gaining momentum in health care. Originally introduced by Rogers (1951), client centred practice has been conceptualized in different ways by various professions. The underlying premise is one of respect for the client and a belief that the client should choose their own goals. The following occupational therapy definition is illustrative:

> 'Client centred practice refers to collaborative approaches aimed at enabling occupation with clients who may be individuals, groups, agencies, governments, corporations, or others. Occupational therapists demonstrate respect for clients, involve clients in decision making, advocate with and for clients in meeting clients' needs, and otherwise recognize clients' experience and knowledge'. (CAOT, 1997, p. 49)

For children, it is especially important to focus on meaningful, purposeful and motivating activities that contribute to their ability to participate in typical childhood occupations. The therapist's role is to work in partnership with clients to facilitate their decision making and to provide them with appropriate information and support. This approach helps to ensure that services are meaningful and appropriate, enabling occupations that clients want to, need to, or are expected to perform (Sumsion, 1999).

International classification of functioning, disability and health (ICF)

Finally, recent changes in the ICF (WHO, 2001) discussed in Chapter 1 have impacted on therapists' intervention approaches. The new ICF model acknowledges the importance of participation and how limitations in activity and participation contribute to disability. The WHO view of health has shifted from a focus on disease and its consequences to health and the factors that contribute to wellbeing at the activity and participation levels. Some bottom-up intervention approaches focused on impairment reduction (for example reducing tone), with little emphasis on activity or participation, whereas top-down approaches focus primarily on activity and participation.

The following case study illustrates how occupational therapists can enable *doing* and incorporate these four features of contemporary intervention approaches.

Matthew

Matthew is an eight-year-old boy with DCD, referred to occupational therapy for difficulties *doing* many functional activities (for example handwriting, tying his shoes, playing ball and bike riding). The therapist completed an initial assessment and determined that Matthew's coordination difficulties were due to problems with bilateral coordination, manual dexterity, self-confidence and inability to remember the steps to perform each activity. First, the therapist asked Matthew and his family what goals were important to them. The therapist obtained Matthew's occupational profile and his treatment goals using the Pediatric activity card sort (Mandich et al., 2004). The therapist then used CO-OP (Polatajko & Mandich, 2004) with Matthew to address his goals (riding a bike and handwriting). CO-OP is a client centred, performance based, problem solving, approach that enables skill acquisition through a process of strategy use and guided discovery. There is an increasing body of research evidence demonstrating the effectiveness of this approach with children with motor problems (for example Polatajko et al., 2001).

CO-OP focuses on enabling children to develop strategies to overcome functional motor problems and promote generalization and transfer. The essential features are client centred, individually tailored intervention; child identified goals which form the motivating focus of intervention; dynamic performance analysis to identify performance breakdown; a global strategy used to frame therapy; domain specific strategies, identified during the treatment to facilitate performance; and generalization and transfer to ecologically appropriate tasks and environments. The first step in the intervention sessions involves teaching the child the global strategy: goal, plan, do, check.

Goal: What do I want to do?
Plan: How am I going to do it?
Do: Do it!
Check: How well did my plan work?

Within this framework, the child discovers which aspects of the task are problematic and how to overcome these problems. This is done by asking questions of the child, such as 'What is going wrong?' 'How did you do that?' 'What do you need to do first?' or 'How might you fix that?' Through this process of guided discovery, the child, in collaboration with the therapist, identifies specific strategies that facilitate task performance.

In keeping with a top-down approach, although the therapist identified some difficulties at the level of body structure and function, she chose to focus intervention at the activity and participation level. First, she observed Matthew *doing* these activities and rated his performance using a behavioural measure such as the Performance quality rating scale (PQRS) (Polatajko & Mandich, 2004). Then she completed a behavioural analysis of where performance was breaking down using dynamic performance analysis (DPA) (Polatajko et al., 2000). This revealed performance breakdown during writing (Matthew's letters are too large, he does not sit properly on the chair when he is writing and at times falls off the chair) and in riding a bike (he does not know how to pedal or to steer the bike).

The therapist structured and graded the practice environment and the tasks and then, by focusing on one thing at a time, she guided Matthew to discover the salient difficult features of the task and plans that would help him address those areas of difficulty. Therapists focusing on enabling *doing* must have the activity as the foreground and the underlying components in the background. If outcomes are targeted at the structure/function level, the therapist may also establish outcome measures that demonstrate to the client how intervening at that level will directly, or indirectly, influence performance at the activity or participation level (that is, increasing range of motion may provide the foundational skills for the individual to don their sweater).

So far in this chapter we have defined *doing*, *being* and *becoming*, addressed the outcomes of occupational engagement, the consequences of not being able to *do* successfully and described one top-down approach that enables *doing*. We now turn our attention to exploring *being*, childhood spirituality, palliative care and children's need for occupational balance.

Let's not forget being

'The very heart of what is important for our children's welfare and for our future is the understanding of ourselves as loving human beings' (Daleo, 1996, p. 10).

Wilcock's (1998) seminal work focused in part on the need for a dynamic balance between *doing* and *being* for healthy living and how *becoming* is dependent on both. She defined *being* as existing or living. It is seen as an inner process of integrating the *doing* and *being* past and present in preparation for the future. Maslow (1968) described it as 'the contemplation and enjoyment of the inner life' and as one of the 'peak experiences in which time disappears and hopes are fulfilled' (p. 214). It could be argued that during these occasions an individual experiences what Csikszentmihalyi (1990) refers to as *flow*. Children can experience flow during many activities, for example during play when all concept of time is lost. Just as children experience flow in the outer, tangible world of *doing* things, so too can they experience flow in their inner world of thoughts, feelings and emotions. Other examples of when such thoughts and emotions can occur include meditation, nature walks and listening to or playing music. Wilcock further stated that *being* is about 'being true to ourselves, to our nature, to our essence, and to what is distinctive about us' (p. 250). During childhood, children develop an increased sense of self-discovery and self-realization, a journey which continues throughout adulthood. So, what does *being* mean for children?

Using Wilcock's definition, *being* means that children need the time to discover who they are, to think, reflect on each day and simply to *be*. In addition, they need to discover their inner nature or *self*. Given discussions in this and previous chapters about the busy, structured and 'hurried' lives of many children in contemporary societies, it is easy to see that many children may not have enough down time, in which they can relax, daydream, and simply *be* themselves. While some adults belittle 'down time' as seemingly unproductive time, in which children daydream, there is no doubt that for all of us, and for children in particular, there is a need to ensure time for restorative and relaxing pursuits. It might be easy to mistake television viewing as down time. However, it is not a process of inner reflection and growth, rather a soaking up of visual and auditory stimulation. The physiological benefits of down time or relaxation include decreased heart rate, lowered blood pressure, decreased respiratory rate, slowing of metabolism and brain waves (Khalsa, 2003). In addition, there are many psychological benefits, including decreased stress, balancing of emotions and increased self awareness.

Maslow's (1968) hierarchy of needs is divided into deficiency needs and *being* needs. Deficiency or D-needs refer to physiological survival needs, safety and security needs; affiliation needs such as acceptance and love; and esteem needs such as approval and recognition. *Being* or B-needs include a need to recognize and comprehend beauty and self-actualization (realizing one's potential). Christiansen (2004) provided examples of occupations that support these B-needs, such as those involving art, music, reflection and creative expression that are relevant to aesthetic/cognition needs. Activities that synthesize experiences such as volunteering, journalizing, and storytelling are relevant to self-actualization needs. Hence, it appears that for both children and adults opportunities to engage in activities which meet *being* needs are important if they are to realize their full potentials. Examples of *being* activities might include: bushwalking, viewing art, listening to or playing music, writing in a diary, creative pursuits in which children become immersed, such as poetry, dance, art and yoga or meditation. While for some children bushwalking might be about *doing*, that is, getting from one place to another, physical exercise or a demonstration of orienteering prowess, for others it may be about experiencing nature, particularly the sounds, smells and sights of the forest. In the latter example, children are experiencing *being* in the moment, *being* mindful of the present and the sensory experiences of *being* alive.

Children may engage in the art of *being* in different ways to adults. However, this does not minimize their need for passive occupational pursuits such as resting while listening to music (see Figure 6.4), or lying on the grass looking at the clouds, or sitting in a tree-house daydreaming. Spending time outdoors and communing with nature, such as walking in forests and parks can enhance feelings of wellbeing, engendering relaxation and restoration. Hence, it is important that children growing up in sprawling, dense cities have ample opportunities to experience

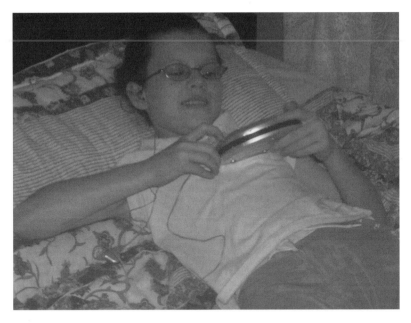

Figure 6.4 Lying on the bed listening to music provides children with downtime to rest and reflect.

nature and outdoor spaces for relaxation, and that these spaces are preserved for future generations.

As advocates for children's health and wellbeing, childhood professionals such as occupational therapists also need to advocate for children having enough down time for relaxation and provide parents with examples of down time pursuits. This may be by advising parents and carers not to over schedule children's lives with too many structured activities, or by providing input into programmes conducted by childcare centres or respite organizations to allow children a balance of *doing* and *being* activities such as time out for their own choice of activities, for rest, for listening to music and other passive pursuits. These have the benefit of allowing children choice and time out from *doing*.

Children and spirituality

'*Let the voice sing out in praise and thanksgiving. Gather together in joyous song. Celebrate the gift of Spirit*'. *(Daleo, 1996, p. 144)*

The importance of spirituality and religious involvement and its impact on people's health has increasingly been recognized within medicine (Mueller et al., 2001). Religion and spirituality are important cultural factors that give structure and meaning to human values, behaviours and experiences. Surveys indicate that most people regard their spiritual and physical health as equally important, and that people have greater spiritual needs during illness (Mueller et al., 2001). Smith

& McSherry (2004) described spiritual beliefs manifested in children as an expression of their development and cognitive thinking and proposed that health care practitioners need to understand these beliefs when caring for hospitalized children.

While the area of human spirituality has recently become a topic of increased awareness and interest for occupational therapists as a component of holistic practice (Belcham, 2004; Christiansen, 1997; Egan & Swedersky, 2003; Howard & Howard, 1997; Kang, 2003), relatively little has been written about spirituality as a childhood occupation. *Being* or *doing* occupations can be spiritual if they are construed as such by the child themself. In the previous example, bushwalking may be *doing* if the focus is on physical activity or orienteering. However, it may be a *being* or spiritual activity if the focus is on experiencing the moment and *being* at one with nature and the universe. Burgman & King (2005) reported that:

> 'Children need access to meaningful occupations in order to connect with their spirituality, finding purpose and meaning in their lives. Spirituality is expressed in the daily activities of children, communicated in their self-care, play, connections with nature, conversations and participation in educational, religious and work contexts . . . Their ability to utilize spiritual qualities such as hope, courage and trust underlies their potential across all aspects of their lives'. (p. 158)

Christiansen (1997) proposed that spirituality should not be ignored by occupational therapists who seek to consider humans as occupational beings. There are indeed parallels between definitions of spirituality and Wilcock's description of *being* in terms of 'being true to ourselves, our nature and our essence' (1998, p. 250). Egan & DeLaat (1994) viewed human spirituality as the essence or true nature of a person expressed in daily actions, which are influenced by values, beliefs and socio-cultural background. While spirituality may be linked to religion for many people, reminders of sacred and spiritual opportunities are found in everyday living (Christiansen, 1997). For some, spirituality stresses the person's subjective perception and experience of something or someone greater than themself (Howard & Howard, 1997). Reading, listening to or playing music, walking in nature, meditating, painting, t'ai chi, dancing, journaling and participating in communities of faith, are all potentially spiritual activities that may nourish the soul by providing opportunities for creating meaning (see Figure 6.5). These spiritual activities and their expression will vary between individuals. Christiansen challenged us to acknowledge that the meaning associated with occupations often has spiritual dimensions. These spiritual occupations can be enacted at both individual and community levels (Kang, 2003). Burgman & King (2005) described children's needs to access healing spaces where they can explore personal meaning of both negative and positive experiences. Such healing spaces and experiences may include play, cultural rituals, daily rituals, nature and connection with their communities, which are meaningful and empowering.

Kang's (2003) construct of psycho-spiritual integration, views spirituality as a harmony of six dimensions (becoming, meaning, being, centredness, connectedness and transcendence). *Becoming* is associated with independence, personal growth,

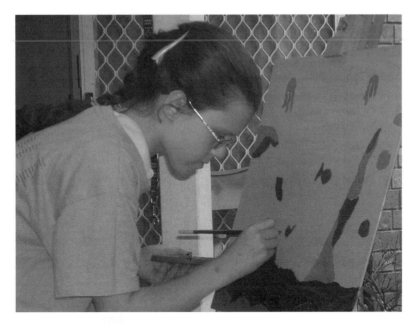

Figure 6.5 Being totally absorbed in painting can lead to an experience of flow.

autonomy, and choice through active *doing*. *Meaning* is the sense of intrinsic purposefulness and vitality that informs the direction of and inspires the process of living. Meaning emerges out of life and shapes it into a unified flow experience. *Being* forms the foundation of our existence as human *beings*. *Being* belongs to the domain of non-doing and pertains to who we really are as people and a species. It includes the creative, intuitive and devotional energies of human consciousness. Kang proposed that within *being* lies the wellspring of our creativity, intuition and love. *Centredness* refers to an inner stability based on knowing and recognizing the core of one's *being*. While some refer to the soul, others refer to a sense of silent clarity at the core of *being* (Kang, 2003). *Connectedness* allows a fullness of *being* to emerge into a profound relationship with all life and the universe. Finally, *transcendence* is the innate drive to find ultimate meaning and happiness. According to Kang's model, spiritual fulfillment exists when most or all of these dimensions are observed in individuals or communities.

It might be argued that if occupational therapists are to be holistic, they must be alert and attentive to spirituality and spiritual occupations in all clients, including children. While *being* can be viewed as one aspect of spirituality, by advocating for children's needs to engage in *being* occupations, we are also acknowledging children as spiritual beings. Experiencing 'being' allows children to tap into their creativity, intuition, motivation and love (Kang, 2003). *Being* occupations are not necessarily passive, but rather involve a quiet activity of an inner kind.

The children with whom we work regularly experience occupational challenges. Many of these relate to problems with various aspects of *doing*, such as acquiring motor, academic or self-care skills. While there is no doubt that we need to focus many of our interventions on helping children *do*, there is a place for supporting and encouraging children to *be*, so that they can connect with their inner selves, their motivation, their sense of meaning and purpose. Many of our clients experience teasing, anxiety and poor self-esteem relating to their skill acquisition difficulties, disfigurement, the nature of their illness or disabling condition. Part of their journey towards self-acceptance and understanding of who they are requires an acceptance of their limitations, as well as *being* aware of their strengths, skills and talents. Occupational therapists and other childhood professionals have an important role in assisting children to discover, acknowledge and accept their strengths and challenges.

Teaching children relaxation and meditation techniques using visual imagery and narrative not only enables children to manage anxiety, but also helps them to experience solitude, connect with their inner *being* and experience calm. The ability to relax deeply is one life skill which all of us benefit from developing. Like all of us, children need opportunities to engage in their own spiritually meaningful activities, in order to provide them with a chance to achieve spiritual harmony or integration. Burgman & King (2005) highlighted that qualities such as resilience, playfulness, enthusiasm, engagement and forgiveness occur when spiritual qualities are expressed through the child themself. Connection with others provides additional support in times of emotional or spiritual need.

Palliative care and being

'Honour the sacred circle of life. Show children the connections between themselves and the world they are part of'. (Daleo, 1996, p. 56)

During terminal care the importance of addressing psychosocial and spiritual concerns, as well as physical symptoms, is recognized, particularly for adults (Mueller et al., 2001). The need for health professionals to acknowledge the impact of culture, spirituality and complementary therapies for children and their families (Kemper & Barnes, 2003) has been documented. For children who have terminal conditions such as muscular dystrophy and end stage cancers, focusing on *being* can be critically important for developing a sense of purpose. Helping to validate the art of simply *being* for these children is vital for their inner wellbeing. According to Burgman & King (2005) in order to assist children who are vulnerable or at risk due to overwhelming circumstances, occupational therapists need to 'assist them to identify and connect with their spiritual qualities, to engage the power of their spirit in the meaning making of their lives' (p. 158).

In the terminal phases of illness, children are usually stripped of their ability to *do*, and their reality often becomes that of *being* truly themselves. Health professionals and parents need to learn to *be* with children during these times, when their greatest ability is *being* their true, quintessential selves. During these times of silent *being*, unspoken communication and *knowing* emerge through connectedness, enabling transcendence described by Kang (2003) as a state of inner freedom and consciousness beyond ego, suffering, pain and action. While the concept of transcendence may sound esoteric to many, particularly in relation to children, it is important not to deny them opportunities and possibilities of striving for an inner peace, even within the context of illness and pain. Adults who spend time with children need to be comfortable with silence, the gift of their presence and the ability to engage with the child in prayer or other culturally relevant spiritual practices. Burgman & King (2005) concur, stating that adults working with these children need to consider and understand their own spirituality and personal values and the impact of these on their relationships with children.

Bailey (2002) reported that religious beliefs are deeply woven into the fabric of family life. In our research on children with disabilities and their families, we interviewed five siblings of a girl who died aged 12, from medical complications related to her severe disabilities. We found that after her death, four of the five siblings viewed their sister as their little angel watching down on them from heaven (Rodger & Tooth, 2004). All of the siblings reminisced about how they used to 'confide in her and tell her secrets' (p. 66). Her brother explained that she 'didn't answer back but she had the loudest presence in the house . . . everyone would come up to her and tell her their problems' (p. 66). By *being* herself, they viewed her as a confidante and as an important support for them as they were growing up. This also provided additional meaning to her life in that one of her roles was that of a listener. Personal, cultural and spiritual beliefs are widely recognized as helpful in coming to terms with disability and bereavement (Rosen, 1996; Siegel & Silverstein, 1994). Spiritual beliefs can provide some sense of meaning and purpose for families and for the presence of a family member with a disability (Siegel & Silverstein, 1994).

Howard & Howard (1997) described disability as affecting an individual's spirituality, sometimes preventing individuals from finding meaning because it separates individual's from their active, creative, reflective potential and prevents individuals from engaging in occupations that create meaning. The resultant unhappiness is related to a sense of loss of either actual or potential ability and the grieving which often accompanies that loss. They described the role of occupational therapists as empowering clients to engage in meaningful activity and connecting clients with their own sense of centredness through occupations grounded in their past and future. This engagement in occupations may be through *being* as much as by *doing* spiritually meaningful activities.

Occupational balance

'Encourage children to live in balance. Bring body, mind and emotions into harmony. Learn to adapt to change with flexibility and strength'. (Daleo, 1996, p. 132)

Christiansen (1997), Kang (2003), Polgar & Landry (2004) and Wilcock (1998), have all used the term *occupational balance*. Christiansen referred to the proper rhythm and change between various modes of *doing*, while Wilcock referred to a harmonious synthesis of *doing*, *being* and *becoming*. Kang proposed that regular engagement in spiritual occupations focused on non-doing or just *being*, enables a healthy sense of inner and occupational balance to emerge. This is counter to our competitive culture that presses people to do more, and to do more 'better and faster'. Polgar & Landry described the need for achieving a balance in occupational participation across the lifespan. The imbalances that they reported may be due to personal choice, external influences (peers, parents, teachers or people in authority), or a person's abilities. So what does occupational balance mean for children?

In the context of this chapter, it can refer to a need to find a balance between *doing* and *being* as the essential processes which enable *becoming*. It can also refer to finding a balance between childhood occupations in terms of productivity (schoolwork), play and leisure, self-care and self-maintenance, and rest and relaxation. In reality the latter refer more to *being*, while the former reflect *doing*. The other aspect to consider is that spiritual activities can provide opportunities for *doing* as well as *being* with the very nature of these being defined by the individual. The balance that is required for all individuals is that there is sufficient engagement in occupations that enhance *being* needs such as aesthetic appreciation and self-actualization. These occupations tend to be ones which epitomize *being* values such as beauty, effortlessness, goodness, playfulness, self-sufficiency, honesty, uniqueness and wholeness (Maslow, 1968). Our job, then, is to assist children to engage in their choice of occupations which encompass *being* as well as *doing* and to recognize children as *spiritual* beings who are on a journey of self-understanding and self-actualization, that involves constructing meaning in their lives.

Summary

Children learn by *doing* and participating in meaningful activities. It is this 'doing' and participating in daily activities that is crucial for normal child development as well as self-actualization. Through participation in the daily occupations of life, children build their occupational repertoire, develop personal independence, become productive and participate in play or leisure activities. Attaining skills enables children to engage in a broad range of occupational roles and in so doing *become* the student, the sports team member, or the friend. Children learn by both *doing* and *being*. By ensuring an appropriate balance of both, they are able to *become* who it is they wish to *become*.

References

Bailey, C. E. (2002). The effect of spiritual beliefs and practices on family functioning: a qualitative study. *Journal of Family Psychotherapy, 13*, 127–144.

Bandura, A. (1997). *Self-efficacy: the exercise of control*. New York: W. H. Freeman.

Baum, C. & Law, M. (1998). Community health: a responsibility, an opportunity, and a fit for occupational therapy. *American Journal of Occupational Therapy, 52*, 7–10.

Belcham, C. (2004). Spirituality in occupational therapy: theory in practice? *British Journal of Occupational Therapy, 67*, 39–46.

Bouffard, M. & Wall, A. E. (1990). A problem solving approach to movement skill acquisition: implications for special populations. In: C. Reid (Ed.), *Problems in movement control* (pp. 119–124). North Holland: Elsevier Science.

Burgman, I. & King, A. (2005). The presence of child spirituality: surviving in a marginalizing world. In: F. Kronenberg, S. Simo Algado & N. Pollard (Eds.), *Occupational therapy without borders: learning from the spirit of survivors* (pp. 157–170). Oxford: Churchill Livingstone.

Canadian Association of Occupational Therapists [CAOT] (1997). *Enabling occupation: an occupational therapy perspective.* Ottawa, Ont.: Canadian Association of Occupational Therapists.

Christiansen, C. H. (1997). Acknowledging a spiritual dimension of occupational therapy practice. *American Journal of Occupational Therapy, 51,* 169–172.

Christiansen, C. H. (1999). Defining lives: occupation as identity: an essay on competence, coherence and the creation of meaning. *American Journal of Occupational Therapy, 5,* 547–58.

Christiansen, C. H. (2004). Occupation and identity: 'becoming' who we are through what we do. In: E. Townsend & C. H. Christiansen (Eds.), *Introduction to occupation: the art and science of living: new multidisciplinary perspectives for understanding human occupation as a central feature of individual experience and social organization* (pp. 121–139). Upper Saddle River, NJ: Prentice Hall.

Clark, F. (1993). Occupation embedded in real life: interweaving occupational science and occupational therapy. *American Journal of Occupational Therapy, 47,* 1067–1078.

Csikszentmihalyi, M. (1990). *Flow: the Psychology of optimal experience.* New York: Harper and Row.

Csikszentmihalyi, M. (1993). Activity and happiness: toward a science of occupation. *Journal of Occupational Science 1,* 38–42.

Daleo, M. S. (1996). *Curriculum of love: cultivating the spiritual nature of children.* Charlottesville, VA: Grace Publishing and Communications.

Davis, J. A. & Polatajko, H. J. (2004). Occupational development. In: C. H. Christiansen & E. Townsend (Eds.), *An introduction to occupation: the art and science of living* (pp. 91–119). Upper Saddle River, NJ: Pearson Education.

Driever, M. J. (2002). Issues in clinical nursing research. Are evidence based practice and best practice the same? *Western Journal of Nursing Research, 24* (5), 591–597.

Egan, M. & DeLaat, M. D. (1994). Considering spirituality in occupational therapy practice. *Canadian Journal of Occupational Therapy, 61,* 95–101.

Egan, M. & Swederksy, J. (2003). Spirituality as experienced by occupational therapists in practice. *American Journal of Occupational Therapy, 57,* 525–533.

Elkind, D. (2001). *The hurried child: growing up too fast too soon* (3rd ed.). Reading, MA: Addison-Wesley.

Erikson, E. H. (1963). *Childhood and society.* New York: Norton.

Fidler, G. S. & Fidler, J. W. (1978). Doing and becoming: purposeful action and self-actualization. *American Journal of Occupational Therapy, 32,* 305–310.

Gentile, A. M. (1992). The nature of skill acquisition: therapeutic implications for children with movement disorders. *Medicine and Sport Science, 36,* 31–40.

Henderson, S. E. & Sugden, D. (1992). *The movement assessment battery for children.* London: Psychological Corporation.

Howard, B. S. & Howard, J. R. (1997). Occupation as spiritual activity. *American Journal of Occupational Therapy, 51,* 181–185.

Kang, C. (2003). A psychospiritual integration frame of reference for occupational therapy. Part 1: conceptual foundations. *Australian Occupational Therapy Journal*, *50*, 92–103.

Kemper, K. J. & Barnes, L. (2003). Considering culture, complementary medicine and spirituality in pediatrics. *Clinical Pediatrics*, *42*, 205–208.

Khalsa, D. S. (2003). The integration of health and spirituality: report on a groundbreaking conference. *Total Health*, *25*, 36–38.

Law, M. & Baum, C. (1998). Evidence-based practice. *Canadian Journal of Occupational Therapy*, *65*, 131–135.

Macnab, J. (2003). *Healthy development in childhood: the role of child factors, family factor, and parenting practices in the prediction of cognitive competence and behavioural dysfunction at schoolage*. Unpublished doctoral dissertation, University of Western Ontario, Western, Ontario, Canada.

Mandich, A., Polatajko, H. J., Macnab, J. J. & Miller, L. T. (2001). Treatment of children with developmental coordination disorder: what is the evidence? *Physical and Occupational Therapy in Pediatrics*, *20* (2/3), 51–68.

Mandich, A., Polatajko, H. & Rodger, S. (2003). Rites of passage: understanding participation of children with developmental coordination disorder. *Human Movement Science*, *22*, 583–595.

Mandich, A., Polatajko, H., Miller, L. & Baum, C. (2004). *The pediatric activity card sort*. Ottawa: Ont.: CAOT.

Maslow, A. (1968). *Towards a psychology of being* (2nd ed.). New York. D. Van Nostrand.

Merriam-Webster Online Dictionary (2005). Retrieved 8 March 2005 from http://www.m-w.com/

Mueller, P. S., Plevak, D. J. & Rummans, T. A. (2001). Religious involvement, spirituality, and medicine: implications for clinical practice. *Mayo Clinic Proceedings*, *76*, 1225–1235.

Piaget, J. (1972). *The psychology of the child*. New York: Basic Books.

Polatajko, H., Mandich, A. & Martini, R. (2000). Dynamic performance analysis: a framework for understanding occupational performance. *American Journal of Occupational Therapy*, *54* (1), 65–72.

Polatajko, H., Mandich, A., Miller, L. & Macnab, J. (2001). Cognitive orientation to daily occupational performance (CO-OP): Part II – the evidence. *Physical and Occupational Therapy in Pediatrics*, *20*, 83–106.

Polatajko, H. & Mandich, A. (2004). *Enabling occupation in children: the cognitive orientation to daily occupational performance approach*. Ottawa: Ont.: CAOT.

Polgar, J. M. & Landry, J. E. (2004). Occupations as a means for individual and group participation in life. In: E. Townsend & C. H. Christiansen (Eds.), *Introduction to occupation: the art and science of living: new multidisciplinary perspectives for understanding human occupation as a central feature of individual experience and social organization* (pp. 197–220). Upper Saddle River, NJ: Prentice Hall.

Reilly, M. (1960). Research potentiality of occupational therapy. *American Journal of Occupational Therapy*, *14*, 206–209.

Rebeiro, K. L. & Cook, J. V. (1999). Opportunity, not prescription: an exploratory study of the experience of occupational engagement. *Canadian Journal of Occupational Therapy*, *66*, 176–87.

Revie, G. & Larkin, D. (1993). Task-specific intervention with children reduces movement problems. *Adapted Physical Activity Quarterly*, *10*, 29–41.

Rodger, S. & Tooth, L. (2004). Adult siblings' perceptions of family life and loss: a pilot case study. *Journal of Developmental and Physical Disabilities*, 16 (1), 53–71.

Rogers, C. R. (1951). *Client centered counselling*. Boston, Mass.: Houghton-Mifflin.

Rosen, E. J. (1996). The family as healing resource. In: C. A. Corr & D. M. Corr (Eds.), *Handbook of childhood death and bereavement* (pp. 223–243). New York: Springer Publishing Company.

Segal, R., Mandich, A. & Polatajko, H. (2002). Stigma and its management: a framework for understanding social isolation of children with developmental coordination disorder. *American Journal of Occupational Therapy*, 56, 422–428.

Siegel, B. & Silverstein, S. (1994). *What about me? Growing up with a developmentally disabled sibling*. New York: Plenum Press.

Sigmundsson, H., Pedersen, A. V., Whiting, H. T. A. & Ingvaldsen, R. P. (1998). We can cure your child's clumsiness! A review of intervention methods. *Scandinavian Journal of Rehabilitation Medicine*, 30, 101–106.

Smith, J. & McSherry, W. (2004). Spirituality and child development: a concept analysis. *Journal of Advanced Nursing*, 45, 307–315.

Sumsion, T. (1999). The client centred approach. In: T. Sumsion (Ed.), *Client centred practice in occupational therapy* (pp. 15–20). Toronto, Ont.: Harcourt Brace.

Thelen, E., Kelso, J. A. & Fogel, A. (1987). Self-organizing systems and infant motor development. *Developmental Review*, 7, 39–65.

Thelen, E. (1995). Motor development: a new synthesis. *American Psychologist*, 50 (2), 79–95.

Turvey, M. T. (1990). Coordination. *American Psychologist*, 45, 938–953.

Virgin, R. & Mandich, A. (2001). *Participation of children with varying abilities*. Proceedings of evidence based practice conference, University of Western Ontario, (p. 10). London, Ontario.

Weinstock-Zlotnick, G. & Hinojosa, J. (2004). Bottom-up or top-down evaluation: is one better than the other? *American Journal of Occupational Therapy*, 58, 594–599.

Wilcock, A. A. (1998). Reflections on doing, being and becoming. *Canadian Journal of Occupational Therapy*, 65, 258–256.

Wilson, A. (1990). *Meditations for women who do too much*. New York: Harper Collins.

Wood, W. (1998). It is jump time for occupational therapy. *American Journal of Occupational Therapy*, 52, 403–411.

World Health Organization (WHO) (2001). *ICF: International classification of functioning, disability and health*. Geneva, Switzerland: World Health Organization.

Zilberbrandt, A. & Mandich, A. (2004). *I am what I do: understanding occupational engagement in children*. Conference proceedings, second Canadian occupational science symposium, (p. 23). Toronto, Canada.

Chapter 7

THE OCCUPATIONAL DEVELOPMENT OF CHILDREN[1]

Jane Davis and Helene Polatajko

Paediatric occupational therapists are keenly interested in human development. Their knowledge of development is fundamental to their practice. Guided by their understanding of normal growth and development they make determinations about the developmental status of a child, the need for and nature of intervention. Paediatric occupational therapists are interested in how a child's growth and development will support their mastery of the occupational world.

Human development has been the focus of study for over a century, leading to a rich and broad literature of the changes humans experience from conception to old age. The vast majority of this literature focuses on the ages and stages through which an individual progresses across the lifespan in specific domains, such as cognitive (Piaget, 1969) and psychosocial development (Erikson, 1950). This literature is essentially devoid of specific information on occupational development, leaving the therapist to infer its course. This is no easy task.

Occupational behaviour is complex. Whether it is discussed in terms of human occupation (Kielhofner, 2002), occupational competence (Polatajko, 1992), or occupational performance (Baum & Christiansen, 2005; Canadian Association of Occupational Therapists (CAOT), 1997), it is considered that the source of occupational behaviour is the interaction of three factors: person, occupation and environment. Since the developmental literature pertains to the person, it is relevant to occupational development; however, on its own it is insufficient.

Occupational development is not only influenced by the developmental status of the person, but also by the demands of the occupation in question and the relevant environmental supports and barriers. For example, when determining a child's readiness to ride a bicycle we must consider not only the physical stature of the child, the child's motor, cognitive and attentional skills, awareness of safety issues and eagerness to ride, but also the style and dimensions of the bike, the neighbourhood in which it will be ridden and parental expectations.

---

[1] Parts of this chapter have been adapted from J. A. Davis & H. J. Polatajko (2004). Occupational development. In: C. Christiansen & E. A. Townsend (Eds.). *Introduction to occupation: the art and science of living*. Upper Saddle River, NJ: Pearson Education. Reproduced with permission.

Occupational development results from the interaction of human beings with their environments. This interaction makes occupational development extremely complex. Therefore it is very difficult for the therapist to predict the course of occupational development from knowledge of person development alone.

The purpose of this chapter is to provide a model to guide therapists in enabling children's optimum occupational development. We will:

(1) Define occupational development
(2) Situate it among and distinguish it from other forms of human development
(3) Present the Interactional model of occupational development (IMOD)
(4) Describe the principles of interactionism and their implications for practice

Occupational development defined

From birth we begin to build our occupational selves. An individual's occupational repertoire is not static but changes throughout life. The progression of change, when characterized by a sequence of ages and stages across the lifespan, is referred to as development. Occupational development has been defined as 'the gradual change in occupational behaviours over time, resulting from the growth and maturation of the individual in interaction with the environment' (CAOT, 1997, p. 40). This definition can be understood in three ways.

First, the gradual change in occupational behaviours can be understood in terms of occupational competence – that is, the progression from novice to mastery, in the performance of given occupation/s. From this perspective occupational development is considered at the *level of the occupation*, with a beginning, a progression, and an endpoint; the expectation being that a child moves through this progression at a rate and in a sequence specific to the occupation. For instance, a child begins to walk by taking a first step, then another, and after a number of tumbles and more practice the child masters walking. Occupational development is an iterative process, with the progression from novice to mastery repeated again and again, with the addition of each new occupation.

Second, the gradual change can also be understood in terms of an individual's occupational repertoire – that is, the set of occupations an individual has at a specific point in the life course. From this perspective, occupational development is considered at the *level of the individual*, with changes having multiple patterns and no specific endpoint. Rather, occupational repertoires change continuously throughout the lifespan, sometimes expanding, sometimes shrinking. There is no a priori determination of the number or specifics of the occupations that constitute an individual's repertoire, either at a particular point in time or across the life course. However, it is anticipated that a repertoire will develop, and that the development is in keeping with the individual's growth and development, and will continue throughout the life course.

Third, gradual change in occupational behaviours can be understood in terms of humankind's occupational possibilities – that is, the set of occupations that exist at any given point in time or place across human evolution. From this perspective, occupational development is considered at *the level of the species* with change occurring constantly across evolution. As with development at the level of the individual, there is no a priori determination of the number or specifics of the occupations that the species will have at any given point in time or place. It is simply anticipated that there will be a continuous development of a large variety of occupations, and that the development is in keeping with the species' needs and possibilities.

Taking all three levels together, occupational development is defined as the systematic process of change in occupational behaviours across time, at the level of occupation, individual and species. At the level of the individual, occupational development is the systematic process of change whereby the individual comes to know the occupational world and becomes competent within it. This will be the primary focus of this chapter.

Occupational development: situated among and distinct from other forms of development

Development is generally described as the ages and stages through which an individual progresses across the lifespan in such domains as cognition, language, perceptual-motor skills and psychosocial behaviour. Historically, there have been four perspectives on how development occurs: preformationist, maturationist, environmentalist and interactionist. The oldest, the *preformationist* view, popular in the Middle Ages, held that children were miniature adults (Aries, 1962) born with all their lifetime characteristics, including body shape and personality, in place. This was moderated by the *maturationist* view which held that heredity dictated what a person was to become; that development was a matter of nature. In the 1700s, John Locke introduced the idea that the individual was born as a tabula rasa (empty slate) and that life experiences alone shaped development. The introduction of this environmentalist view, with its perspective that environment alone impacts development, heralded the nature/nurture debate, which raged for a significant portion of the twentieth century. These opposing views were brought together in the interactionist view, which holds that development occurs as a result of the interaction of nature and nurture.

Interactionism is built on the premise that there is a reciprocal interactive relationship between people and their environments that determines the course of development. Thus, the changes observed to occur across time, are the expression of '. . . progressive, mutual accommodation, throughout the lifespan, between a growing human organism and the changing immediate environments in which it lives . . .' (Bronfenbrenner, 1977, p. 514). The nature/nurture question is no longer concerned with determining which one drives development, rather with understanding how they interact to produce the developmental changes humans experience.

The evidence being accumulated, suggests that the interaction between the developing individual and the environment, between nature and nurture, is not simply additive (Plomin, 1994), but operates in complex ways. Interesting work is emerging, describing this interaction. For example, Macnab (2003) applied multi-stage generalized linear regression to data from the National longitudinal survey of children and youth of Canada. She found a variety of direct and indirect (mediated) effects, (for example neonatal status and family environment), each contributing directly and independently to school-age competence. She also found that positive parenting was a direct contributor to outcome while hostile/ineffective parenting mediated the association between preschool behaviour and school competence.

The nature of the interaction between nurture and nature, and their relative contribution to development, is domain specific. For example, heredity has a large (almost exclusive) role in eye colour, less in cognitive development and perhaps least in moral development. Further, there is a dynamic interaction between the domains themselves (Cole & Cole, 1996), with physical, cognitive, psychosocial and moral each affecting the other. This is particularly the case for occupational development.

At the level of the individual, the systematic change in occupational behaviour occurring over time results in the individual's active participation in the world, through occupation. From the *International classification of functioning, disability and health* (ICF) (WHO, 2001), it can be seen that the status of the individual is only one determinant; person factors interact with environmental factors in complex, multidirectional ways.

Micro-occupational development: developing occupational competence

The most frequently discussed level of occupational development is development of competence in a single occupation, or in the component skills that subtend occupational competence (for example mature grasp). The key focus of micro-occupational development is on how domain specific development establishes the capacity for occupational performance. Much of the developmental literature describes the occupations that can be expected at various ages and stages and the skills required for their performance. Frequently, the behaviours noted for each age and stage are occupational in nature. The infant explores objects in many different ways, mouthing, banging, dropping and throwing. The toddler develops independence in self-care tasks such as self-feeding and hand washing. The preschooler rides a tricycle.

There have been some attempts made to theorize the development of occupational competence in children. Case-Smith (2005) created a model of the development of child occupations, which is conceptualized as the interaction among individual abilities, occupations and environments. She used this model as an outline to discuss the qualitative changes in the play occupations of children during infancy, early and middle childhood. She discussed the child's development in the cognitive, psychosocial and sensorimotor domains, and how these interact with the play environment, describing children's developing occupational competence in play (see Table 7.1).

Humphry (2002) drew on dynamic systems theory to create a model of developmental processes, which explicates the interaction between person and environment

Table 7.1 Development of play occupations: 0 to 10 years.

Age/stage	Developing competence in and through play
Infancy/toddlers	
0 to 6 months	*Exploratory play* – grasps, mouths and examines objects *Social play* – smiles and coos
6 to 12 months	*Functional play* – rolls a ball; pushes a car in a track *Social play* – imitates simple gestures
12 to 18 months	*Functional play* – pretends to eat; stacks blocks, scribbles with a crayon *Gross motor play* – explores all spaces in room *Social play* – begins peer interaction
18 to 24 months	*Functional play* – strings beads; turns pages of a book; draws circles with crayon *Pretend/symbolic play* – feeds baby doll; uses play hammer *Gross motor play* – sits on and pushes ride-on toys; climbs on jungle gyms *Social play* – participates in groups of children
Early childhood	
24 to 36 months	*Symbolic play* – bathes doll then dresses it in pyjamas and puts it to bed *Constructive play* – builds puzzles; colours in pictures *Gross motor play* – jumps; rough and tumble play; rides tricycle *Social play* – takes turns; plays with peers
3 to 4 years	*Complex imaginary play* – acts out roles and uses abstract objects in scripted play *Constructive play* – cuts out simple shapes; draws a face *Rough and tumble play* – does playground activities; runs *Social play* – participates in circle time, games, art time with peers
4 to 5 years	*Games with rules* – participates in simple games, such as, 'duck, duck, goose' *Constructive play* – builds complex block structures; builds ten-piece puzzle *Social play/dramatic play* – plays 'dress up' with peers; tells stories
5 to 6 years	*Games with rules* – plays board and computer games *Dramatic play* – role plays real world stories *Sports* – participates in ball play *Social play* – plays games with friends; enjoys singing and dancing
Middle childhood	
6 to 10 years	*Games with rules* – plays computer and card games that require abstract thinking *Crafts and hobbies* – has hobbies such as drawing; collects stamps, coins, dolls *Organized sports* – competes in sports, such as soccer/football, basketball, hockey *Social play* – talks and jokes with friends; belongs to clubs, such as choir, scouts and guides

Based on information found in Case-Smith (2005).

in developing occupational competence. She identified four fundamental aspects of occupational development:

(1) Intentional actions
(2) Mechanisms for generating occupational behaviours
(3) Socio-cultural niche – children are more inclined to imitate culturally relevant occupations
(4) Engagement in occupation as conditions for developmental changes

Edwards & Christiansen (2005) discussed occupation as both a product of development and a facilitator of the process of development. Growth, maturation and learning are three key factors in development. Occupation and the domains of development act in a reciprocal, interactive manner to further changes in the individual across the lifespan. Occupational behaviour shapes development and vice versa. They identified theorists whose work can inform our understanding of occupational behaviour changes across the lifespan: Freud, Piaget, Kohlberg, Havighurst, Erikson, Levinson, Watson, Bandura and Baltes. The work of each theorist is proposed to contribute to our understanding of micro-level occupational development. However, these theories tend to overemphasize the association between intrinsic changes of the individual and the development of new behaviours, and therefore are inadequate to explain fully the complexities of occupational development at the other levels, that is, meso- and macro-levels.

Meso-occupational development: developing an occupational life course

The constellation of occupations an individual accumulates across the lifespan, their life course occupational repertoire, represents the meso-level. Marked by the changes in the specific occupations that an individual can and does perform over the course of life, meso-occupational development is governed by the principles underlying the occupational trajectories and transitions that occur across the life course, and the process whereby these occur. Davis & Polatajko (2004) combined knowledge from sociology, human geography, anthropology and psychology to create an interactionist perspective on occupational development.

The interactional model of occupational development (IMOD)

The IMOD describes the nature of the change across the life course, whereby the individual comes to know and become competent in the occupational world. The IMOD holds that the systematic change in occupational behaviours, across time, is the outcome of the interactions of persons with their occupations in the context of their environments. The IMOD is based on the premise that since interactionism underlies both individual development and occupational behaviour, it is a key

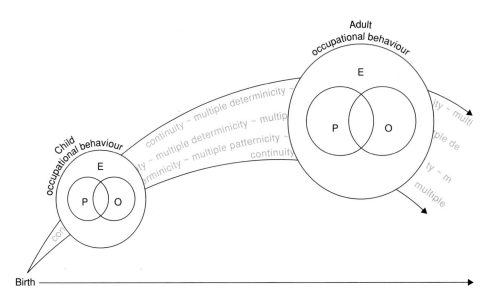

Figure 7.1 Interactional model of occupational development.

mechanism of occupational development. The three variables of interactional occupational development are:

(1) Occupational behaviour is defined as the interaction of the person and occupation in the context of the environment
(2) Time, referring to the lifespan of an individual, many of which comprise the span of human evolution
(3) Interaction between occupational behaviour and time (see Figure 7.1)

The first is depicted as three circles composed of two intersecting circles, representing person and occupation, inside a third circle, which represents the environmental context. Growth and development are represented by the expanding arc in which the principles of interactionism appear as a backdrop. The occupational behaviour circles are shown at points in time, the one on the right larger than the one on the left, indicating growth and development, over time. The meter for time in the figure is the individual life course, the meso-level of occupational development.

Evidence for the IMOD has existed for some time. The story from the 1790s of Victor, in *The Wild Boy of Aveyron* (Itard, 1962), depicts the pervasive negative effect on all aspects of development from being raised apart from civilization. The more recent story of Genie, a young girl who was confined to a crib for most of her 13 years (Curtiss, 1977), shows a similar negative developmental effect from severe prolonged deprivation. The stories from Romanian orphanages have demonstrated that less severe deprivation of shorter duration also has detrimental effects on development. However, these experiences also demonstrate that the effects are influenced by the duration of the deprivation and can be reversed through exposure to richer occupational environments (Rutter et al., 1998). These observations provide supporting evidence for the interactional nature of occupational development. Further, they suggest that classic stage theory alone, is not sufficient to account for occupational development.

The principles of interactionism[2]

Many domains of human development are governed by classical stage theory. This makes it possible not only to describe an individual's stage of development, but also to predict what will come next. For example, Piaget's stages of cognitive development can be used to describe the level of development of a particular individual, describe it as normal, advanced, or delayed and even predict what is likely to happen next. Because occupational development is the result not only of the growth and development of the person but also of their occupations and environments, it is not governed by stage theory alone.

Stage theory applies to occupational development only to the extent that it governs the development of the person; it does not govern the development of the person's occupation or environment. Consequently, stage theory is of considerable value when considering the development of occupational competence, at least in children, but is of much less value when considering the development of an individual's occupational repertoire and of even less value when considering the development of the species' occupations across evolution. Drawing from lifespan development (Baltes, 1987; 1997; Baltes et al., 1999), life course (Elder, 1998; 1999) and ageing literature (Atchley, 1999), three principles have applicability to the interactional development of human occupation: staged continuity, multiple determinicity and multiple patternicity.

Staged continuity

Staged continuity, originally referred to as continuity by Davis & Polatajko (2004), holds that the development of a life course occupational repertoire is a continuous process of accumulation of occupational behaviours commencing at birth. It is influenced by the ages and stages of human development, but no specific age or stage is dominant. It is based on continuity theory (Atchley, 1999), which asserts that development does not end in childhood; rather, adults continue to adapt to changes in themselves and their life situations throughout the lifespan. Staged continuity combines the concepts of classic stage and continuity theory, acknowledging the influence of development on the interaction among person, occupation and environment.

The changes in occupational behaviour across the lifespan are influenced by developmental changes. Thus, it can be expected that the infant will lie on their back

---

[2] Parts of this section are taken and/or adapted from Davis & Polatajko, 2004, pp. 97–109.

mouthing objects; the toddler will cruise around furniture, refining gross motor skills; and the preschooler will play with crayons, honing fine motor skills. Nevertheless, generalities aside, environmental influences, occupational exposure and unusual aptitudes can result in occupational behaviours that are beyond the expectations of the age and stage of the individual.

Multiple determinicity

Multiple determinicity holds that many factors play a role in occupational development. Expanding on this principle of multiple determinicity, as initially proposed by Davis & Polatajko (2004), the IMOD is comprised of four key determinants of occupational development: person, occupation, environment and interaction.

Determinant: person

There are three person determinants for occupational development: genes/ heredity, learning/plasticity and active participation/motivation. Many of an individual's innate abilities and their temperament are *genetically predetermined* (Saudino & Eaton, 1991). Scarr & McCartney (1983) suggested that genes influence an individual's development in two ways: through their expression as phenotypes and through their direct influence on individual environmental choice. Thus, an infant's genetic make-up may be expressed through certain occupational abilities and interests, and through temperament that influences occupational, developmental, environmental interactions.

Scientists have recently mapped the human genome and have begun to determine the role of over 30 000 genes in the unfolding of human life (International Humane Genome Sequencing Consortium, 2001). For example, the work on Williams syndrome, a rare genetic condition, demonstrates the variable influence of genetics on occupational development. While individuals with Williams syndrome cannot tie their shoes, write their name, or perform simple addition, they are avid readers and have extraordinary music abilities. These individuals demonstrate a great love of music, a wider range of emotional responses to music than typically noted, a higher incidence of perfect pitch and strong musical rhythm (Don et al., 1999; Lenhoff et al., 2001; Williams Syndrome Foundation, 2004).

Child prodigies also demonstrate exceptionally mature abilities in the performance of specific occupations at a young age (typically before the age of ten). Both innate mental and physical capacities, and temperament and personality factors, such as persistence, passion and commitment, influence their occupational development. Often seen as precocious, child prodigies are most commonly found to have superior abilities in music (such as playing the violin or piano, and singing), chess and visual arts (Feldman & Goldsmith, 1986). As Plomin (1994) pointed out, although genes influence development, they cannot do it alone. Without the influence of learning, active participation, an enabling environment and occupational exposure, an individual will not develop these skills.

Learning governs how genes are expressed through interaction with the environment, and regulates the course of development (Conger & Galambos, 1997).

It 'is the process by which behaviour or the potential for behaviour is modified as a result of experience' (Conger & Galambos, 1997, p. 31). The ability to learn is a function of *neural plasticity*, a term referring to the ability of the central nervous system to adapt structurally or functionally in response to environmental demands (Jacobs, 1999). The degree of change that the central nervous system can undergo is age dependent. Learning occurs more readily in early life when plasticity is greatest (Leakey & Lewin, 1992).

Individuals must learn how to do any occupations that they choose to perform in their life. Over the lifespan, as human abilities develop, they learn to feed themselves, protect themselves from the elements, navigate their environments, express their individuality and be creative. Children learn to bring together their developing capacities to reach a desired occupational outcome (Humphry, 2002). Cultural systems and social structures are created for the transfer of occupational information and possibilities from adults to children (Newman & Newman, 1997), to allow for development of occupational behaviours that *fit* with societal expectations. Thus, the developing capacities of the child, guided by adults, are brought together within the performance of new culturally relevant occupations (Humphry, 2002). This occupational performance leads to the development of further physical, cognitive and affective capacities, which are subsequently used by the child to perform current occupations with increased competence, as well as to develop new occupations (Edwards & Christiansen, 2005; Humphry, 2002). Since each child is born with different capacities, the development of competence in each occupation will be unique. The ease of learning signifies the 'fit' among the child's innate and developing capacities, the child's environments, and the occupations being learned. These occupations will form the basis for their occupational repertoire.

Individuals are *active participants* in their own development, shaping and directing their life course occupational repertoire from birth. Active children, with their innate and unique predispositions, affect the environments in which they interact, thus acting as an agent in their own development by selecting the pathways they wish to follow (Elder, 1998).

Since occupation is doing, it follows that occupational development demands *active participation* of the individual. Across the life span, individuals act on their environment and are active in other's environments (Rutter et al., 1997). In the absence of opportunity for active participation or human agency, occupational development is stunted or becomes abnormal. Unfortunately, there are many true life examples of this situation, such as the children in the Romanian orphanages. The effects of these depriving environments result in decreased ability of children to actively participate in constructing their life course occupational repertoire. Active participation remains essential throughout life, even in the later stages of life, where it has been shown that engagement in occupation can help maintain capacities and slow deterioration (Schaie, 1994).

An important factor in active participation is *motivation*. An individual's motivation toward initiating a behaviour, which refers to an individual's 'needs, goals and desires that provoke them to action' (Conger & Galambos, 1997, p. 35), also impacts development, by influencing acquisition of additional behaviours.

Without a motive or motivation to act, stagnation could occur in certain areas of individual development, affecting health and wellbeing. Active occupational participation is influenced by the individual's motivation to engage in that occupation, and leads to the development of occupational competence and the development of an occupational repertoire. The stronger the motivation an individual has for an occupation, the more likely it is that they will engage in the occupation and acquire the necessary competencies for the occupation to develop. From early on, very young children show motivation to engage in occupation, beyond simple imitation. Although it is difficult to know what is motivating the very young child to do, each appears to strive for an individual occupational outcome (Humphry, 2002). This desired outcome motivates them to learn to perform an activity by gaining an understanding of the intent of the occupation. Children often construct new ways of reaching their intended outcome, demonstrating their active participation in their occupational development.

Although it is commonly believed that children are primarily motivated to do *fun* things, studies have shown many other motivators for children's active occupational participation. In her analysis of historical literary works, Davis (2000) found 12 themes of motivating factors leading children to participate in occupations such as wanting to know everything about everything, trying to outdo one another, sense of accomplishment, pleasing and assisting one another and wanting to be a grown-up. Many of these themes were supported in a study by Wiseman et al. (2005), which examined the factors that influenced why children do (or stop doing) the occupations they do. They interviewed eight children and their parents and uncovered numerous motivating factors for the children: feels good, positive reinforcement, being good at *it*, curiosity, desire to teach or help others, feeling of responsibility and competition.

Determinant: occupation

Largely, what makes humans distinct from other species are the things we do. Historically, occupations were focused on immediate survival needs (Wilcock, 1998). However, as occupations evolved, their purposes expanded to encompass other human needs (for example creativity, socialization, relaxation and accumulation of material goods). New occupations are constantly being formed, due to technological advances and cultural and societal demands, expanding humankind's occupational possibilities.

Two factors which influence a child's uptake of occupational possibilities are *occupational exposure* and *occupational expectations*. As children grow, they are exposed to occupations by the people around them (see Figure 7.2). Children see what others do and this may provide them with the motivation to develop those occupations. This motivation occurs when there is a fit among the child's abilities, their environment and the occupation. In some instances, children appear to have an innate drive to do certain things regardless of exposure (Wiseman et al., 2005); however, for the most part, children are not likely to develop occupations unless they are exposed to them. Although children might be exposed to many different occupations, society's occupational expectations limit their ability to participate in

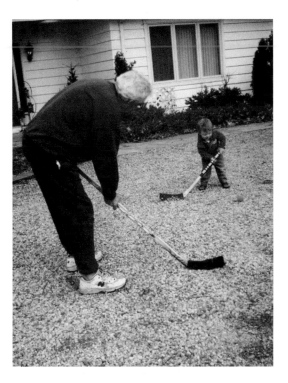

Figure 7.2 Grandfather and grandson playing road hockey.

all of them. Occupational expectations are constructed by a society or culture and pertain to who should be engaging in what occupations at what age, and which occupations are culturally and socially sanctioned. These three interrelated occupational determinants, (for example possibilities, exposure and expectations), play a central role in the development of the child's occupational repertoire.

Determinant: environment

Enabling and depriving environments have a considerable influence on the occupational development of individuals. These environments include: physical, social, cultural and historical aspects.

All humans live in *physical and social environmental contexts* and interact with these contexts through their participation in occupations across the lifespan. Individuals gain knowledge and develop their occupational competencies and repertoires within these environments. From birth, the size of the individual's world increases. When infants are born their physical and social environments are understood by what they can see, hear, taste, smell and touch, in their immediate vicinity. Although many environments influence their care, an infant's interaction with their environment is restricted to the immediate context. Toddlers begin to explore space with their newly developed mobility, developing new occupations, such as climbing and running. In middle childhood, as independence increases, children begin to use newly developed occupations, such as biking, to move into their neighbourhoods and communities, but still stay close to home. Once they enter high school, children spend increasingly more time away from home, at increasingly greater distances. They begin participating with peers in clubs and after school sports and games.

The natural and built physical environments enable individuals to do what they need, want, or are expected to do. *Social environments* provide individuals with support, norms, education and resources that enable performance. Infants are born with limited capacity to survive; they are dependent on care-givers to enable their required occupations of eating, sleeping, dressing, bathing and playing. As young children learn, they no longer require the same level of physical support to engage in their occupations, although emotional support remains crucial. By middle childhood, the physical support required by children for occupational participation shifts to, for example, being driven to community events and lacing up ice skates. Emotional support remains a crucial aspect of the social environment throughout the lifespan, and deprived environments can have substantial influences on occupational development. Morison et al. (1995), studying children in an orphanage, found that a child's exposure to toys and attention from care-givers help to mediate the negative effects of the depriving environment. Once children are removed from deprived environments they are able to develop a certain level of occupation competence and establish an occupational repertoire (Rutter et al., 1998). This evidence suggests that the environment interacts with the maturational stage of the child in determining occupational development.

The physical and social environments in which humans live are constructed by their *historical and cultural contexts*. Pioneers such as Margaret Mead and Vygotsky have made us aware of the importance of society and culture on development (Damon, 1989; Harkness, 1992; Vygotsky, 1978). Two studies examining the influence of culture on children's occupational participation found that Mayan and Ugandan children's occupations were different from North American children's occupations (Bazyk et al., 2003; Gaskins, 1999; Sedgwick et al., 2003). Sedgwick and colleagues provide an example of the influences of cultural environments on occupational development in childhood. They found that children in Uganda performed different occupations from those children in North America, at different ages and in different ways. At very young ages, Ugandan children helped with chores around the home, including selling vegetables, sweeping, collecting water and caring for younger siblings. Children played with toys made from old containers and tyres that had been discarded. Bazyk and colleagues found that Mayan culture had very different values and expectations associated with play from those of North American culture, demonstrating how culture influences the development of these occupations.

Historical trends and circumstances shape culture and impact on the individual's development of values, beliefs, preferences, lifestyles and skills. 'Cultures define what is desirable to be learned, what is to be believed, and how to behave' (Scarr, 1993, p. 1335); in other words, cultures shape human occupation. The extent to which history influences human development was recognized by Bronfenbrenner (1994) when he added the chronosystem to his general ecological model, which 'encompasses change or consistency over time not only in the characteristics of the person but also of the environment' (Bronfenbrenner, 1994, p. 1646). By examining children's occupations over a 340-year period using literary works, Davis et al. (2002) provided evidence that the dominant socio-cultural discourse of different historical periods influenced what children did.

Determinant: interaction

Considering interaction as a determinant brings into focus that the interaction of person, occupation and environment is, in itself, a determinant of development. The person and environment 'inter-penetrate one another in such a complex manner that any attempt to unravel them tends to destroy the natural unity of the whole and to create an artificial distinction between organism and environment' (Hall & Lindzey, 1970, p. 316). The person and environment come together through the performance of occupation. This determinant is considered so important in the occupational developmental process that it names the perspective, as a whole.

Discussing the interaction between person and environments, Scarr & McCartney (1983) hypothesized that 'people make their own environments' based on their genetic make-up. Scarr & Ricciuti (1991) proposed the notion of 'a good enough environment' (p. 19), which they feel is the *typical* environment available to most children in most cultures. It is proposed that the typical environments in which most children are raised contain many variables that provide the basics for 'normal' human development, and therefore, normal development takes place. According to Scarr & Ricciuti, the 'good enough environment' provides individuals with environments from which they can choose experiences that *match* their genetic make-up. However, they noted that this theory requires that the environment be varied and allow opportunities that match the individual's genotype.

Scarr & McCartney (1983) suggested that if the genotype and environment do not match, the effects of either could be greatly diminished. For example, a child prodigy who has innate talent for drawing will never fully develop occupational competence in drawing unless they are exposed to a rich and supportive artistic environment, including expert instruction, emotional support, strict personal discipline and a commitment to occupational competence development (Feldman & Goldsmith, 1986). This would suggest the need for a goodness of fit between the individual's genotype and the environment, and demonstrates the importance of individuals being exposed to and engaging in diverse occupations. Wiseman et al. (2005) found that occupational exposure was one of two initial steps in establishing occupations.

Without occupational exposure, many children and adults will never realize their innate talents unless the individual uncovers them on their own. This is akin to the concept of a 'just right challenge', where it is proposed that the environment and occupation must present the appropriate challenge to be engaging (Yerxa et al., 1989), to allow *flow*, or enjoyment (Csikszentmihalyi, 1975). Extrapolating this concept into the realm of development, it would seem likely that there needs to be a 'just right environment' that matches the individual's genotype, to allow for, and to support and enable the development of each individual's optimal occupational competence and life course occupational repertoire.

Multiple patternicity[3]

Multiple patternicity holds that an individual's occupational life course is marked by periods of both growth and decline, expansion and contraction, with occupations emerging at various points throughout the individual's life, involving different skills and developing at different rates. Two patterns mark the development of an occupational repertoire: multiple variations and changing mastery.

Multiple variations

The multiple variations pattern holds that growth and development is neither smooth nor unidirectional, involving both decline and growth. Different aspects of development show different patterns at different times. Adapted from the principles of *multidirectionality* and *trajectories and transitions* found in the literature on adult development and ageing, the principle of multiple variations describes the pattern of gains and losses, and the variations in rate, characteristics, quality, quantity, complexity and specialization involved in life course occupational development.

The occupational life course is seen as following a trajectory modified by various transitions. Trajectories are continuations of development, while transitions are periods of change or disruption in the trajectory. There are numerous potential times for transition in the course of a life. Some are related to the developmental milestones that mark the ages and stages of the domains that are foundational for occupational behaviours (for example cognitive, affective and physical). Others relate to life events, such as getting that first tricycle, starting kindergarten, going on a first trip away from home, graduating, getting a first job, having a baby, losing a loved one and retiring. Thus, it is difficult to characterize the pattern of occupational life course development, a priori.

Muir (1999) suggested four developmental patterns: *continuous*, gradually increasing with age (for example height, weight); *step*, increasing in a stop and start manner (for example mobility, cognition); *inverted U-shape*, first increasing, then reaching a plateau, and then decreasing (for example visual acuity, coordination); and *U-shaped*, first decreasing, then being absent, and then increasing. Using in-depth interviews to examine the occupations that children do, Wiseman et al. (2005) found that the pattern of occupational engagement varied widely among children. In some cases children as young as six years of age had abandoned occupations that other older children were still continuing. Also, some children had continued with such occupations as drawing and painting pictures since toddlerhood. Thus, none of the patterns described by Muir completely characterize the occupational life course. Hence, the occupational life course is described as having multiple variations.

Changing mastery

Changing mastery holds that an individual's proficiency in occupational performance changes over time. The concept of mastery refers to the change in levels of

---

[3] This section is taken from Davis & Polatajko, 2004 pp. 105–109, with modifications.

proficiency in skill performance, as a result of maturation and experience. People are thought to have a natural drive for mastery, which 'requires an individual to integrate his behaviour and develop skill in performing certain tasks' (Osipow, 1968, p. 92). Mastery is not static, rather proficiency changes across the lifespan, sometimes increasing, sometimes decreasing.

The development of mastery begins in infancy, when behaviours are very global in their intent. For example, infants use crying as a general form of communicating discomfort, hunger, tiredness or boredom. With time and experience and as the child gains control of primitive reflexes and develops voluntary movement patterns, these behaviours become more specialized and distinct in nature. The skills that are first developed in infancy, appear to be *virtually released* through interaction with the environment and are quickly and easily mastered (Bruner, 1973), while mastery of learned skills is dependent on the development of these *pre-wired* skills, and proceeds at a much slower rate. Increasingly, skills are performed to meet specific goals, showing greater intent. For example, as children develop language and other communication skills, their crying becomes more specialized in its form, intention and usefulness.

Along with the notion of specialization, behaviours also become more complex. The discrete features of children's behaviours increase in quantity, and become more refined and skilled, behaviour becomes more proficient. The increased quality is due, in part, to the increased integration of the cognitive, affective and physical components of occupational behaviour. As children develop, these components show greater interplay. This can be seen in children's increasing sophistication in toy use (for example banging blocks on a table top compared to constructing a fort of blocks). Each phase of development across the lifespan sees the emergence and disappearance of mastery of a variety of occupational skills. When an individual masters a skill they achieve control or power over a task or situation (Osipow, 1968).

At birth, babies are totally dependent on care-givers for basic necessities. Through interactions with their developing child, care-givers provide opportunities for learning and adaptation. In infancy, primitive reflexes are reorganized into simple voluntary movement patterns. Preschool children are focused on mastering foundational skills required for occupational competency in their elementary school years. Throughout adolescence, the number of occupations over which mastery is achieved increases, as does the quality and complexity of the occupations.

Macro-occupational development: the evolution of human occupations

Humans have always engaged in occupations. These have changed in concert with the evolving human and the evolving world. Consequently, there is a vast array of occupations that humans have engaged in at various points in history; some persist today, while many have changed. The development of these occupations across the course of human history is referred to as macro-occupational development. The occupations of humans across evolution have been of considerable interest to scholars, particularly anthropologists, and there are countless descriptions of macro-occupational development available, albeit not under that rubric. Nonetheless, the study of the evolution of the human species has been tied to occupation, so much so that evolutionary eras have been named in terms of the key occupations of the time such as hunters/gatherers, agrarians. Thus, there is a wealth of information available on the development of occupation at the species level.

An interest in the macro-level of occupational development emerged with the advent of occupational science. One of the key proponents of understanding human occupation across time was Wilcock (1998), who published a comprehensive study of human history from an occupational perspective. Wilcock described occupational changes that occurred at each evolutionary age (see Table 7.2). She showed that human biological and occupational evolution have a reciprocal relationship, which is influenced by environmental context. The evolution of

Table 7.2 The evolution of human occupations.

Evolutionary age	Human occupations

Hunters/gatherers	• Humans hunt, gather and scavenge for food.
	  — simple stone tools developed to help with survival
	  — sharing or social interaction does not occur
	• As groups get larger food sharing develops and occupations are divided among group members.

Agriculture	• Shift from hunting/gathering to farming occupations.
	• Farmers begin to plant own food, remain in one place with larger groups of people.
	• Both women's and men's occupations change to accommodate farming.
	• Possible reasons for this shift:
	  — climatic changes that produced physical environments conducive to agriculture
	  — increases in population requiring different means of sustainability
	  — development of occupational capacity or competence, which led to increases in skills, development of new occupations

Industrialization town and city workers	• Producing goods for others' consumption. • Occupations are still about survival needs. However, many individuals receive remuneration for their work and services. • Paid work is valued. • More social occupations emerge as groups became larger. • Occupational specialization occurs, whereby the individual does small parts of a larger occupation, repetitively.
Post-industrialization	• Work becomes primarily something you do so that you can earn money to buy food and material things. • Occupations change from those of production to service. • Technological development begins to drive occupational development instead of human nature and needs.

Based on information found in Wilcock (1998).

human occupation has matched the evolution of human biological capacities and they, in turn, have provided humans with the capability to create further occupational possibilities and construct the necessary tools and materials to enact those occupations.

Davis et al. (2002) added to this literature with their study of literary works written between 1650 and 1990. They found evidence of both change and continuation. Over this 340-year period some childhood occupations, such as coal collecting, essentially disappeared. New occupations emerged, such as playing computer games and some remained throughout, such as playing with balls or dolls. Most significantly, the change in occupations over time was influenced by dominant socio-cultural beliefs and values. Similarly, Bing (2005), describing the evolution of occupations as they relate to historical beliefs, argued that numerous variables contribute to macro-level occupational development. He stated that historical beliefs alone have not determined occupational behaviour; technological advances have also altered the amount of time spent in work and leisure occupations.

Implications for practice

Staged continuity implies that children have a continuous, innate tendency towards doing or being occupied. Specific occupations will change across the life-span, in concert with their age and stage of development. However, other factors, namely previous occupations, may also influence a child's occupational repertoire. The occupational behaviour of a child who is not occupied or not occupied with occupations that are consistent with their age or developmental stage may indicate a problem. However, the principle of multiple determinicity, would suggest that more than the developmental status of the child needs to be investigated.

The principles of multiple determinicity and patternicity show that the occupational behaviour of an individual cannot be predicted from age and stage alone. Thus, a child's occupational repertoire cannot be inferred from knowledge of the child's age and stage of development alone. Nor can it be inferred that a child beyond a particular age will no longer acquire occupations that are typical of that age or stage. To carry out a comprehensive evaluation of the occupational developmental status of a child, the therapist goes beyond assessing the child's developmental level in the components of occupational behaviour (for example cognitive, affective and physical). The therapist also determines the particular occupations the child can do, did in the past, does now, and wants to, needs to or is expected to do, using such tools as the Canadian Occupational Performance Measure (Law et al., 1998). The therapist also determines the child's occupational opportunities and the barriers and supports present in the child's environment. Based on stage theory, when a therapist finds that a child has an occupational competence that is incongruent with their developmental status, the therapist may consider that the child has developed a splinter skill. If working from a sensory integrative therapy framework, the child may be taken back to earlier stages of development in therapy (Ayres, 1972). Within the context of multiple determinicity and patternicity, splinter skills are better understood as evidence of the influence of interaction-ism on occupational development. Thus, when attempting to promote a child's occupational development a therapist using these principles would consider a number of strategies that could be used to improve a child's occupational competence, including performance based treatments, such as, the cognitive orientation to daily occupational performance approach (Polatajko & Mandich, 2004), or environmental adaptations or modifications (Letts et al., 2003).

Summary

Paediatric occupational therapists are keenly interested in human development, not for its own sake but for its role in supporting mastery of occupations across the life course. Occupational development is defined as the systematic process of change in occupational behaviours across time, at the level of the occupation, the individual and the species. Occupational development is not only influenced by the developmental status of the person, but also by the occupations and environments with which they interact. The Interactional Model of Occupational Development (IMOD) describes the nature of this interaction. It is based on the premise that interactionism is a key mechanism of occupational development, underlying both individual development and occupational behaviour. The principles that govern occupational development are staged continuity, multiple determinicity and multiple patternicity. Each of these helps to explain and predict the course of occupational development and has implications for practice.

References

Atchley, R. C. (1999). *Continuity and adaptation in ageing: creating positive experiences.* Baltimore, MD: The Johns Hopkins University Press.

Aries, P. (1962). *Centuries of childhood: a social history of family life* (R. Baldick, Trans.). New York, NY: Alfred Knopf.

Ayres, J. (1972). *Sensory integration and learning disorders.* Los Angeles, CA: Western Psychological Services.

Baltes, P. B. (1987). Theoretical propositions of lifespan developmental psychology: on the dynamics between growth and decline. *Developmental Psychology, 23* (5), 611–626.

Baltes, P. B. (1997). On the incomplete architecture of human ontogeny: selection, optimization and compensation as foundation of developmental theory. *American Psychologist, 52* (4), 366–380.

Baltes, P. B., Staudinger, U. M. & Lindenberger, U. (1999). Lifespan psychology: theory and application to intellectual functioning. *Annual Review of Psychology, 50,* 471–507.

Baum, C. M. & Christiansen, C. H. (2005). Person–environment–occupation performance: an occupation based framework for practice. In: C. H. Christiansen, C. M. Baum & J. Bass-Haugen (Eds.), *Occupational therapy: performance, participation, and wellbeing* (3rd ed., pp. 243–266). Thorofare, NJ: Slack Inc.

Bazyk, S., Stalnaker, D., Llerena, M., Ekelman, B. & Bazyk, J. (2003). Play in Mayan children. *American Journal of Occupational Therapy*, 57 (3), 273–283.

Bing, R. (2005). The evolution of occupation. In: C. H. Christiansen, C. M. Baum & J. Bass-Haugen (Eds.), *Occupational therapy: performance, participation, and wellbeing* (pp. 24–40). Thorofare, NJ: Slack Inc.

Bronfenbrenner, U. (1977). Toward an experimental ecology of human development. *American Psychologist*, 32, 513–531.

Bronfenbrenner, U. (1994). Ecological models of human development. In: T. Husen & T. N. Postlethwaite (Eds.), *The international encyclopedia of education* (2nd ed., pp. 1643–1647). New York, NY: Elsevier Science Inc.

Bruner, J. S. (1973). Organization of early skilled action. *Child Development*, 44, 1–11.

Canadian Association of Occupational Therapists (CAOT) (1997). *Enabling occupation: an occupational therapy perspective*. Ottawa, Ont.: CAOT Publications ACE.

Case-Smith, J. (2005). Development of childhood occupations. In: J. Case-Smith (Ed.), *Occupational therapy for children* (5th ed., chap. 4). St. Louis, MO: Mosby, Inc.

Cole, M. & Cole, S. R. (1996). *The development of children* (3rd ed.). New York, NY: W. H. Freeman and Company.

Conger, J. J. & Galambos, N. L. (1997). *Adolescence and youth: psychological development in a changing world* (5th ed.). Don Mills, Ont.: Addison-Wesley Educational Publishers Inc.

Csikszentmihalyi, M. (1975). *Beyond boredom and anxiety*. San Francisco, CA: Jossey-Bass, Inc. Publishers.

Curtiss, S. (1977). *Genie: a psycholinguistic study of a modern day 'wild child'*. New York, NY: Academic Press.

Damon, W. (1989). Introduction: advances in development research. In: W. Damon (Ed.), *Child development today and tomorrow* (pp. 1–13). San Francisco, CA: Jossey-Bass Inc.

Davis, J. A. (2000). *Historical development of children's occupations during late childhood from the 1650s to the 1990s*. Unpublished master's thesis, University of Western Ontario, London, Ontario, Canada.

Davis, J. A., Polatajko, H. J. & Ruud, C. (2002). Children in context: influence of history on the development of the predominant occupations of children. *Journal of Occupational Science*, 9 (2), 54–64.

Davis, J. A. & Polatajko, H. J. (2004). Occupational development. In: C. Christiansen & E. Townsend (Eds.), *An introduction to occupation: the art and science of living* (pp. 91–119). Upper Saddle River, NJ: Pearson Education.

Don, A., Schellenberg, G. & Rourke, B. (1999). Music and language skills of children with Williams syndrome. *Child Neuropsychology*, 5, 154–170.

Edwards, D. & Christiansen, C. (2005). Occupational development. In: C. H. Christiansen, C. M. Baum & J. Bass-Haugen (Eds.), *Occupational therapy: performance, participation and wellbeing* (pp. 42–70). Thorofare, NJ: Slack Inc.

Elder, G. H. Jr. (1998). The life course as developmental theory. *Child Development*, 69 (1), 1–12.

Elder, G. H. Jr. (1999). *Children of the great depression: social change in life experience*. Chicago, IL: University of Chicago Press. (Originally published 1974).

Erikson, E. (1950). *Childhood and society*. New York, NY: Norton.

Feldman, D. H. & Goldsmith, L. T. (1986). *Nature's gambit: child prodigies and the development of human potential*. New York, NY: Basic Books.

Gaskins, S. (1999). Children's daily lives in a Mayan village: a case study of culturally constructed roles and occupations. In: A. Göncü (Ed.), *Children's engagement in the world: socio-cultural perspectives* (pp. 25–61). New York, NY: Cambridge University Press.

Hall, C. S. & Lindzey, G. (1970). *Theories of personality* (2nd ed.). New York, NY: Wiley.

Harkness, S. (1992). Human development in psychological anthropology. In: T. Schwartz, G. M. White & C. A. Lutz (Eds.), *New directions in psychological anthropology* (pp. 102–122). Cambridge, UK: Cambridge University Press.

Humphry, R. (2002). Young children's occupations: explicating the dynamics of developmental processes. *American Journal of Occupational Therapy*, 56, 171–179.

International Humane Genome Sequencing Consortium (2001). Initial sequencing and analysis of the human genome. *Nature*, 409, 860–921.

Itard, J. M. G. (1962). *Wild boy of Aveyron*. New York, NY: Meredith Publishing Co.

Jacobs, K. (1999). *Quick reference dictionary for occupational therapy* (2nd ed.). Thorofare, NJ: Slack Inc.

Kielhofner, G. (2002). Dynamics of human occupation. In: G. Kielhofner (Ed.), *Model of human occupation* (3rd ed., pp. 28–43). Baltimore, MD: Lippincott, Williams & Wilkins.

Law, M., Baptiste, S., Carswell, A., McColl, M. A., Polatajko, H. & Pollock, N. (1998). *Canadian occupational performance measure* (3rd ed.). Toronto, Ont.: CAOT Publications ACE.

Leakey, R. & Lewin, R. (1992). *Origins reconsidered: in search of what makes us human*. Toronto, Ont.: Doubleday.

Lenhoff, H., Perales, O. & Hickok, G. (2001). Absolute pitch in Williams syndrome. *Music Perception*, 18 (3), 491–503.

Letts, L., Rigby, P. & Stewart, D. (Eds.) (2003). *Using environments to enable occupational performance*. Thorofare, NJ: Slack Inc.

Macnab, J. (2003). *Healthy development in childhood: the role of child factors, family factors and parenting practices in predicting cognitive competence and behavioural dysfunction at school-age*. Unpublished doctoral dissertation, University of Western Ontario, London, Ontario, Canada.

Morison, S. J., Ames, E. W. & Chisholm, K. (1995). The development of children adopted from Romanian orphanages. *Merrill-Palmer Quarterly*, 41 (4), 411–430.

Muir, D. (1999). Theories and methods in developmental psychology, In: A. Slater & D. Muir (Eds.), *The Blackwell reader in developmental psychology* (pp. 3–16). Malden, Mass.: Blackwell Publishers Ltd.

Newman, P. R. & Newman, B. M. (1997). *Childhood and adolescence*. Pacific Grove, Calif.: Brooks/Cole Publishing Company.

Osipow, S. H. (1968). *Theories of career development*. New York, NY: Meredith Corporation.

Piaget, J. (1969). *The psychology of the child* (H. Weaver, Trans.). New York, NY: Basic Books.

Plomin, R. (1994). *Genetics and experience: the interplay between nature and nurture*. Thousand Oaks, CA: Sage Publications.

Polatajko, H. J. (1992). Muriel Driver Lecture 1992: naming and framing occupational therapy: a lecture dedicated to the life of Nancy B. *Canadian Journal of Occupational Therapy*, 59 (4), 189–200.

Polatajko, H. J. & Mandich, A. (2004). *Enabling occupation in children: cognitive orientation to daily occupational performance (CO-OP) approach*. Ottawa, Ont.: CAOT Publishing ACE.

Rutter, M., Dunn, J., Plomin, R., Simonoff, E., Pickles, A., Maughan, B., et al. (1997). Integrating nature and nurture: implications of person–environment correlations and interactions for developmental psychopathology. *Development and Psychopathology, 9,* 335–364.

Rutter, M. & the English and Romanian Adoptees (ERA) study team (1998). Developmental catch-up and deficit, following adoption after severe global early privation. *Journal of Child Psychology and Psychiatry, 39* (4), 465–476.

Saudino, K. J. & Eaton, W. O. (1991). Infant temperament and genetics: an objective twin study of motor activity level. *Child Development, 62,* 1167–1174.

Scarr, S. (1993). Biological and cultural diversity: the legacy of Darwin for development. *Child Development, 64,* 1333–1353.

Scarr, S. & McCartney, K. (1983). How people make their own environments: a theory of genotype–environment effects. *Child Development, 54,* 424–435.

Scarr, S. & Ricciuti, A. (1991). What effects do parents have on their children? In: L. Okagaki & R. J. Sternberg (Eds.), *Directors of development: influences on the development of children's thinking* (pp. 3–23). Hillsdale, NJ: Lawrence Erlbaum Associates, Inc.

Schaie, K. W. (1994). The course of adult intellectual development. *American Psychologist, 48* (1), 304–313.

Sedgwick, A., Polatajko, H. J. & Davis, J. A. (2003). *Children's occupations: a naturalistic study of Ugandan children.* Poster presented at Canadian Association of Occupational Therapists Conference, Winnipeg, Manitoba. 26 May 2003.

Vygotsky, L. S. (1978). *Mind in society: the development of higher psychological process.* M. Cole, V. John-Steiner, S. Scribner & E. Souberman, (Eds.). Cambridge, MA: Harvard University Press.

Wilcock, A. A. (1998). *An occupational perspective of health.* Thorofare, NJ: Slack Inc.

Williams Syndrome Foundation (22 June 2004). *Nightline transcript: two fathers, two scientists: a father's love: when everything you do is not enough.* (Televised on Friday 9 October 1998). Retrieved 24 January 2005, from http://williamssyndrome.org/multimedia/niteline.htm

Wiseman, J. O., Davis, J. A. & Polatajko, H. J. (2005). Occupational development: understanding why children do the things they do. *Journal of Occupational Science, 12* (1), 26–35.

World Health Organization (2001). *The World Health Organization's International Classification of Function, Disability and Health.* Geneva: World Health Organization.

Wright, L. (1997). *Twins and what they tell us about who we are.* Toronto, Ont.: John Wiley & Sons, Inc.

Yerxa, E. J., Clark, F., Frank, G., Jackson, J., Parham, D., Pierce, D., et al. (1989). An introduction to occupational science: a foundation for occupational therapy in the twenty-first century. *Occupational Therapy in Health Care, 6* (4), 1–17.

Chapter 8

COMMUNICATION AND SOCIAL SKILLS FOR OCCUPATIONAL ENGAGEMENT

Gail Woodyatt and Sylvia Rodger

The communication and social skills acquired during childhood are fundamental to the formation of friendships and provide the mechanism for meaningful interactions with peers and adults. These skills are as critical to successful occupational engagements as motor, cognitive and academic skills. Through adult imitation and modelling, play and curriculum experiences, children learn and practise the social and conversational skills necessary for occupational engagement.

Occupational engagement refers to the child's meaningful involvement in the range of occupations required by their life roles. For example, as part of her role of sister, five-year-old Mary plays with her three-year-old sister, Julia. This requires sharing toys, taking turns, waiting, talking, leading and following. Mary enjoys building cubby houses with draped sheets. She arranges her dolls under the table with Julia. They negotiate where their soft toys can be seated and the positioning of props. Julia enjoys following Mary's lead, but likes to assert herself by moving her doll's cot under the table as well. They do not always negotiate the space well and Julia often ends up in tears as Mary pushes the cot outside the cubby house. Mary likes to 'read' books to Julia and the dolls. Both Mary and Julia are learning about playing together, cooperating, developing the same play theme, negotiating conflict, having conversations, taking turns and sharing.

This scenario reflects an opportunity through everyday occupations in which communication and social skills are learned. The sisters' skills are developmentally different. However, they manage the interaction positively most of the time. When children have difficulties with these basic communication and social skills, they often have less satisfying and productive occupational engagements. They may avoid social situations and become withdrawn, missing out on additional opportunities to develop these skills.

The aims of this chapter are to:

(1) Provide an overview of major developmental milestones in children's acquisition of communication skills between birth and 12 years
(2) Outline the critical social skills acquired during childhood that are necessary for social interaction and the development and maintenance of friendships

(3) Demonstrate how these communication and social skills are integral for occupational engagement
(4) Provide an overview of how occupational therapists and speech pathologists can work together to help children develop and utilize communication and social skills

Acquisition of communication skills

In the previous scenario, various communication and social skills were observed. Mary and Julia's play interactions are not only precursors to later social situations but result from the interaction of physical and cognitive developmental factors and past experiences. Bruner (1973) divided these cognitive skills into *thing* and *people* skills. Children learn how to understand their physical world of *things*, and gain such concepts as object permanence, means–end, and cause–effect (Piaget, 1952). In addition, children need to understand their social world and develop their *people* skills via language and speech.

Communication is a two-way interaction and refers not only to the words and sentences used but also to an individual's understanding of what is spoken. Communication is more than the expressive and receptive nature of the spoken word, but also relates to non-verbal aspects. Effective communicators understand, interpret and use facial expressions, gestures, nuances of intonation and also incorporate their understanding of the context. These communication behaviours or linguistic skills continue to develop into adulthood and are modified through experience. Certain behaviours cluster and are usually referred to as developmental milestones, such as the infant's first words.

Some definitions

Skills in all the aspects of communication are essential to the development of the social competence necessary for occupational engagement. A brief summary of various terms is needed before we continue a discussion on the development of these skills. Speech, voice and fluency will not be considered in much detail in this chapter, yet a brief description of each aspect is necessary to ensure a clear understanding of communication (see Table 8.1).

The main focus in this chapter, however, is language. Language is a vital and integral part of communication. It can be words or deaf signs, symbols or pictographs, and by sharing the meaning of these linguistic features, we can communicate intentionally with others. Language is interactive, evolving, and can be as simple as a 'yes' or 'no' answer to a question, or as complex as a Shakespearean tragedy. The majority of this chapter will focus on the three basic linguistic aspects of semantics, syntax and pragmatics (see Table 8.2).

In this chapter, we are considering only the development of and the use of the English language. However, components of language (see Table 8.2) are particular to cultural groupings as all languages have their own vocabulary, grammar, pragmatic aspects and sound rules. Different cultural groups have different pragmatic

Table 8.1 Aspects of communication and their definitions.

Aspects of communication	Definitions
Language	Shared systems of meaning among a group of people. These systems may be spoken, written, or gestural (as in the sign language of the deaf community)
Speech	The production of sounds by the organs of speech (for example lips and tongue)
Voice	The output of our air stream, modified by the vibration of the larynx, the movement of the soft palate and the resonating sinus cavities
Fluency	Smooth production of speech and language output without excessive repetitions, hesitations, or prolongations

Table 8.2 Components of language and their definitions.

Components of language	Definitions
Phonology	The rules of sound combinations in speech
Semantics	The knowledge of words and their meanings; vocabulary
Syntax/morphology	The structural aspects of language; the grammatical rules that allow us to combine words efficiently, correct order of nouns and verbs and the other parts of speech in our sentences. Morphology is the knowledge of the smaller meaningful elements of our words (such as -s for plurals, -ed for the past tense)
Pragmatics	Why we use language (for example requesting, greeting) and how we use our language (for example conversational skills such as eye contact, turn taking, appropriate intonation, topic initiation)

features and these need to be considered when working with children from different ethnic backgrounds. The various aspects of language have to be learned through many interactions for individuals to be successful communicators within their own culture.

Social interactional perspective

Individuals may have difficulties in any of the components of communication and these can affect their ability to communicate effectively and efficiently. As health professionals working with children we need to know how language skills develop, when they develop and the impact of problems on occupational performance.

Due to the breadth, depth and interrelatedness of communication features, communication development has been investigated in many different ways. It can be investigated from a bottom-up perspective; from the structural and psychological processes involved; from the activity level which considers the linguistic frameworks of what is said; or from a more top-down perspective, when a person's participation and life roles are considered. The approach taken in this chapter is from the participatory or social interactional perspective. Many children are disadvantaged in their daily occupations because they are operating without a well developed, intricate communication system.

Individuals communicate for different purposes. The words we hear are usually mapped onto our social intentions. We develop language so that we can interact with someone about something we share (Bruner, 1976; Warren et al., 2002). Communication, as a process, also involves the realization that we can affect others in our environment (McLean & Snyder-McLean, 1993). Difficulties in any of the myriad aspects of communication will be expressed differently in the children with whom we work and explains why some children struggle in everyday life.

From a social interactional perspective, learning to communicate starts from a baby's first days, or even whilst in utero, and is reliant on the two-way interactions of both communicative partners. That is, changes in an infant's or toddler's behaviour change the behaviour of the communicative partners, which then support and facilitate the development of the child's communicative behaviours (Warren et al., 2002). For example, a child's developing interest in objects in the environment, such as looking up at a noise in the sky causes the communicative partner to say 'plane', increasing the child's vocabulary.

Stages of communication

The development of communication can be outlined in many ways. The pragmatics perspective (Austin, 1962) describes spoken words as speech acts with a linguistic form (locution), an intended function (illocutionary force) and its effect on the listener (perlocution) (Hoff, 2001). Bates et al. (1975) adapted Austin's work into developmental stages (see Table 8.3).

In the locutionary stage, children use their first words, which can refer to objects and/or actions, but it is only when we know what the child's intentions are that we can determine the meaning of what they are trying to say (McLean & Snyder-McLean, 1999). Nine different communicative functions were noted by Dore (1975) for a child at the single word level (that is labelling, repeating, answering, requesting action, requesting information, calling, greeting, protesting and practising). Ninio & Wheeler (cited in Ninio et al., 1994) expanded this list, noting that by 22 months, a child could express up to 65 different intents, including exclamations of disapproval, distress, or surprise, agreeing or disagreeing with a proposition, or correcting an utterance. By this early age, a typically developing toddler is becoming a sophisticated communicator, if not yet sophisticated in their ability to express these intents linguistically.

By the time a child has learned about 50 words and understands almost 200, the first word combinations begin to appear (Bates et al., 1979; Bochner et al., 1997). These combinations are not true grammatical structures but tend to be semantic strings of single words chunked together to help the child better describe the world.

Table 8.3 Description of developmental stages of communication.

Speech act developmental stages	Descriptions
The perlocutionary stage (birth to 10 months)	People assign meaning to an infant's reactive motor actions or noises without any evidence that the infant is knowingly trying to influence another.
The illocutionary stage (10–12 months)	Children use gestures or eye gaze to deliberately signal their desires. These gestures include open-handed requests, showing an object to an adult, waving bye-bye, and finally finger pointing to an object, perhaps to encourage the adult to give it to the child, or for the adult to name it, or comment upon it.
The locutionary stage (12 months +)	Communicative intentions are expressed using traditional linguistic forms such as the spoken word, word combinations and complex utterances.

Adapted from Bates et al. (1975); McLean & Snyder-McLean (1987, 1999); Sugarman-Bell (1978).

Again, we need to know the child's intended meaning before we can interpret what they are saying. Unless we know the context, can hear the child's intonation and see their expression and accompanying gestures, we may have difficulty interpreting the child's spoken words.

By this stage, children's ability to learn language seems magical to their parents, as they quickly amass a large vocabulary and begin combining words into true grammatical forms. Children learn to understand at least nine words daily (Carey, 1978), and learn to say at least 2–5 words daily from about 18 months to 6 years (Owens, 1996). They quickly *map* words onto their experiences, their actions and gradually develop a greater understanding of the meaning.

True grammatical constructions develop around the age of two years. Children still use the semantic constructions but now scaffold them into longer syntactic constructions: 'Mummy eat', and 'eat apple' quickly become 'Mummy eat apple'. Once the child has a mean length of utterance (or MLU) of approximately 2.5 words, the use of the smaller meaningful parts of words or grammatical morphemes appear. Most children develop their use in approximately the same order over the next 24 to 30 months (Brown, 1973). The early morphemes tend to be the use of 'ing' as in 'jumping', the prepositions 'in' and 'on', the plural 's' as in 'cats'. The later developing morphemes include the use of the article 'a' and 'the', the regular past tense 'ed' as in 'jumped', the uncontractible copula 'is' as 'Is it red?' and the contractible auxiliary 'is' as in 'He's running'. By the age of three or four years, most typically developing children use grammatically correct simple sentences. Between three and five years children gradually learn to ask questions correctly by reversing the verb order, for example, 'What is he doing?' as well as use more complicated constructions such as 'Will Mummy let me go on that ride?' Younger children start to string sentences together by using 'and' and 'then'. Later, they begin to use conjunctions such as 'because', 'if', 'so', 'when' and 'after'.

Children learn these constructions to help them make sense of their world, to ask appropriate questions, to express their intentions, and to have conversations. By five years of age most children are competent communicators, even if lacking absolute adult forms or vocabulary. They are also becoming competent social beings involved in complex peer interactions. Nevertheless, children are still learning about how to communicate events happening around them, and from their past. They need to develop their narrative skills (that is link more than one sentence about the same topic). Their worlds are expanding and they need to be able to tell their parents the details of what happened in their preschool day (albeit often unwillingly), and their teachers about what has happened at home. Adults still play a large role in sustaining these conversations by asking questions and keeping the child on topic. They do this by following the child's lead, responding to previous statements and requesting further information (Hoff, 2001).

With their friends and peers, however, children need to enter into and maintain a range of social interaction skills without adult scaffolding. They need to join in play, direct the play, share materials, ask for assistance, offer suggestions, find out what other children like or want to do and assert themselves. To do this children require a solid language base, but they also need the pragmatic conversational competencies such as appropriate eye contact, turn taking skills; they need to know not only what to say, but when they should say it; and they need to know how to say something using suitable intonation and with the appropriate facial expressions and body gestures. They also have to be able to read others' non-verbal gestures and expressions, a skill we know that some children, especially those with autism spectrum disorders (ASD) fail to develop.

Development of socio-dramatic play

One important aspect of the daily occupations of children is that of socio-dramatic play. Play is the avenue by which children refine and practise their social skills, as well as the medium for emotional expression (Patterson & Westby, 1998). The relationships between the development of play and language have been identified (McCune-Nicolich, 1981; Westby, 1988; 1991). These relationships are not unidirectional or causative, but instead are thought to be homologous – that is, certain play behaviours are thought to appear at the same time as certain language behaviours due to the child's underlying cognitive development (Roth & Clark, 1987).

Play and language development milestones provide us with glimpses of preschoolers' worlds as they introduce props into play, develop themes, organize their play and take on roles (Patterson & Westby, 1998; Westby, 1988). Between 12 and 18 months, as children start to play symbolically (such as pretending to drink from an empty cup), they also begin to use their first words. By 24 months, as they begin to combine play schemas, such as pretending to pour a drink, put in the sugar, stir, and then drink from the empty cup, they start to combine words. By the age of three years, as they combine more complex play schemes, such as following through all the actions of preparing a meal, they are able to provide an ongoing commentary with highlights of what they have done, are doing and are planning to do.

Prior to three and a half years, children share roles with peers, but by this age they begin to share roles with dolls and puppets. The child typically is the adult, and the doll the 'baby'. They also begin to consider emotions, and attribute these to the dolls (Patterson & Westby, 1998). Then, by the age of four years, socio-dramatic play is fully expressed. Children now use their language to set the scenes from their imagination or familiar themes from television or movies. They plan events, find the props and organize each other. Unless children have sufficient language to support this play, however, they can find themselves either ostracized from the play situations, or playing the role of the 'baby' or character 'acted upon'.

By five to six years, children play out their own plots and events with several sequences of action, and the scenes are constantly evolving according to the players' imagination and whims. Children's language is now able to support such play, with their receptive vocabulary now around 13 000 words (Gard et al., 1993) and their syntax more adult-like (Paul, 2001). Further, their social behaviours with peers are both comprehensive and relatively competent (Brown & Conroy, 2002).

Communication skills of the school-age child

An interactional perspective persists through to middle childhood. It acknowledges that while communication skills improve within the context of social interactions, children's communication abilities further help them become more socially competent (Kaczmarek, 2002). Social competence refers to the consequences of a person's interactions with other people (Spence, 1995) leading to peer acceptance, friendships and membership of social networks (Kaczmarek, 2002). Children with poor language skills, including those with ASD, have difficulty in all these areas and may need to be directed in ways to become involved in peer activities (Beilinson & Olswang, 2003).

The world of the school-age child, however, is also broadening into educational environments and children now interact with teachers as well as peers and family members. These environments are increasingly structured, with new social skills required in each. A child's speech and language skills, particularly in the pragmatic aspects of communication, are vital to achieving positive outcomes.

Of course, a child's language skills are not fully developed by school entry, nor are their social skills. As noted by Hoff (2001), communication development is a 'long process with no single endpoint' (p. 311), neither as the communicator nor the listener. Further, the influences on the child after the age of 5–6 years are also broadening. Children are now becoming exposed to the written word in books, on computers and in their environment. Children learn from these new exposures to words and their meanings about combining and using words in reading and writing. We communicate in writing and in speech for many reasons – to pass on information, to retell events, to create new stories, to tell our life stories, to lighten the seriousness of life with some humour. This last aspect of humour develops as we grow. An infant can be entertained by a funny face, a preschooler by funny words, young schoolchildren with puns and riddles, and older children by sophisticated play on words.

The development of humour is paralleled by the growing child's ability to understand abstractions of language and non-literal language, the knowledge that words can have multiple meanings, and to learn about antonyms, synonyms and homonyms. Children with ASD, for example, frequently fail to understand jokes and subtle humour. Children also have to learn to monitor their own understanding. Hoff (2001) reported various studies that tell how five-year-olds are still not able to realize how much they don't know. As they progress through the school years they develop expertise in asking for clarification, and in making sure they understand what is being said. In oral communication situations, children become more expert in picking up non-verbal information from their communicative partners. They learn to recognize environmental clues, facial expressions and body gestures. Most changes in conversation skills are made between second and fifth grades (ages approximately seven to ten years), although fifth graders (ten-year-olds) are still more likely to respond to the content of the conversation. With the exception of those with ASD, by late adolescence, most teenagers are more receptive to the feelings and attitudes of their communicative partners (Hoff, 2001).

Social competence and social skills: inter-professional management

In this section, we will look at how professionals understand social skills from their different but complementary perspectives; how they understand the importance of these skills; and how they work together when children experience difficulties in this domain. Two brief case studies will be used to illustrate the presentation and management of these difficulties.

Defining social competence and social skills

Social competence is the ability to obtain successful outcomes from interactions with others (Spence & Donovan, 1998). It is generally accepted that social skills form a subset of skills within the broader domain of social competence. Social skills refer to discrete, observable behaviours that occur in a particular situation, while social competence refers to a global and evaluative judgement of an individual's performance (Gresham, 1998). Gresham & Elliot (1990) defined social skills as 'socially acceptable learned behaviours that enable a person to interact effectively with others and to avoid socially unacceptable responses' (p. 1). These skills are sometimes referred to as micro- and macro-level skills (Spence, 2003). Micro-level skills include pragmatic linguistic components related to communicative aspects, such as tone of voice, volume, rate and clarity of speech, and the quantity and quality of non-verbal skills such as eye contact, facial expression, posture, social distance and use of gesture. These are modified according to the demands of social situations and impact on the success of social interactions. At a macro-level, the micro-level skills are integrated with appropriate strategies for different pragmatic social tasks such as starting conversations, greeting people, requesting help or information, offering assistance, joining in and offering invitations (Spence, 2003).

Developing social skills to enable successful relationships is one of the most important accomplishments of childhood. When a child does not have these social skills in their repertoire, this is referred to as an acquisition deficit. By contrast, performance deficits occur when the person possesses the skills, yet fails to demonstrate them in specific situations. Affective factors (for example arousal caused by anxiety or anger), cognitive deficits (for example depression) or competing/ interfering problem behaviours (for example positive reinforcement of inappropriate behaviour from a peer group) may lead to performance difficulties (Gresham, 1997). Deficits in interpersonal problem solving may also result in inappropriate or problematic social responses. Fluency deficits in social skills (Gresham, 1998) (not related to fluency problems in communication) result from a lack of exposure to sufficient role models, insufficient skill rehearsal or inconsistent reinforcement. Essentially, lack of social skills practice leads to fluency deficits. Analysis of the type of social skill deficit experienced is important to ensure targeted interventions.

Friendships

The development of friendships is an important childhood task. Friendship is a 'dynamic, reciprocal relationship between two individuals' (Burk, 1996, p. 283). While friendships develop as a result of children being together and learning about one another, they are not guaranteed. As children become friends they negotiate boundaries for functioning, requiring cooperation, mutual liking and trust. Friendships are influenced by a psychologically safe environment that promotes social interaction (Burk, 1996). Children learn to develop friendships, associate, negotiate, empathize and cooperate with others. This requires development of skills such as sharing and turn taking, an appreciation of others' viewpoints (theory of mind), empathy and social rules such as manners (Newman, 2004). Children need friends to ensure their emotional wellbeing and stability. Children with friends feel they have self-worth and are more secure. Good friends are also able to assist children to deal positively with life's stresses and support them through difficult times (Petersen, 2002). Hence, it is important to help children to develop the underlying social skills that assist with the formation of friendships.

Children and adolescents with poor social skills have been shown to be at greater risk of delinquency, depression, social withdrawal, poor academic performance, substance abuse and serious emotional/behavioural disturbances (for example Petersen, 2002) and social phobia (for example Spence et al., 1999). Social skills deficits lead to a lack of successful social interactions, resulting in expectancies of poor outcomes and negative thoughts. Subsequent avoidance reduces the opportunity for practising social skills and perpetuates the cycle (Spence et al., 1999).

Children with social skills deficits

Children seen by occupational therapists and speech pathologists known to have significant social skill difficulties include those with:

(1) Learning disabilities with poor peer acceptance, who are more likely to be aggressive, immature and inattentive (Swanson, 1996; Swanson & Malone, 1992); and to have difficulties with social perception, behaviour, problem solving and verbal communication (Cermak & Aberson, 1997)
(2) Speech and language impairments, who have poor peer relationships, in particular poor access and dispute resolution skills, low responsivity and ineffective interaction styles (Craig, 1993)
(3) ASD who have difficulty forming relationships, developing conversational skills and reading subtle interpersonal responses (Gutstein & Sheely, 2001)

Let us look at two case scenarios. These will be used to describe how team members can work together to assess and treat social skills difficulties.

Ethan

Ethan is a four-and-a-half-year-old only child referred by his preschool teacher due to concerns with lack of socializing and empathy, and suspected speech and language skills deficits. He presented with intelligible speech, but inconsistent delayed phonological processes (for example 'poon' for 'spoon', 'took' for 'chook'). He was chatty during speech pathology assessment but had a short attention span. His auditory comprehension and expressive communication were mildly delayed. He had weak reasoning skills and significant word finding difficulties. For example, the speech pathologist said, 'What is this part for?' pointing to the windscreen on a picture of a car. Ethan said, 'Maybe I don't know, maybe I can't remember, maybe something to look out the window, maybe glass'. He is very interested in dinosaurs!

Hannah

Hannah is an attractive 12-year-old who has attended speech pathology intermittently since three years of age. She has low average intelligence (WISC verbal IQ 85, performance IQ 86). She attended occupational therapy from the age of ten for assistance with visual memory and visual motor integration. Her receptive and expressive language skills are below average. She lacks speech fluency (repeats words and hesitates), and has word finding and organizational difficulties. She has a flat monotone voice and was diagnosed with Asperger's Syndrome when she was nine years old. Her goals are to be better at conversations at school, to make friends and do public speaking at school.

Social skills assessment

Prior to embarking on any social skills intervention, appropriate assessment of a child's social skills deficits is critical (Bracegirdle, 1990). The choice of the most appropriate method of assessment will depend on the purpose of the assessment, the age of the child and the context. During assessment, information should be gathered from multiple sources and take into account the child's performance across multiple contexts. Table 8.4 provides a brief summary of assessment methods. In addition, the environments in which the child functions should be addressed (Sheridan et al., 1999) in order to promote treatment utility and social validity. Comprehensive assessment of the environment also enables careful planning of generalization strategies (for example involvement of peers, parents, teachers and contexts for intervention).

With Ethan, the speech pathologist and occupational therapist had the opportunity to directly observe him at preschool during inside and outdoor sessions and at lunch time. They observed that he played on his own, and did not engage with others, unless facilitated by a teacher. It became obvious that the other children found him difficult to understand and that they often gave up, after they had tried several times to interact with him. His play skills were delayed and more characteristic of those of a two-and-a-half- to three-year-old. His short attention span meant that he moved from activity to activity, not remaining long enough to develop play themes or interactions. He was disruptive at group time when listening to stories, frequently wandering off or losing interest. He annoyed other children around him when distracted. An interview with his mother about his skills at home, confirmed these observations. His status as an only child may also have led to fewer opportunities for play interactions at home. His mother reported that they seldom had other children home to play. The teacher completed the 'School Social Behavior Scales' (Merrell, 1993). The multiple sources of information confirmed that Ethan's delayed language and play skills, short attention span and distractability contributed to his difficulty in socializing with other children.

In Hannah's case, the speech pathologist used the Social Skills Questionnaire (Spence, 1995) completed by her mother. This identified problems with nonverbal skills, such as looking at the speaker's face, standing too close to others, lack of facial expressions, conversational issues (for example difficulties with choosing the right time and place to talk, starting conversations, taking turns, asking questions, knowing when the listener does not understand), emotional regulation (for example expressing anger, showing consistent body language with emotions), problem solving (for example self calming, predicting consequences, working out solutions), and making friends. She also interviewed Hannah's class teacher regarding her perspectives on Hannah's social skills at school. Discussions with Hannah revealed concerns regarding her lack of friends, difficulties having conversations and desire to do some public speaking.

Social skills intervention

Social skills programmes are based on the premise that poor peer relationships are due to social skills deficits and that these can be improved through training. It is also recognized that naturalistic environmental contexts (such as school, home, community) are integral to effective programs (Cermak & Aberson, 1997). It is

Table 8.4 Types of social skills assessment.

Type of assessment	Details
Primary methods	First line choices
Direct/naturalistic observation (classroom, playground, group)	Behavioural observation requires: (1) Observation and recording of behaviours in natural settings (2) The use of trained, objective observers (3) Objective rating or behaviour coding system to minimize rater bias and subjectivity While this is the preferred method of observation in classes and playgrounds, it is time consuming and requires a large number of observations for reliable measurement. For example Peer Social Behaviour Code (PSBC), part of the Systematic Screening for Behaviour Disorders (SSBD) (Walker & Severson, 1992).
Behaviour rating scales or questionnaires (child, parent, teacher)	A widely used method of assessing children's behaviour because they are: (1) Less expensive than observation in terms of time and training (2) Capable of providing data on low frequency behaviour that may not be easily seen (3) Objective and reliable (4) Used to obtain information from parents and teachers when young children cannot provide information themselves (5) Able to capitalize on informants' observations over a period of time in natural settings (6) Able to capitalize on the expert judgements and observations of persons familiar with the child's behaviour Examples: School Social Behavior Scales (SSBS) (Merrell, 1993) (kindergarten – end of year 12), the Social Skills Rating System (SSRS) (Gresham & Elliot, 1990) comprises three domains of social skills, problem behaviours, and academic competence. The social skills scale includes cooperation, assertion, responsibility, empathy and self-control. Walker-McConnell Scale of Social Competence and School Adjustment (SSCSA) (Walker & McConnell, 1995) designed specifically for teachers and school based professionals focuses on social competence. Social Skills Questionnaires (Spence, 1995) 8–18 years; this also has parent, teacher and student versions.
Secondary methods	Second line choices
Sociometric measures	Sociometric assessment techniques, for example peer nomination and peer ranking, measure peer acceptance or social reputation rather than social skills. These techniques fail to provide any information about why a child is liked or disliked by peers. Sociometric techniques can range from highly structured interview schedules to unstructured formats.
Interviews (child, parent, teacher)	Interviewing provides relevant and functional information about the environments in which behaviour problems occur. Interviewing also provides the possibility for children to role-play various social situations, providing an avenue for observation.
Tertiary methods	Third line choices
Projective-expressive techniques	Examples include drawing and sentence completion tasks, can be used for rapport building and hypothesis generation.
Self-report instruments	Self-report instruments useful for evaluating internalizing problems. However, there is limited evidence for the effectiveness of self-report assessments for social skills. One of the most researched self-report instruments is the Social Skills Rating System (SSRS) (Demaray et al., 1995; Gresham & Elliot, 1990).

Adapted from Merrell (2001).

best when skills are acquired in the actual physical context in which they are used (for example playground with practical relevance for recess) and are adaptable to various social situations. Physical characteristics of the setting (such as place, space, equipment, layout), the environmental demands (such as rules, norms, behavioural expectations) and contingencies (social rewards and punishers) need to be considered for intervention procedures to be valid.

Social skills training (SST) has been conducted with children and adolescents with a range of behavioural, emotional and mental health difficulties for several decades. Occupational therapists and speech pathologists have complementary professional knowledge, which places them in an ideal position to co-facilitate social skills groups. Speech pathologists have in-depth knowledge of the development of communication and conversation and how to support children's speech and language skills, while occupational therapists have knowledge of group dynamics, skill acquisition, facilitating play, childhood activities and occupations, and goal setting with individuals and groups (Cermak & Aberson, 1997). Both professions have shared knowledge in the areas of social learning, behavioural reinforcement, facilitating role-play and appropriate modelling of social skills. These skills enable therapists to modify commercially available social skills training programmes as required, to meet the needs of specific individuals within groups. In addition, they are able to utilize play and activity groups as an appropriate arena for the enhancement of social skills. Activity groups can be incorporated into classrooms and playgrounds, enabling children with special needs to integrate social skills in naturalistic settings. Effective SST needs to be individualized for specific children even if the training does occur in groups. So now we consider how we might assist Ethan and Hannah.

Ethan is a preschooler with delayed speech and language skills. In consultation with his mother and teacher it was decided that the first priority should be some individual speech pathology sessions to address his phonological difficulties with substitutions and blends, to assist his intelligibility and to work on his delayed receptive and expressive language. Following this, the occupational therapist and speech pathologist identified several preschool children in their school district who had difficulties with social interaction secondary to delayed communication and play skills. They decided to run an intensive group twice a week for four weeks at a preschool (enabling use of an appropriate, naturalistic context). Preschoolers like Ethan have occupational roles as friends, siblings and preschool students. All of these require the development of adequate social skills to ensure optimal occupational engagement to enable play at home and preschool, when visiting friends, and for them to engage maximally with the early educational curriculum, which requires small and large group activities.

The social skills group focused on a different play theme each week with, an identified micro- and macro-level social skill that supported their engagement in play and educational occupations. For example, one week the play theme was dinosaurs. Hence, activities were developed around the micro-skills of volume and rate of speech and the macro-skill of greetings. Speech volume and rate could be incorporated with the activities with adult and baby dinosaurs (who speak loudly

Table 8.5 Overview of social skills session for preschoolers.

Week number and play theme (two sessions per week)	Micro-social skill	Macro-social skill
(1) Dinosaurs – play in sand tray with plastic dinosaurs.	Voice volume (loud, soft, just right). Speech rate (fast, slow, just right).	Greetings (such as hello, goodbye, how are you?). Pretend greetings with dinosaurs meeting, practise role play in group.
(2) Mr Men (such as Mr Happy, Miss Grumpy). Painting expressions on Mr Men faces in painting area with easels. Use of story books, mirrors, photos of expressions.	Facial expressions (recognizing emotions and facial expressions attached to various emotions).	Starting conversations (such as questions: how are you today? commenting on painting or colours of paint). Practise in group and while painting.
(3) Playing with favourite toys in small groups (round robin – with children taking turns to play in the different groups).	Social distance (how far apart to stand, recognizing when others are busy).	Joining in. (for example questions: What are you doing? How about we . . . ? Let's . . .).
(4) Playing shops (shopkeepers and customers), shop corner with cash register, pretend food items, empty boxes and packets from real food items.	Gesture. Posture.	Requesting information, help (such as asking pretend shopkeeper how much things cost, where to find item.)

and softly respectively), and rate around fast and slow moving (and talking) dinosaurs. Each session involved elements of direct instruction, practice and role-playing. Time for incidental practice during playing with plastic dinosaurs in a large sand tray was arranged with a focus on dinosaurs greeting one another (for example saying hello and goodbye). Role-playing greetings with each other was also incorporated at the beginning (with group members) and end of the session (with parents who arrived to pick them up). Table 8.5 provides a brief overview of the four week programme.

In Hannah's case, the therapists also ran a social skills group for 12–14-year-olds. It was held at a local municipal hall. Eight children attended this group for two hours once a week over eight weeks. During each session, one of the therapists withdrew two children for half an hour each to work on specific goals. Each child therefore received two half-hour individual sessions over the eight weeks. All the children in the group had goals involving making and keeping friends, conversations and learning to join in at school. Pre-adolescent children have occupational roles including those of school student, friend, sibling, team member (for example sports or debating). These roles require children to develop increasingly sophisticated social skills so that they can function appropriately within these social and educational roles. The group programme therefore needed to address the social skills required by children in this age group who are becoming increasingly social beings in environments outside the home, and in contexts in which parents have less influence (as facilitators of children's social engagements). Children of this age are also able to identify their own intervention goals, which can be prioritized in terms of group and individual goals.

Each child also had specific goals, for example in Hannah's case, confidence with public speaking. The speech pathologist therefore worked individually with Hannah on speech clarity, volume, rate and expression to assist her with speaking in front of the class. Videotaping of her presentations with both the clinician and Hannah working through the tapes together helped self-reflection. Hannah also revealed that she became anxious when ordering food at the school canteen, when there was a long queue of people waiting behind her and lots of background noise.

In addition to the group sessions, the children and therapists also engaged in two social outings to a nearby shopping centre, where they ate together so that they had practice ordering food in a busy environment (to incorporate one of Hannah's goals) and then practising appropriate manners and conversational skills (goals relevant to all group participants), while eating a meal together. With the group situated in the community, the therapists could utilize appropriate environments for practising skills learnt in the group situation.

Being aware of the evidence based literature, the two therapists incorporated best practice strategies in their planning of the social skills group. For example, effective programmes are known to incorporate both cognitive behavioural training and emotional affective or motivational skills (Peterson, 2002). Cognitive behavioural approaches incorporate knowledge of prosocial strategies for friendship making, generating, considering and choosing strategies for solving social problems, as well as practising solutions. Addressing emotional motivational factors requires helping children to gain emotional control of angry, aggressive feelings and anxiety, and practising more socially constructive interactions. Motivational techniques such as goal setting, self-monitoring, evaluation, positive feedback and peer group training are also critical (Peterson, 2002).

The SST programme described by Spence (1995) was used as a basis for the sessions developed for Hannah's group. It aims to teach a range of fundamental social skills and strategies to deal with commonly presenting social situations. The programme comprises behavioural social skills training incorporating discussion, modelling, role-playing, rehearsal, feedback and reinforcement; social perception skills training involving correct interpretation of social cues from others and the context; self-instructional/self-regulation techniques such as self-monitoring, self-talk, and self-reinforcement; social problem solving (identifying the problem, generating alternative solutions, predicting consequences, planning appropriate responses); and reduction of competing inappropriate responses (including cognitive restructuring, relaxation training and parent training).

Various topics covered over the eight weeks included: starting conversations, joining in, offering invitations, asking for and offering help, using appropriate facial expression, listening skills, assertion, negotiation and conflict resolution. Another essential feature of successful social skills groups is providing adequate liaison with parents and teachers to support the skill learning of attendees (Macdonald et al.,

Table 8.6 Strategies for promoting long-term and generalized outcomes from social skills training (SST).

- Selection of social skills for training based on empirical evidence of their social validity.
- Attention to skills that are culturally appropriate for children, based on cultural context.
- Maximum participation of all children in social skills groups.
- Adequate duration of SST.
- Booster sessions to facilitate maintenance of learned skills.
- School level training in addition to specific social skills group to ensure daily training versus time limited groups.
- Extension of SST into the child's naturalistic settings at school and home.
- Use of token economy and contingency management methods to enhance practice and group participation.
- Involvement of teachers, parents and peers within and between training sessions.
- Inclusion of socially competent peers in SST groups to provide models of target behaviour.
- Ensure the fidelity of training by trainers and programme adherence.
- Inclusion of adjunct interventions and management techniques to minimize competing/inhibiting responses that reduce the use of socially skilled behaviour.

Adapted from Spence (2003) p. 93.

2003). Not only do parents value the dialogue with professionals and gain support from them, but also the contact enables parents to support their children's practice of newly learnt skills at home. Teacher liaison is important to ensure full knowledge of the children's behaviour and transfer of skills to school.

As evidence based practitioners the therapists reviewed the evidence on SST prior to embarking on planning for the group. They only found a few meta-analyses, which had been conducted with mixed results (for example Beelman et al., 1994; Kavale et al., 1997; Schneider, 1992; Swanson & Malone, 1992). These studies show that the impact of SST varies according to the type of intervention, measures used and length of follow-up. The effectiveness of SST also appears to vary as a function of the child's presenting problems, although meta-analyses are not necessarily consistent with one another (Spence, 2003). Gresham (1997) noted that meta-analyses had not yet addressed issues of participant characteristics, type of measures, type of participants, short versus long-term effects and impact on generalization to real life contexts. In the absence of any clear pattern of results from these meta-analyses, Spence (2003) recommended increasing SST efficacy by addressing long-term and generalized outcomes. Strategies to support these outcomes are identified in Table 8.6.

Summary

This chapter has described the major milestones in the acquisition of language and communication skills, many of which are necessary for the development of conversational and social skills. In addition, social skills also require the subtle understanding of non-verbal skills, social contexts, self-monitoring and recognition and understanding of emotions. Children with ASD and other speech and language difficulties, as well as those with acquired conditions such as traumatic brain injury, frequently have social skills difficulties which need intervention. Together with educators, and school counsellors or psychologists, occupational therapists and speech pathologists can provide assessment as well as individual and/or group intervention to address social skill deficits. These programmes need to be individualized for group members, held in natural contexts, involve parents and ensure sufficient practice with peers in supportive natural settings. Development of communication and social skills enables children to participate optimally in the social contexts which are so much a part of their everyday worlds. This, in turn, enables engagement in their occupational roles and in the daily social activities which are critical to their happiness and quality of life.

References

Austin, J. L. (1962). *How to do things with words*. Oxford, UK: University Press.

Bates, E., Camaioni, L. & Volterra, V. (1975). The acquisition of performatives prior to speech. *Merrill-Palmer Quarterly, 21*, 205–226.

Bates, E., Benigni, L., Bretherton, I., Camaioni, L. & Volterra, V. (1979). *The emergence of symbols: cognition and communication in infancy*. New York: Academic Press.

Beelman, A., Pfingsten, U. & Loesel, F. (1994). Effects of training social competence in children: a meta-analysis of recent evaluation studies. *Journal of Clinical Child Psychology, 23*, 260–271.

Beilinson, J. S. & Olswang, L. B. (2003). Facilitating peer-group entry in kindergarteners with impairment in social communication. *Language, Speech, and Hearing Services in Schools, 34*, 154–166.

Bochner, S., Price, P. & Jones J. (1997). *Child language development: learning to talk*. London, UK: Whurr Publishers.

Bracegirdle, H. (1990). Developmental social skills training programmes: are they effective? *British Journal of Occupational Therapy, 53* (5), 195–196.

Brown, R. (1973). *A first language: the first stages*. Cambridge, MA: Harvard University Press.

Brown, W. H. & Conroy, M. A. (2002). Promoting peer-related social-communicative competence in preschool children. In: H. Goldstein, L. A. Kaczmarek & K. M. English (Eds.), *Promoting social communication: children with developmental disabilities from birth to adolescence*. Baltimore, MD: Paul H. Brookes Publishing.

Bruner, J. (1973). Organization of early skills action. *Child Development, 44*, 1–11.

Bruner, J. (1976). From communication to language: a psychological perspective. *Cognition, 3*, 155–187.

Burk, D. (1996). Understanding friendship and social interaction. *Childhood Education, 72*, 282–285.

Carey, S. (1978). The child as word learner. In: M. Halle, J. Bresnan & G. Miller (Eds.), *Linguistic theory and psychological reality* (pp. 264–293). Cambridge, MA: MIT Press.

Cermak, S. A. & Aberson, J. R. (1997). Social skills in children with learning disabilities. *Occupational Therapy in Mental Health, 13*, 1–24.

Craig, H. K. (1993). Social skills of children with specific language impairment: peer relationships. *Language, Speech and Hearing Services in Schools, 24*, 206–215.

Demaray, M. K., Ruffalo, S. L., Carlson, J., Busse, R. T., Olson, A. E., McManus, S. M., et al. (1995). Social skills assessment: a comparative evaluation of six published rating scales. *School Pyschology Review*, 24, 648–671.

Dore, J. (1975). Holophrases, speech acts and language universals. *Journal of Child Language*, 2, 21–40.

Gard, A., Gilman, L. & Gorman, J. (1993). *Speech and language development chart* (2nd ed.). Austin, TX: Pro-Ed.

Gresham, F. M. (1997). Social competence and students with behavior disorders: where we've been, where we are and where we should go. *Education and Treatment of Children*, 20, 233–249.

Gresham, F. M. (1998). Social skills training with children. In: T. S. Watson & F. M. Gresham (Eds.), *Handbook of child behavior therapy* (pp. 475–497). New York: Plenum Press.

Gresham, F. M. & Elliot, S. N. (1990). *Social skills rating system*. Circle Pines, Minn.: American Guidance Service.

Gutstein, S. E. & Sheely, R. K. (2001). *Relationship development intervention with young children*. London, UK: Jessica Kingsley Publishers.

Hoff, E. (2001). *Language development* (2nd ed.). Belmont, CA: Wadsworth Thomson Learning.

Kaczmarek, L. A. (2002). Assessment of social-communicative competence: an interdisciplinary model. In: H. Goldstein, L. A. Kaczmarek & K. M. English (Eds.), *Promoting social communication: children with developmental disabilities from birth to adolescence* (pp. 55–115). Baltimore, MD: Paul H. Brookes Publishing.

Kavale, K. A., Mathur, S. R., Forness, S. R., Rutherford, R. B. & Quinn, M. M. (1997). Effectiveness of social skills training for students with behaviour disorders: a meta-analysis. In: T. E. Scruggs & M. A. Mastropieri (Eds.), *Advances in learning and behavioural disabilities*. (Vol. 11, pp. 1–26). Greenwich, CT: JAI.

Macdonald, E., Chowdury, U., Dabney, J., Wolpert, M. & Stein, S. (2003). A social skills group for children. *Emotional and Behavioural Difficulties*, 8, 43–52.

McCune-Nicolich, L. (1981). Toward symbolic functioning: structure of early pretend games and potential parallels with language. *Child Development*, 52, 785–797.

McLean, J. & Snyder-McLean, L. (1987). Form and function of communicative behaviour among persons with severe developmental disorders. *Australia and New Zealand Journal of Developmental Disabilities*, 13, 83–98.

McLean, J. & Snyder-McLean, L. (1993). Communication intervention for adults with severe mental retardation. *Topics in Language Disorders*, 13, 47–60.

McLean, J. & Snyder-McLean, L. (1999). *How children learn language*. San Diego, CA: Singular Publishing.

Merrell, K. W. (1993). *School social behavior scales*. Iowa City: assessment-intervention resources. Retrieved 24 March 2005 from http:www.assessment-intervention.com

Merrell, K. W. (2001). Assessment of children's social skills: recent developments, best practices and new directions. *Exceptionality*, 9, 3–18.

Newman, S. (2004). *Stepping out: using games and activities to help your child with special needs*. Chapter 7 Social development (pp. 207–241). London: Jessica Kingsley Publishers.

Ninio, A., Snow, C. E., Pan, B. A. & Rollins, P. R. (1994). Classifying communicative acts in children's interactions. *Journal of Communication Disorders*, 27, 157–187.

Owens, R. E. (1996). *Language development: an introduction* (4th ed.). Boston, MA: Allyn & Bacon.

Patterson, J. L. & Westby, C. E. (1998). The development of play. In: W. O. Haynes & B. B. Schulman (Eds.), *Communication development: foundations, processes and clinical applications* (pp. 135–163). Baltimore, MD: Williams & Wilkins.

Paul, R. (2001). *Language disorders from infancy through adolescence: assessment and intervention*. St Louis, MO: Mosby Inc.

Petersen, L. (2002). *Social skills training: primary years of schooling Years 8–12*. Melbourne: Australian Council for Educational Research.

Piaget, J. (1952). *The origins of intelligence*. New York: Norton.

Quinn, M. M., Kavale, K. A., Mathur, S. R., Rutherford, R. B. & Forness, S. R. (1999). A meta-analysis of social skills interventions for students with emotional and behavioural disorders. *Journal of Emotional and Behavioural Disorders*, 7, 54–64.

Roth, F. P. & Clark, D. M. (1987). Symbolic play and social participation abilities of language-impaired and normally developing children. *Journal of Speech and Hearing Disorders*, 52, 17–29.

Schneider, B. H. (1992). Didactic methods for enhancing children's peer relations: a quantitative review. *Clinical Psychology Review*, 12, 363–382.

Sheridan, S. M., Hungelmann, A. & Maughn, D. P. (1999). A contextualized framework for social skills assessment, intervention and generalization. *School Psychology Review*, 28, 84–103.

Spence, S. (1995). *Social skills training: enhancing social competence with children and adolescents*. Windsor, UK: The NFER-NELSON Publishing Company Ltd.

Spence, S. (2003). Social skills training with children and young people: theory, evidence and practice. *Child and Adolescent Mental Health*, 8, 84–96.

Spence, S. & Donovan, C. (1998). Interpersonal problems. In: P. J. Graham (Ed.), *Cognitive behaviour therapy for children and families* (pp. 217–245). New York: Cambridge University Press.

Spence, S., Donovan, C. & Brechman-Toussaint, M. (1999). Social skills, social outcomes and cognitive factors of childhood social phobia. *Journal of Abnormal Psychology*, 108, 211–221.

Sugarman-Bell, S. (1978). Some organizational aspects of pre-verbal communication. In: I. Markova (Ed.), *The social context of language* (pp. 49–66). Chichester, UK: John Wiley & Sons.

Swanson, H. L. (1996). Meta-analysis, replication, social skills and learning disabilities. *The Journal of Special Education*, 30, 213–221.

Swanson, H. L. & Malone, S. (1992). Social skills and learning disabilities: a meta-analysis of the literature. *School Psychology Review*, 21, 427–443.

Walker, H. M. & Severson, H. (1992). *Systematic screening for behavior disorders*. Longmont, CO: Sopris West.

Walker, H. M. & McConnell, S. (1995). *Walker-McConnell scale of social competence and social adjustment, elementary version*. San Diego, CA: Singular.

Warren, S. F., Yoder, P. J. & Leew, S. V. (2002). Promoting social competence in infants and toddlers. In: H. Goldstein, L. A. Kaczmarek & K. M. English (Eds.), *Promoting social communication: children with developmental disabilities from birth to adolescence* (pp. 121–149). Baltimore, MD: Paul H. Brookes Publishing.

Westby, C. E. (1988). Children's play: reflections of social competence. *Seminars in Speech and Language*, 9, 1–13.

Westby, C. (1991). A scale for assessing children's pretend play. In: C. Schaefer, K. Gitlin & A. Sandgrund (Eds.), *Play diagnosis and assessment*. New York, NY: John Wiley.

Chapter 9

DEVELOPING AS A PLAYER

Patty Rigby and Sylvia Rodger

This chapter focuses on the occupational role of player from infancy until the end of middle childhood. During this time, children develop many play skills and engage in a range of play experiences. During childhood, many important play transitions occur, such as the transition from early self-focused exploratory and sensorimotor play to more social and cooperative forms of play. These more complex and socially engaging types of play require the development of communication and social skills discussed in Chapter 8, and provide important opportunities for the development of friendships.

Throughout childhood children develop their own play style (Sturgess et al., 2002), engage in functional, object related and constructional play, the nature and complexity of which changes with the acquisition of motor and cognitive skills. Imaginative/ pretend and symbolic play manifests and reinforces the development of cognitive, social and language skills. Later in childhood, children engage more in games with rules, such as board, computer and outdoor games, which lead into specific sports, recreational or leisure interests and involvement with sports clubs or neighbour-hood games. It is beyond the scope of this chapter to provide comprehensive details of developmental stages with respect to play skills during infancy, early and middle childhood. However, it is important for occupational therapists and early childhood professionals to understand play development as a foundation for working with children to enable their participation as players in appropriate contexts.

In addition to providing an avenue for skill development, play has a unique value for its own sake. Threats to children's play, discussed in Chapters 1 and 4 include parents spending more time working and less time with their children, academic pressures, diminished understanding of the value of play, urban environments with less play space, parental fears when children are not adequately supervised, fewer natural environments for play, excessive safety regulations in playgrounds (Sturgess, 2003), increased involvement in electronically mediated and virtual playscapes (Provenzo Jr, 1998). This chapter addresses the impact of these threats on play and the need for occupational therapists to advocate for children's right to play (Canadian Association of Occupational Therapists, 2002a; 2002b; Guddemi et al., 1998; Sturgess, 2003), and to assume an important role in enabling play. The benefits of play and the importance of encouraging playfulness and playful opportunities throughout children's lives are highlighted. This chapter also focuses on the critical role of the environment in enabling children's play and playfulness (both for children with and without disabilities). Occupational supports for play are described, focusing on the play activity itself and ways of ensuring the 'just right' challenge for children. The person–environment–occupation (PEO) model (Law et al., 1996; Strong et al., 1999) will be used to illustrate ways of optimizing children's play experiences and enhancing their participation in play.

The aims of this chapter are to:

(1) Define play and its functions from an occupational perspective
(2) Address the value of play for its own sake
(3) Highlight the occupational role of player
(4) Promote the concept of a goodness of child–play–environment fit to optimize participation
(5) Discuss both environmental and occupational supports as enablers of children's play

Definitions of play

In any discussion of play, irrespective of the disciplinary background of the author, a number of common issues arise. The most pervasive of these relates to the definition of play (Bundy, 1993; 1997; Canadian Association of Occupational Therapists, 2002b; Ferland, 1997; Manning, 1998; Sturgess, 2003). While most clinicians and researchers claim that they recognize play when they see it, the development of a universally accepted definition of play has been elusive. Authors (such as Sturgess et al., 2002) even challenge this assumption, arguing that whether an activity is play or not, lies fairly in the eyes of the player, that is the child themself. Despite the lack of a universally accepted definition, a number of characteristics of play are considered critical and separate it from other occupations. These are:

(1) Intrinsic motivation
(2) Attention to means rather than ends (that is play is process- rather than product-oriented)
(3) Organism rather than stimulus dominated (that is play involves toys and objects)
(4) Non-literal, simulative behaviour (that is pretending)
(5) Freedom from externally imposed rules
(6) Requiring active participation of the player (Rubin et al., 1983)

Several occupational therapists have drawn on these characteristics in an attempt to define play from an occupational perspective. Bundy (1991), reflecting an interactionist perspective, proposed a working definition of play: 'the transaction between an individual and the environment that is intrinsically motivated, internally controlled and free of many of the constraints of objective reality' (p. 59).

The practices and activities commonly referred to as *play* in childhood and youth, are typically referred to as *leisure* in adulthood. However, there is little agreement on the comparability of these constructs (Freysinger, 1998). There is no doubt that the meanings, motivations, forms and opportunities of play/leisure change across the lifespan. Bundy (1993) claimed that play and leisure warrant special attention as they differ from the other major occupations (productivity and self-care). These differences arise from the fact that:

(1) Play is a transaction or activity engaged in freely by individuals
(2) Play is determined by the players such that they are in control, and become absorbed in the activity
(3) Play allows the suspension of real life consequences
(4) Play is a style (playfulness) used when problems or situations are approached flexibly

Bundy postulated that without playfulness, all activities become work.

Ferland (1997) described play as 'a subjective attitude in which pleasure, interest and spontaneity are combined and which is expressed through freely chosen behaviour in which no specific performance is expected' (p. 20). Both Bundy (1993) and Ferland (1997) refer to an inherent quality of play which lies within the individual. Bundy referred to this trait as *playfulness*, while Ferland used the term 'ludic or playful attitude'. Playfulness was also considered by Lieberman (1977) as a personality trait that manifests throughout adult life. Ferland described a number of essential components often associated with play, such as pleasure, discovery, mastery, creativity and self-expression. Bundy (1993; 1997) viewed playfulness as a 'flexible style or approach' in which creativity and flexibility are used to address challenges and to problem solve.

Sturgess (2003) proposed a model to describe play as a child chosen occupation. She described play as being predominant in children but lasting across the lifespan as a combination of playfulness and leisure, expressed in behaviours such as games, jokes and recreation. According to Sturgess, play is:

'essentially non-literal, opportunistic and episodic, engaging, imaginative/creative, fluid and active, predominantly for the moment, and therefore concerned more with means than ends, and joyful. It focuses on a playful or "as if" attitude and must be intrinsically motivated.' (p. 104)

She contended that play occurs when adequate developmental and prerequisite skills have been acquired over time and an immediate opportunity to be playful arises. Physical resources and enough time are essential support circumstances for play. Any play episode is influenced by the individual child's personal play style (for example play and toy preferences, preference for individual versus group play). In her model, both the child's personality and genetic endowment, as well as the richness, support and safety of the environment influence play. Finally, she postulated that play is only play when it is viewed as play by the child themself. This highlights the concept of play as being a subjective attitude of the player, not just an observable behaviour, about which the three authors, Bundy, Ferland and Sturgess, agree.

All these occupational perspectives of play are consistent with contemporary occupational therapy practice, which focuses on client centredness; occupational performance as the transaction between the person, environment and occupation (Canadian Association of Occupational Therapists, 2002b; Law et al., 1996); and current views of health, disability and the influences of the environment on functioning (World Health Organization, 2001). Occupational therapists are concerned with the occupation of play and the child developing as a player.

Valuing play: the functions of play

Play matters in the lives of children. Play may have been considered frivolous and unimportant in the past and in some cultures it continues to lack value where the development of specific skills is favoured. Today, in western culture in particular, the importance of play is more widely recognized and play has become greatly valued in the daily lives of children.

Play is recognized as a universal right for every child in the *United Nations convention on the rights of the child* (Save the Children Canada, 2000). UNICEF (2002) identified the need for strategies and actions to provide access to appropriate, user-friendly services and opportunities to promote physical, mental and emotional health amongst children through play, sport and recreation. Play is particularly important for children in countries plagued by poverty, conflict and humanitarian crises.

Play is what young children do and it is the preferred occupation of young children. It is common knowledge that learning through play contributes to cognitive, physical, social, emotional and language development (for example Bredekamp & Copple, 1997; Freysinger, 1998; Gagnon & Nagle, 2004). Children are active learners who construct their knowledge and understanding of the world through play experiences (Shipley, 2002; Sturgess, 2003). Through play children gain mastery about how their body works in relation to the demands of activities and environments and gain knowledge about the world around them. Not only do they learn what they are capable of doing, they learn how to do things and how things work. Play challenges children, stretching their abilities and imagination. Competence developed through play enables children to feel confident about what they can and can't do, and confident to avail themselves of similar future opportunities and activities (Bredekamp & Copple, 1997; Hanline, 1999).

Through play, children learn about occupational roles and behaviours, and how to interact safely and appropriately within their environment. For example, children engage in interactive pretend play with peers, by imitating various roles within familiar domestic and community scenarios, such as pretending to cook a meal and feed a doll, or playing fire fighters and police. These scenarios allow them to explore role related behaviours, helping them to make sense of their world. They learn to problem solve, share and negotiate, and take turns. They develop their abilities to read and to give socially appropriate cues in order to join others in play, and gain an understanding of norms and expectations to guide socially appropriate behaviours (for example, obeying rules, sharing, being sensitive to others and their property and being trustworthy). Play influences the development of social competence and relationships with adults and peers (Guralnick et al., 1995; McArdle, 2001). Play also provides a major means for emotional regulation (Sroufe, 1996) enabling experimentation with actions and their emotional consequences.

The occupational role of player

Occupational therapists are concerned with the occupation of play and the child developing as a lifelong player. A case study illustrates the importance of the role of player and play as occupation, and describes some of the different contexts in which children engage in this dynamic role. Success in the player role provides meaningful occupational engagement, enhancing quality of life. Using an occupation based perspective, the occupational therapist observes, assesses, interprets and intervenes in the child's role performance as a player (Burke, 1998). While the occupational role of player remains throughout childhood, its expression, the time spent engaging in it and its function alters, as illustrated by the following case study.

Henry

For three-and-a-half-year-old Henry the role of player is his primary occupational role. As a player at home, in his high-rise inner city apartment, he enjoys building with Duplo™ blocks, playing with his train set, and playing with his cars in his toy garage set. At childcare, which he attends three days a week while his parents work, he is also a player and engages in different activities and games as part of the occupation of play. In this setting, he loves to be outside in the sandpit with the diggers and trucks, playing at the water trough and riding the tricycles. Sometimes he plays alone, or in parallel with others. He enjoys riding tricycles with the other boys and racing around the race track. Henry and his friends also dress up as super heroes, racing on the tricycles to various imaginary rescue scenes. When he visits his grandparents, his role of player is shaped by the games they play with him and the affordances of the physical environment. His grandfather bought a toy golf set which Henry plays with in the back garden. He imitates his grandfather's golf swing and places the plastic golf ball on small tees, while he watches Granddad practise his swing. There is also an old tree with low branches that he likes to climb, and some bushes which his grandmother lets him drape with old towels to make a 'cubby house'. His grandmother brings him snacks to eat in the cubby house with his favourite toy rabbit. She often squeezes in and has a tea party with him.

Across these three environments Henry's primary occupational role is player. In each, he engages in the occupation of play; however, he plays differently in each setting. There are different types of play – alone and with others (solitary, parallel, associative), as well as gross motor/physical, constructional, functional, object play and pretence. The role of player is important as it enables him to connect with peers at childcare (while learning social and communication skills) and grandparents (learning to relate to adults and learning through imitating and being provided with playful opportunities by play valuing adults). The role of player at home provides him with the opportunity to play alone, creating his own games, solving problems and learning how to amuse himself.

Throughout childhood the role of player also changes as play takes on different forms as a result of ongoing maturation and as the contexts change. In addition, the time spent in play changes as other occupational roles such as that of student dominate. At ten years for example, Henry is still an only child. He plays at home with his PlayStation™ and with computer games. He occasionally reads a book before bed, and sometimes listens to music. He collects and paints little toy soldiers, which he sets up in armies on a battlefield on the dining room table. Henry has a best mate, Jack, with whom he plays at school. Usually they go down to the oval at lunch-time to play football. Sometimes he and Jack go to the library to play chess on the computer. He goes to after school care every afternoon where he plays in the school playground. In particular, he enjoys shooting hoops at basketball, playing chasing games and handball. Henry's grandparents have moved to a retirement village. When he visits, he often takes over toy soldiers to paint or toys to fix in his grandfather's little workshop. He is making a small wooden boat, which is an ongoing project he works on with his grandfather. He plays basketball at the weekends in a club team.

This case study has illustrated how the type of play, the environments for play and choice and availability of playmates change throughout childhood. Occupational therapists must understand the personal and environmental factors, the role of player, the time required to engage in play themes and the occupation of play for a particular child at any given point in time, if they are to facilitate children's playful experiences and mastery of the role of player.

Many children experience challenges and barriers to their participation in play. The difficulties experienced by children with physical and developmental disabilities are well known (Brown & Gordon, 1987; Holaday et al., 1997; King et al., 2003; Mulderij, 1997; Richardson, 2002). There are, however, numerous other groups, such as children who live in poverty, children from orphanages, and children who are 'at risk' for academic and school adjustment difficulties who also may be deprived of play opportunities and experiences, and/or experience difficulties participating in play (Gagnon & Nagle, 2004; Taneja et al., 2002).

Enabling goodness of child–play–environment fit: optimizing participation

The occupational therapist addresses play performance issues in a systematic manner by using a frame of reference such as the PEO model (Law et al., 1996; Strong et al., 1999). The occupational performance of playing involves a complex, transactional relationship of the player (the person), the play activity (the occupation) and the context (the environment). There must be a goodness of fit or congruence in the person–environment–occupation (PEO) transaction to achieve optimal performance, such as an engaging playful experience. The role of the occupational

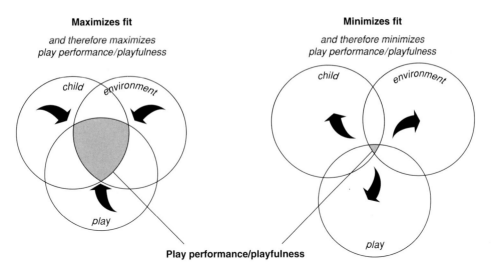

Maximizes fit

*and therefore maximizes
play performance/playfulness*

Minimizes fit

*and therefore minimizes
play performance/playfulness*

Play performance/playfulness

Figure 9.1 How the goodness of child–environment–play fit can optimize or minimize play performance and playfulness. Adapted from M. Law, B. Cooper, S. Strong, D. Stewart, P. Rigby & L. Letts (1996). The person–environment–occupation model: a transactive approach to occupational performance. *Canadian Journal of Occupational Therapy, 63,* 9–23. Reprinted with the permission of CAOT Publications ACE.

therapist, therefore, becomes one of developing children's abilities and potential for play, enabling participation in play, and advocating for cultural, social, temporal and physical environments that support play for children with or without disabilities (Rigby & Huggins, 2003). If the ultimate goal of intervention is to enable the child to achieve successful participation in play, therapists should focus on achieving goodness of child–play–environment fit.

Development of the PEO model was influenced by the Canadian occupational therapy guidelines for client centred practice (Canadian Association of Occupational Therapists, 2002b), theories of human ecology and person–environment behaviour, and by the theory of flow (Csikszentmihalyi, 1990). Three interacting spheres represent the main dimensions of the model (person, environment and occupation), and when the spheres overlap there is a goodness of PEO fit to optimize occupational performance. When the PEO fit is poor, occupational performance is hindered and is less than optimal. This is illustrated in Figure 9.1, which shows how these concepts are applied to a child's play performance and playfulness. We can assume that a child's play performance, like performance of other occupations, will be influenced by the relationship of the child's skills and interests, the barriers and supports in the play environment, and the challenges and appeal of the play activities.

The environment is broadly defined in this model to include institutional, socioeconomic, cultural, social and physical domains (Law et al., 1996). Each of these domains can be considered from the perspective of the individual, the household and the community. Occupational performance is influenced by and cannot be separated from the influences of the environment (Rigby & Letts, 2003). The PEO

model assists the occupational therapist to analyse problems in occupational performance, to plan and evaluate interventions, and to communicate occupational
therapy practices (Strong et al., 1999). Examples are provided in this section to
illustrate how the PEO model guides assessment and intervention practice to
enable children's participation in play and their expression of playfulness.

Using assessment to guide intervention

The selection of a play assessment will vary depending upon the purpose of the
assessment. Five assessments of play are described in Table 9.1. The assessment of
play is most often performed by observation in a familiar play environment.
Observation is considered to be an ecologically valid approach for collecting
information about a child's natural behaviours (Pellegrini, 2001). Play is what children like to do and they expend considerable social, cognitive and motor resources
while playing, therefore play assessment may provide very meaningful insights
about a child's interests, functional abilities and behaviours (Pellegrini, 2001).
Two scenarios are presented that describe typical applications of play assessments
to guide intervention.

Suzie: assessing development through play

Suzie is a recently adopted four-year-old who started attending an early childhood school
programme. Her adoptive parents are concerned about her play development, especially her social and symbolic play. One common purpose for selecting a play assessment is to assess play from a developmental perspective. The Knox preschool play scale
(PPS) (Knox, 1997) was used by the occupational therapist to gain a developmental
description of Suzie's play at nursery school. Suzie engaged in simple repetitive
sensorimotor play, preferring toys providing simple cause–effect. The summary of Suzie's
scored PPS was based on the following play observations at school.

In the space and material management section of the PPS, her interests, manipulation, construction and purpose in play were at a 12–18 month level, with a longer
attention span at an 18–24 month level. At the water play station, Suzie splashed
the water and watched her hand movement for several seconds, then picked up a
small bottle floating in the water and poured it out. She began to repeatedly
submerge the bottle to fill it with water and to pour it out again. After about five
minutes at the water table she moved over to the book centre and picked up a book
lying on the floor. She began flapping the pages holding it close to her face and
smiling. When Suzie moved to the playhouse, she began stacking plates and
moving them from one counter to the other. She played alongside two peers without initiating interaction; however, she paused several times to watch the actions
of the girl across from her. When she moved to the toy microwave, she opened
the door and removed a pot with a lid. She began putting it in and out of the
microwave, alternating with lifting the lid from the pot and peering inside. The

Table 9.1 Assessments of play.

Title	Author and source	Age and population	Purpose	Clinical utility
Knox preschool play scale	Available to copy from Knox (1997).	Any child; 0–6 years.	To describe child's play skills across four dimensions (space management, material management, pretence/symbolic and participation) from a developmental perspective.	Observations made during indoor and outdoor play; scored in six month increments from 0–3 years and yearly increments from 3–6 years.
Assessment of ludic behaviours	Included in Ferland (1997).	Preschool children with physical disability with or without cognitive disability.	To examine characteristics of a child's ludic attitude, play interests, skills and difficulties.	Uses both observation of child during free play, and structured parent interview.
Play history	Takata (1974); Behnke & Fetkovich (1984). Available to copy from Bryze (1997).	Infancy through adolescence; any diagnosis.	To explore child's play experiences and opportunities.	Semi-structured interview with parent or care-giver; covers current and previous play experiences.
Test of playfulness	Bundy et al., (2001). Available to copy from Bundy (1997).	All children, infancy through 15 years.	To examine four elements of playfulness: motivation, control, suspension of reality and framing play.	Observations made during free play; recommended to videotape 2 × 15–30 minute play segments (indoors and outdoors).
Trans-disciplinary play-based assessment	Included in Linder (1993).	0–6 years; developmental delays.	To utilize play observations for the purposes of assessing underlying developmental skills, learning style, interaction patterns and other behaviours.	Observations made by interdisciplinary team of developmental experts over 60–90 minutes. Play session has six phases including structured and unstructured play.

occupational therapist joined her there to explore her social participation and symbolic play further. The occupational therapist modelled a domestic scenario of stirring soup in another pot, scooping it into one of the bowls and pretending to eat the soup, saying 'Mmm hmm, good soup'. She scooped soup into a bowl and offered it to Suzie. Suzie set the bowl down and continued with her own actions. After a second attempt by the therapist, Suzie awkwardly imitated her actions and made appropriate mealtime sounds and verbal requests (for example, 'more soup'). The therapist offered soup to the girl Suzie had shown interest in, and she brought her doll over and began to feed it. The occupational therapist then facilitated an inter-active pretend scenario involving making food, feeding dolls and themselves. This scenario demonstrated that Suzie's pretence/symbolic play and participation were most like the 12–18 month level of the PPS, with emerging skills at the 18–24 month level.

The PPS provided a developmental description of Suzie's play, which helped in the selection of appropriate play activities and materials for Suzie at home and at school, to match her developmental play skills and provide a goodness of child–play–environment fit. The PPS also allowed the occupational therapist to use the concept of 'a zone of proximal development' (ZPD), introduced by Vygotsky (1978). He believed that children benefit from learning opportunities provided through interactive play with an adult who can model new play behaviours to help the child progress. In this case, the therapist used the ZPD to explore Suzie's capacity to interact socially with an adult and peer, and to use imitation and pretence. This approach focuses on the child's learning potential, and requires an awareness of emerging skills and interests, challenging the child to develop new and expanded competencies.

Kaisa: assessing and enabling playfulness

Another common purpose for play assessment is to assess the child's playfulness. Bundy operationally defined four key elements of playfulness in the test of playfulness (ToP) (Bundy, 1997; 1998; Bundy et al., 2001). In order for a child to express a playful attitude and approach, the play experience must allow a combination of intrinsic motivation, internal control, freedom to suspend reality, and success in reading and giving social cues, which frame the play, as shown in the playfulness profile in Figure 9.2. A desirable outcome for occupational therapy is to enable a child to express playfulness.

Kaisa is a five-year-old girl with cerebral palsy. She uses a walker for mobility. When the occupational therapist first used the ToP to assess Kaisa during designated playtime in her integrated kindergarten programme, she found that Kaisa's play performance was not playful (see Figure 9.2). Kaisa's aide had been directing her to play at a table with puzzles and blocks. She did not appear very interested in these activities. She kept turning her head to watch the play of a few girls at the doll centre. When some music was started, the aide brought Kaisa over to join a group of children who were marching in a circle, and singing and doing actions with the song. Kaisa initially sang along, but struggled to keep pace with her walker and soon collapsed on the floor and sat watching. She stopped singing, and was largely ignored by her peers.

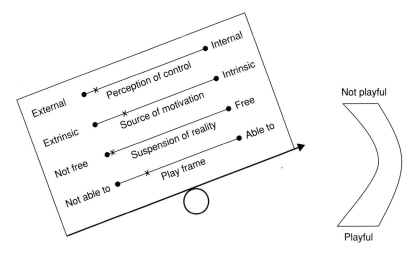

Figure 9.2 Playfulness profile for Kaisa. Reproduced from A. G. Fisher, E. A. Murray & A. C. Bundy (1991) (Eds) *Sensory integration: theory and practice.* Philadelphia: F. A. Davis Company. Reprinted with the permission of F. A. Davis Company.

The occupational therapist also used the form, Observations of Factors Influencing Playfulness (Rigby & Huggins, 2003), to analyse factors influencing Kaisa's playfulness, as shown in Figure 9.3. Based on this analysis of PEO fit in relation to the ToP domains and Kaisa's ToP score, she worked with the kindergarten teacher and the aide to try strategies in the classroom during play to better support Kaisa's playfulness. The goal was to achieve better PEO fit during play. The primary focus was to change the social environment to make it more responsive to what was interesting and motivating to her, and to foster Kaisa's initiative and self-direction during play. The occupational therapist modelled to the aide how to read Kaisa's social cues and to follow her lead, giving Kaisa choices and opportunities to engage in activities in which she appeared interested. This involved making play materials and activities more accessible to Kaisa and modifying some activities so that they better matched her abilities; these being changes to both the physical environment and to the play activities themselves. Using the role of play partner, the occupational therapist also modelled socially interactive play to Kaisa by first assisting her to physically access the doll centre, then by playing alongside Kaisa and her peers and facilitating social exchanges within a pretend play scenario.

When the ToP was readministered a few months later, Kaisa's playfulness profile and PEO fit analysis indicated that she was more playful at kindergarten and that the goodness of PEO fit had improved. The occupational therapist observed that Kaisa was free to choose where she wanted to play. Initially she watched three children playing at a toy garage. After several minutes she joined them, picked up a small doll and pretended that her doll was the 'child' and the doll of the girl beside her was the 'mum'. The girl was responsive and began interacting with Kaisa and her doll. The play theme at the garage shifted to be inclusive of the domestic family scenario that Kaisa had initiated. Three girls, including

Name of child: Kaisa
Where is play: Kindergarten classroom
Age: 6 years, 3 months
Who supervized play: Teacher aide
Date: 13 September, 2004
Time of day: 11:00–11:20 am

Brief description of context of play (the setting, the players, the activities and any occurrences preceding the play observation): Play takes place during free play time in the kindergarten curriculum. An educational aide is assigned to work with Kaisa throughout the morning and provides her with constant one:one assistance, direction and attention.

ToP elements	Factors influencing person-environment-occupation fit	Promote playfulness	Hinder playfulness
Intrinsic motivation (engaged; process; affect; persists; obj; interaction)	— Kaisa watched peers play at doll centre and appeared interested in their play. — Peers ignored Kaisa while they marched to music. — Kaisa struggled with walker during marching and collapsed to sit and watch peers march.	✓	✓✓
Internal control (decides; safe; modifies; challenges; initiates; enters; supports; negotiates; shares)	— Aide directed Kaisa to play with puzzles and blocks. — Aide took Kaisa to march to music with children in circle. — Kaisa was an onlooker of the play and activities of other players. She did not initiate joining them.		✓✓✓
Suspension of reality (mischief; tease; clowns/jokes; pretends; unconventional)	— More potential for suspension of reality with block play than with puzzles. — Aide took approach of instructing Kaisa through completion of puzzles and block construction; focus was on structured learning. — Activity of marching to music has potential to allow suspension of reality. — Kaisa's focus was on physical aspect of this activity.	✓ ✓	✓
Framing play (transitions; responds; gives cues)	— Aide ignored or was not aware of Kaisa's cues that she was interested in the play at the doll centre. — Peers did not give Kaisa any cues that were welcoming or encouraging during the marching activity.		✓

Summary:
Recommendations:

Figure 9.3 Factors influencing Kaisa's play performance using the Observations of Factors Influencing Playfulness Form. Reproduced from L. Letts, P. Rigby, & D. Stewart (Eds.) (2003). *Using environments to enable occupational performance*. Thorofare, NJ: Slack Incorporated.

Kaisa, became very engaged in the doll interactions. The girls shared a close physical proximity, the dolls were easy to manipulate, and the garage involved a range of skills, enabling Kaisa to participate to the extent of her physical abilities, while the other girls challenged themselves to manipulate the small parts to further the actions within the pretend scenario. The aide was less directly involved in Kaisa's play and provided physical help as needed, and acted as a play partner from time to time to bridge or further the play.

Parents, who have the resources to do so, can be invited to videotape their child during play time at home (including both indoor and outdoor play) or in the community, to bring in for analysis by the occupational therapist with an assessment such as the ToP and/or the Knox PPS, and the PEO analysis of the play transactions. The therapist would provide the parent(s) with instructions for the taped play sessions, based on the criteria for the play session described in the chosen play assessment. Using videotape(s) made by parents is a useful strategy as this can open a dialogue with the parents about their observations of the child–play–environment fit together with the therapist's observations, which can lead to collaboration in examining what is helping and hindering play, and how to better support the child's play participation.

Ensuring the right conditions for play: assessing barriers and supports

Playfulness is not a stable trait of the child, and the expression of playfulness, through behaviours observed during play, can differ considerably from one setting to the next (Rigby & Gaik, in press [a]). In a study involving 16 children with cerebral palsy, playfulness scores varied significantly across three different environments (Rigby & Gaik, in press [a]). Many of these children demonstrated the capacity to be quite playful in one or more settings, while they were not playful in others. They were more playful at home and least playful during playtime at school. The tapes made for this study were viewed again for the purposes of a qualitative analysis of the child–play–environment relationship (Rigby & Gaik, in press [b]). The thematic analysis highlighted that the children's play was influenced by the goodness of fit between the child's interests and abilities, and characteristics of the play activity and the environment. Figure 9.4 illustrates how the child–environment–play relationship varied across the three settings.

These findings suggest that some settings and play activities can provide a better match with a child's abilities and interests. The child–environment–play analysis would naturally lead to the identification of strategies for interventions to enable the child's play participation. The occupational therapist can identify what is engaging a child in play, and what is supporting the play in one setting and apply this knowledge to another. Intervention (for example making accommodations for the child; removing barriers; utilizing assistive technologies) can enhance play performance and participation.

Occupational therapists can use their occupational performance analysis skills, which includes analysis of the steps of an activity, and the physical, cognitive and

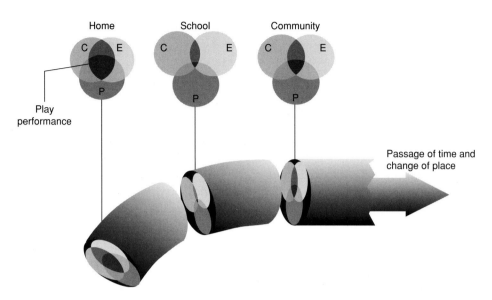

Figure 9.4 Variations in goodness of child–environment–play fit across three different settings: home, school and community. Adapted from M. Law, B. Cooper, S. Strong, D. Stewart, P. Rigby, & L. Letts (1996). The person–environment–occupation model: a transactive approach to occupational performance. *Canadian Journal of Occupational Therapy*, 63, 9–23. Reprinted with the permission of CAOT Publications ACE.

social demands of the activity, to conduct this analysis. Some therapists refer to this process as 'task' analysis (for a good resource on task analysis see Watson & Wilson, 2003). *Observations of factors influencing playfulness* (Rigby & Huggins, 2003) is a useful tool for organizing and focusing this analysis of play. This form contains questions such as:

- What does the child appear interested in?
- What appears to be motivating for the child? Motivating factors are typically social, sensory, or object-related.
- What is hindering the child's participation?
- Do the child's skills match the demands and challenges of the play activities?
- Is the child able to access play activities and play materials that they are interested in, that are integral to the play theme and that can extend and further the play theme?
- Are there choices and opportunities available to the child? How is the play theme supported? How are the players supported?

Enabling optimal child–environment–play fit

The child
The goodness of child–environment–play activity fit is crucial to a successful play exchange (Rigby & Gaik, in press [b]; Rigby & Huggins, 2003). The child's level

of developmental maturity, skills, abilities and emotional self-regulation (to moderate behaviours) are important components of the fit equation. Equally important is the child's motivation to participate in the play activity. The child must show interest and want to participate for play to happen. Motivation can arise from the child's curiosity and desire to explore the setting and the play possibilities, and it can be based on the child's familiarity with the other players and play activities. There are many aspects of the play activity itself and the play context that can be motivating for the child and enhance the child's eagerness to engage in play. Bundy considers motivation as a key element of playfulness and central to the test of environmental supportiveness that examines the characteristics of the play environment (including temporal aspects) in relation to the child's experience of playfulness (Bronson & Bundy, 2001; Bundy, 1999).

The play environment

Key examples of strategies to support children's participation in play are presented at various environmental levels in Table 9.2. First, play must be valued and supported at a societal and systems level so that children of various backgrounds, ages and abilities have access to motivating and appealing play opportunities. The document, *A world fit for children*, developed by UNICEF (2002) outlined a number of policy recommendations to ensure that play is central among the needs and rights of children everywhere. Ensuring that children have ready access to safe, supported play opportunities can be enormously challenging, particularly in times of war, poverty and natural disasters. In post-industrial societies, urban growth creates increased traffic, housing density, longer parental absences (for commuting and demanding jobs) and increased risk of crime, all of which can reduce adequately supervised, safe residential play spaces (McArdle, 2001). Thus, governments and communities must make commitments to increase resources for children's play. The occupational therapist can be involved in community planning as well as advocacy roles at the institutional level.

Child centred, play based programmes have been widely adopted at an institutional level (Bredekamp & Copple, 1997; Shipley, 2002). Programmes adopting a child centred approach, in which care providers were sensitive and responsive to children, were associated with more sociable and attentive children who displayed better thinking skills (Peisner-Feinberg et al., 2001), independence and playfulness (Mahoney & Powell, 1998; Rigby & Gaik, in press [a]). In play settings children need to know the rules and expectations for their behaviours, and to feel safe, accepted, and encouraged to explore and to actively engage in interactive play.

In terms of the *cultural environment*, some authors have suggested that while the content and themes of play may differ across cultures, the type of play may not be that different (for example Ramsey, 1998). Some types of play may be more culturally sensitive. For example, socio-dramatic play is more likely to reflect these differences due to the shared language or cultural knowledge which is reflected in play themes. Gender and socio-economic status also interact with culture to influence the way in which children play. Most research and writing about play espouses a western perspective. The primacy of the occupation of play in

Table 9.2 Using the environment to support the play of children with varying abilities.

Environmental level	Examples of strategies that support children's participation in play
Systems level: policy	From *World fit for children* (UNICEF, 2002): — Make commitment to value play, acknowledging that: (a) Play is central among the needs and rights of children (b) It is integral to family and community life Ensure that children have daily access to safe, stimulating play opportunities; establish programmes for professionals and parents about the benefits of play and how to create opportunities for play. — Design physically accessible play spaces. — Develop recreational games and activities that are inclusive of all children and their needs, respecting that children of various ages will have different interests and abilities. — Provide resources and support to programmes to enable them to facilitate the participation of all children. — Create infrastructure in communities in order to build and maintain play spaces and recreational opportunities that are safe and accessible (such as in urban environments, there is need for traffic control and supervision of play spaces) (McArdle, 2001).
Institutional rules and practices	— Adopt a child centred approach; instruct care-providers on how to be sensitive and responsive to children's needs and play cues. — Create rules and boundaries for play, so children clearly understand what they have permission to do and to use in their play. Create an environment that is safe, accepting, respectful and encouraging of play. Allow enough time so children can develop play themes and interactive relationships (this often takes more than 30 minutes). — Design play spaces, play and recreational programmes to ensure all children have access to developmentally appropriate play opportunities, and have experiences tailored to individual differences (Brazelton & Greenspan, 2000).
Cultural environment	— Creating attitudes that play is valued and an important part of a child's daily life, thereby making time in child's schedule for child centred, child directed play (Bredecamp & Copple, 1997). — Ensure that children feel safe, welcomed and have permission to use play materials and play equipment, and direct their own play.

Social environment: adults	— Adult play partners can provide scaffolding for play by making play space and resources available, and by playing alongside children to facilitate social exchanges and development of play theme. Adults must be observant of the children's play cues and the development of the play theme, and provide assistance unobtrusively, so as not to disrupt play interactions and the developing play theme. Adults can enable social interactions amongst groups of children by facilitating and supporting the reading and giving of social cues during group play and by modelling appropriate social behaviours.
	— Adults should get down to child's level and play alongside child; follow child's lead and pace, play to child's tempo, giving child time to respond and interact before helping child.
Social environment: peer players	— Create opportunities for peers to play together or alongside each other and in close physical proximity; create opportunities for integration of children with special needs with their typically developing peers (Richardson, 2002).
	— Create opportunities for children with special needs to reciprocate and provide help to peers, rather than only receiving assistance from others (Richardson, 2002).
	— Create opportunities for children of same gender to play together.
Physical environment	— Create safe physical settings in which dangerous, unsafe furniture, equipment and materials are removed (play materials must be repaired, maintained or replaced to ensure that they are safe).
	— Create play spaces with appropriately sized furniture, equipment and materials for targeted age groups (for example what's appropriate for toddlers or preschool-aged children will differ from what school-aged children use).
	— Use diverse types of equipment that support various forms of play, with graduated levels of challenge, and those that afford numerous opportunities for social interaction (for example materials that support sensory exploration, construction, dramatic and social play) (Barbour, 1999).
	— Use assistive technologies and adapted or modified play equipment/materials to support play.
	— Use enclosed space, or structure the space with physical barriers to enable children with physical disabilities to remain physically proximal to their peers during play. Materials that don't roll or slide away are preferred.
	— Children with special needs may prefer familiar toys and activities in unfamiliar environments and new, novel play materials are better introduced in familiar environments (Rigby & Gaik, in press [b]).

childhood may well be a western-held belief. Some recent studies (for example Bazyk et al., 2003) have challenged occupational therapists' widely held belief that 'play is a child's major occupation', in relation to the play of children from various minority cultures. Their study of Mayan children demonstrated that parental values and customs of child rearing and views of the primacy of adult work influenced children's occupations. In this society, parents did not encourage play but permitted it if it did not interfere with work. Despite this, children found ways to integrate play activities and playfulness into their daily occupations. This study highlighted the need to be aware of parents' and teachers' cultural beliefs and the impact of this on the physical and social settings and experiences provided.

With respect to the *social environment*, it is preferable that other children are included, to provide opportunities for interactive, social play. Adults, however, have important roles for facilitating play. They provide play opportunities by structuring time and places to play, and providing resources for play. They provide supervision without intruding or directing, and can support play through their role of play partner (Rigby & Huggins, 2003). The play partner plays with the child or group of children with the goal of facilitating play and social interaction. Some strategies about doing this have been described already and will be developed further in the next section when describing flow (Csikszentmihalyi, 1997). Care providers can also be taught how to be successful play partners (Rigby & Huggins, 2003).

Environments that encourage interactive peer play are developmentally important. Gagnon & Nagle (2004) established that there is a relationship between peer play and social-emotional development. Preschool children who played together with or alongside and proximal to peers, demonstrated higher levels of positive social relations and less teacher reported behaviour problems (van den Oord & Rispens, 1999). Occupational therapists can facilitate peer relationships in play through adopting the role of play partner and through intervening with groups of children, rather than working exclusively with individuals. For example, when providing direct service to a child with a disability, the occupational therapist could invite the child's sibling(s) or another child with similar abilities (and interests) to join in.

Physical features of the environment can be either barriers or resources for play. Ideally, the space and play materials should be accessible to the children for whom the play setting was designed. Barbour (1999) discovered a number of playground/playroom features that supported children with varying abilities to play together. These included: diverse types of equipment that supported various forms of play, those that had graduated levels of challenge, and those that afforded numerous opportunities for social interaction (for example materials that supported sensory exploration and construction, dramatic and social play). Rigby & Gaik (in press [b]) found that it was easier for children with physical disabilities to play in close proximity with their peers in enclosed spaces. In open spaces, they had difficulty keeping up with the movement of their typically developing peers. Adaptive play materials, equipment and assistive technologies designed for children with disabilities can be modified by occupational therapists to meet the specific needs of children with varying abilities (Rigby & Huggins, 2003).

Play activities

Features of play activities themselves are also critical to the child–play–environment fit equation. Features that can be manipulated, adapted and modified allow for better child – activity fit. Toys and play materials that are multi-purpose (can be used in many ways) and unstructured (for example blocks, boxes, dolls, play dough, paper and crayons) encourage play that children can control and shape to express their creativity and problem solving abilities. Children can use toys repeatedly in many different ways without getting bored. It is important to choose play activities that are appropriate to the child's age or developmental level. A child's play is creative when it grows out of their daily life, and reflects their experiences (for example playing house, imitating familiar characters from movies and TV).

Csikszentmihalyi's construct of flow (1990; 1997) is useful to apply to the child–play environment analysis. Flow happens when one is immersed and totally absorbed in what one is doing, and is an experience of harmony. This description is consistent with the concepts of PEO fit enabling optimal occupational performance. In order to experience flow, there must be goodness of fit between the challenges of the activity and the skills of the individual (Csikszentmihalyi, 1997). When challenge is high in relation to low skills, anxiety is experienced. When challenge is low, in relation to high skills, boredom may be experienced. An important concept of flow is the benefit of achieving arousal, or increased concentration, focus and involvement with what one is doing. This happens when challenges slightly exceed skills. This will enable the child to achieve a sense of control in the doing. When the level of play skill matches the level of challenge we call this the 'just right challenge' for facilitating play skills.

The occupational therapist is well equipped to grade the level of challenge of activities to ensure goodness of child–activity fit and to enable flow. Occupational analysis can help the occupational therapist to identify how to grade the activity appropriately to match the skill set, interests and motivations of the child. The occupational therapist may introduce a modified approach to the play activity, or strategies to allow for compensation, or assistive technologies to support the child's participation in play. As the child engages in the play and gains confidence as a player, challenges can be introduced to keep the play stimulating and enable further mastery.

Summary

This chapter has focused on the importance of childhood play and examined child–environment–play fit to optimize children's participation. Play is a primary occupation of childhood and we have emphasized the critical role occupational therapists have in enabling children to play and be playful. A systematic approach to the assessment and development of intervention strategies has been presented with reference to the PEO model (Law et al., 1996). Clinical reasoning enables integration of assessment with intervention to ensure better child–environment–play fit. The physical, social, cultural environment and expectations must be considered when both assessing and supporting children's play. Modifying barriers, helping the child to acquire play skills or compensate for specific deficits, and providing appropriate play activities and materials may all be required to enable children's development as players.

References

Barbour, A. C. (1999). The impact of playground design on the play behaviours of children with differing levels of physical competence. *Early Childhood Research Quarterly, 14* (1), 75–98.

Bazyk, S., Stalnaker, D., Llerena, M., Ekelman, B. & Bazyk, J. (2003). Play in Mayan children. *American Journal of Occupational Therapy, 57,* 273–283.

Behnke, C. & Fetkovich, M. M. (1984). Examining the reliability and validity of the play history. *American Journal of Occupational Therapy, 38,* 94–100.

Brazelton, T. B. & Greenspan, S. I. (2000). *The irreducible needs of children: what every child must have to grow, learn and flourish.* Boulder, CO: Perseus Pub.

Bredekamp, S. & Copple, C. (Eds.) (1997). *Developmentally appropriate practice in early childhood programs serving children from birth through age eight* (Rev. ed.). Washington DC: National Association for the Education of Young Children.

Bronson, M. J. & Bundy, A. (2001). A correlational study of a test of playfulness and a test of environmental supportiveness for play. *Occupational Therapy Journal of Research, 21,* 241–259.

Brown, M. & Gordon, W. A. (1987). Impact of impairment on activity patterns of children. *Archives of Physical Medicine and Rehabilitation, 68,* 828–832.

Bryze, K. (1997). Narrative contributions to the play history. In: L. D. Parham & L. S. Fazio (Eds.), *Play in occupational therapy for children* (pp. 23–34). St Louis, MO: C. V. Mosby.

Bundy, A. (1991). Play theory and sensory integration. In: A. G. Fisher, E. A. Murray & A. C. Bundy (Eds.), *Sensory integration: theory and Practice* (pp. 46–68). Philadelphia: F. A. Davis.

Bundy, A. C. (1993). Assessment of play and leisure: delineation of the problem. *American Journal of Occupational Therapy, 47* (3), 217–222.

Bundy, A. C. (1997). Play and playfulness: What to look for. In: L. D. Parham & L. S. Fazio (Eds.), *Play in occupational therapy for children* (pp. 52–66). St Louis, MO: Mosby-Year Book Inc.

Bundy, A. C. (1998). *Test of playfulness (ToP): research version 3.5.* Ft Collins, CO: Colorado State University, Department of Occupational Therapy.

Bundy, A. C. (1999). *Test of environmental supportiveness.* Ft Collins, CO: Colorado State University.

Bundy, A., Nelson, L., Metzger, M. & Bingaman, K. (2001). Validity and reliability of a test of playfulness. *Occupational Therapy Journal of Research, 21* (4), 276–292.

Burke, J. (1998). The life role of the infant and young child. In: J. Case-Smith (Ed.), *Pediatric occupational therapy and early intervention* (2nd ed., pp. 189–206). Boston, MA: Butterworth-Heinemann.

Canadian Association of Occupational Therapists (2002a). *Enabling occupation: an occupational therapy perspective.* Ottawa, Ont.: CAOT Publications ACE.

Canadian Association of Occupational Therapists (2002b). *Profile of occupational therapy practice in Canada* (2nd ed.). Ottawa, Ont.: CAOT Publications ACE.

Csikszentmihalyi, M. (1990). *Flow: the psychology of optimal experience*. New York: Harper Perennial.

Csikszentmihalyi, M. (1997). *Finding flow: the psychology of engagement with everyday life*. New York: BasicBooks.

Ferland, F. (1997). *Play, children with physical disabilities and occupational therapy: the Ludic model*. Ottawa, Ont.: University of Ottawa.

Freysinger, V. J. (1998). Play in the context of lifespan human development. In: D. P. Fromberg & D. Bergen (Eds.), *Play from birth to twelve and beyond* (pp. 14–22). London: Garland Publishing, Inc.

Gagnon, S. G. & Nagle, R. J. (2004). Relationships between peer interactive play and social competence in at-risk preschool children. *Psychology in the schools*, 41 (2), 173–189.

Guddemi, M., Jambor, T. & Moore, R. (1998). Advocacy for the child's right to play. In: D. P. Fromberg & D. Bergen (Eds.), *Play from birth to twelve and beyond* (pp. 519–529). London: Garland Publishing, Inc.

Guralnick, M. J., Connor, R. T., Hammond, M., Gottman, J. M. & Kinnish, K. (1995). Immediate effects of mainstreamed settings on the social interactions and social integration of preschool children. *American Journal on Mental Retardation*, 100 (4), 359–377.

Hanline, M. F. (1999). Developing a preschool play-based curriculum. *International Journal of Disability, Development and Education*, 46, 289–305.

Holaday, B., Swan, J. H. & Turner-Henson, A. (1997). Images of the neighborhood and activity patterns of chronically ill school age children. *Environment and Behavior*, 29 (3), 348–373.

King, G., Law, M., King, S., Rosenbaum, P., Kertoy, M. K. & Young, N. L. (2003). A conceptual model of the factors affecting the recreation and leisure participation of children with disabilities. *Physical and Occupational Therapy in Pediatrics*, 23 (1), 63–90.

Knox, S. (1997). Development and current use of the Knox preschool play scale. In: L. D. Parham & L. S. Fazio (Eds.), *Play in occupational therapy for children* (pp. 35–51). St. Louis, Mo.: Mosby-Year Book Inc.

Law, M., Cooper, B., Strong, S., Stewart, D., Rigby, P. & Letts, L. (1996). The person-environment-occupation model: a transactive approach to occupational performance. *Canadian Journal of Occupational Therapy*, 63 (1), 9–23.

Letts, L., Rigby, P. & Stewart, D. (Eds.) (2003). *Using environments to enable occupational performance*. Thorofare, NJ: Slack Incorporated.

Lieberman, J. N. (1977). *Playfulness: its relationship to imagination and creativity*. New York: Academic Press.

Linder, T. W. (1993). *Trans-disciplinary play-based assessment: a functional approach to working with young children* (Rev. ed.). Baltimore, MD: Paul H. Brookes.

McArdle, R. (2001). Children's play. *Child: Care, Health and Development*, 27 (6), 509–514.

Mahoney, G. & Powell, A. (1998). Modifying parent–child interaction: enhancing the development of handicapped children. *Journal of Special Education*, 22, 82–96.

Manning, M. L. (1998). Play development from ages eight to twelve. In: D. P. Fromberg & D. Bergen (Eds.), *Play from birth to twelve and beyond* (pp. 154–161). London: Garland Publishing, Inc.

Mulderij, K. J. (1997). Peer relations and friendship in physically disabled children. *Child: Care, Health and Development*, 23, 379–389.

van den Oord, E. J. C. G. & Rispens, J. (1999). Differences between school classes in preschoolers' psychosocial adjustment: evidence for the importance of children's interpersonal relations. *Journal of Child Psychology and Psychiatry*, 40 (3), 417–430.

Peisner-Feinberg, E. S., Burchinal, M. R., Clifford, R. M., Culkin, M. L., Howes, C., Kagan, S. L., et al. (2001). The relation of preschool childcare quality to children's cognitive and social developmental trajectories through second grade. *Child Development, 72,* 1534–1553.

Pellegrini, A. D. (2001). Practitioner review: the role of direct observation in the assessment of young children. *Journal of Child Psychology and Psychiatry, 42* (7), 861–869.

Provenzo Jr, E. F. (1998). Electronically mediated playscapes. In: D. P. Fromberg & D. Bergen (Eds.), *Play from birth to twelve and beyond* (pp. 513–518). London: Garland Publishing, Inc.

Ramsey, P. G. (1998). Diversity and play: influences of race, culture, class and gender. In: D. P. Fromberg & D. Bergen (Eds.), *Play from birth to twelve and beyond* (pp. 23–33). London: Garland Publishing, Inc.

Richardson, P. K. (2002). The school as social context: social interaction patterns of children with physical disabilities. *American Journal of Occupational Therapy, 56,* 296–304.

Rigby, P. & Huggins, L. (2003). Enabling young children to play by creating supportive environments. In: L. Letts, P. Rigby & D. Stewart (Eds.), *Using environments to enable occupational performance* (pp. 155–175). Thorofare, NJ: Slack Incorporated.

Rigby, P. & Letts, L. (2003). Environment and occupational performance: theoretical considerations. In: L. Letts, P. Rigby & D. Stewart (Eds.), *Using environments to enable occupational performance* (pp. 17–32). Thorofare, NJ: Slack Incorporated.

Rigby, P. & Gaik, S. (in press [a]). Stability of playfulness across environmental settings: a pilot study. *Physical and Occupational Therapy in Pediatrics.*

Rigby, P. & Gaik, S. (in press [b]). An exploration of child–play–environment fit for children with physical disabilities. Manuscript submitted for publication.

Rubin, K. H., Fein, G. G. & Vandenberg, B. (1983). Play. In: P. Mussen & E. M. Hetherington (Eds.), *Handbook of child psychology. socialization, personality and social development* (4th ed., Vol. 4). New York, NY: John Wiley.

Save the Children Canada (2000). *United Nations convention on the rights of children, articles 2, 3, 12, 23, 31.* Retrieved 10 February 2005 from http://www.savethechildren.ca/en/whoweare/whounrights.html

Shipley, D. (2002). *Empowering children: play-based curriculum for lifelong learning* (3rd ed.). Toronto: Thomson Nelson.

Sroufe, L. A. (1996). *Emotional development: the organization of emotional life in the early years.* New York: Cambridge University Press.

Strong, S., Rigby, P., Law, M., Cooper, B., Letts, L. & Stewart, D. (1999). Application of the person–environment–occupation model: a practical tool. *Canadian Journal of Occupational Therapy, 66* (3), 122–133.

Sturgess, J. (2003). A model describing play as a child-chosen activity: is this still valid in contemporary Australia? *Australian Occupational Therapy Journal, 50* (2), 104–108.

Sturgess, J., Rodger, S. & Ozanne, A. (2002). A review of the use of self-report assessment with young children. *British Journal of Occupational Therapy, 65,* 108–116.

Takata, N. (1974). Play as a prescription. In: M. Reilly (Ed.), *Play as exploratory learning* (pp. 209–246). Beverly Hills, CA: Sage.

Taneja, V., Sriram, S., Beri, R. S., Sreenivas, V., Aggarwal, R., Kaur, R., et al. (2002). 'Not by bread alone': impact of a structured 90-minute play session on development of children in an orphanage. *Child: Care, Health and Development, 28,* 95–100.

UNICEF (2002). *A world fit for children.* Retrieved 10 February 2005 from http://www.unicef.org/publications/files/pub_wffc_en.pdf

Vygotsky, L. S. (1978). Mind in society: the development of higher mental processes. In: M. Cole, V. John-Streiner & S. S. E. Souberman (Eds.), *Mind in society*. Cambridge MA: Harvard University Press.

Watson, D. E. & Wilson, S. A. (2003). *Task analysis: an individualized and population approach* (2nd ed.). Bethesda, MD: AOTA Press.

World Health Organization (2001). *International classification of functioning, disability and health*. Geneva: World Health Organization.

Chapter 10

I CAN DO IT: DEVELOPING, PROMOTING AND MANAGING CHILDREN'S SELF-CARE NEEDS

Sylvia Rodger and G. Ted Brown

During the first decade of life, children develop from being totally dependent on their parents/care-givers for all their self-care needs to becoming independent in looking after themselves. In fact, by five to six years of age most children are able to look after their own self-care needs sufficiently to manage on their own at school for approximately six hours a day. At school entry, most typically developing children can manage their toileting and personal hygiene routines, eat lunch on their own, and dress and undress for physical education or swimming lessons.

By the end of middle childhood (that is by 12 years of age) parents are usually no longer involved with any of the self-care routines of typically developing children. Most children at this age start to assert their right to privacy when completing self-care tasks. For the most part, they are choosing their own clothes, have decided what they like and do not like to eat, and have established their own personal hygiene routines.

Self-care activities can be divided into basic activities of daily living, known as BADL, and instrumental activities of daily living, known as IADL (American Occupational Therapy Association, 2002). BADL refer to personal care activities that are oriented to taking care of one's own body (including eating, drinking, dressing, grooming/hygiene, functional mobility, sleep/rest and toileting) (Perr, 2004). IADL refer to those activities undertaken to look after oneself in one's family, the community and at school. These activities are oriented towards interacting with the environment, and are frequently complex (Law et al., 2001). Children complete IADL as they become involved as part of a family and learn to take responsibility for chores and household maintenance, such as taking out the garbage, shopping, making their own beds, caring for pets, completing yard work, clearing up and washing dishes, placing laundry in the hamper, using the telephone and other communication devices, catching public transport, financial management (pocket money) and making themselves a snack (Christiansen & Matuska, 2004).

As a result of increased independence in looking after and taking responsibility for themselves, children develop a sense of autonomy and self-efficacy. Autonomy refers to the individual's self-efficacy, self-identity, independence and ability to manage their own care (Porr & Rainville, 1999). Developing this ability to look after one's own needs enables children to master the important occupational roles of self-carer and self-maintainer (Canadian Association of Occupational Therapists, 1997).

Many disorders experienced by children impact on their ability to develop and master self-care tasks and routines (such as developmental coordination disorder, cerebral palsy, spina bifida, Down's syndrome, autism spectrum disorder, muscular dystrophy, limb deficiency, juvenile idiopathic arthritis). Difficulty with self-care is frequently a reason for referral of children for occupational therapy services in medical, educational and community settings (Hong & Howard, 2002). Occupational therapists are recognized for their ability to problem solve self-care difficulties (Christiansen & Matuska, 2004). In this chapter we aim to highlight the occupational therapy process of assessment and management of children's self-care issues. A case study will be used to illustrate the potential self-care challenges present for children at various developmental levels between infancy and the end of middle childhood using the *International Classification of Functioning, Disability and Health* (ICF) (World Health Organization, 2001) model as a framework. The objectives of this chapter are as follows:

(1) To describe children's self-care skills (both BADL and IADL)
(2) To provide a brief overview of the typical development of children's self-care skills from 0–12 years of age
(3) To apply the ICF model to one health condition which impacts on children's self-care skills from the toddler years through to early adolescence
(4) To demonstrate how occupational therapy management of self-care challenges enables children's optimal participation
(5) To describe the importance of self-management of BADL and IADL for the development of autonomy, self-efficacy and life satisfaction

Children's self-care skills

Activities of daily living refer to tasks related to personal care and self-maintenance. BADL refers to 'activities at home and in the community designed to enable basic survival and wellbeing' (Christiansen & Matuska, 2004, p. 3). They are often related to the care of one's own body and include bathing/showering, bowel and bladder management, dressing, eating, feeding, functional mobility, personal device care, personal hygiene and grooming, sleep, rest and toilet hygiene. IADL involve tasks related to interacting with the environment and are optional in nature, inferring that they can be delegated to another individual (American Occupational Therapy Association, 2002).

It has been reported that adults spend approximately 10% to 15% of their total waking day completing BADL and IADL (Harvey & Pentland, 2004). Children, and more specifically children with disabilities, spend a larger proportion of their waking hours than adults participating in or being assisted to complete their BADL and IADL (Barnes & Case-Smith, 2004). The younger the child, the more assistance and supervision required. As children develop, the level of sophistication and expectations of their BADL and IADL will also increase. It is beyond the scope of this chapter to provide detailed lists of specific self-care milestones. The paediatric occupational therapy textbook edited by Case-Smith (2002) and the book chapter by Barnes & Case-Smith (2004) provide overviews of the development of self-care skills in children. Readers are also referred to *Vineland Adaptive Behavior Scales* (Sparrow et al., 1984), *Pediatric Evaluation of Disability Inventory* (Haley et al., 1992), *Hawaii Early Learning Profile* (Furuno et al., 1985), and *Battelle Developmental Inventory* (Newborg et al., 1984) for detailed overviews of children's self-care skill development. Specific types of BADL and IADL in which children engage, as well as examples at three age levels (toddlerhood, early school-age, and pre-adolescence), are listed in Tables 10.1 and 10.2.

Managing ADL challenges: optimizing children's self-care participation

When dealing with children's self-care skills, it is essential for occupational therapists to be knowledgeable about normal development and how performance skills and patterns develop within childhood contexts. Two other important elements in relation to self-care skills are the social and cultural context of a child's family (including structure, values, roles, routines) and a child's physical living environments of childcare, home, school and community (American Occupational Therapy Association, 2002). Other factors that impact on children's self-care skills include a child's sensory, motor, cognitive and psychosocial abilities (Barnes & Case-Smith, 2004). These need to be considered when assessing and planning intervention related to children's self-care needs.

Before implementing any intervention strategy, it is important to establish a baseline of a child's self-care skills through assessment. There are a variety of methods for obtaining relevant information, including parental/care-giver or teacher interview, informal clinical observations and using standardized evaluation tools. Establishing what is important to the child and their parents in terms of the child's self-care participation will facilitate their engagement in the assessment and intervention process. This is one of the hallmarks of client and family-centred practice (Canadian Association of Occupational Therapists, 1997).

A number of self-care instruments with established psychometric properties, consistent with the ICF framework, that measure BADL and IADL are available for use with children. These include the Pediatric Evaluation of Disability Inventory (PEDI) (Haley et al., 1992), the Functional Independence Measure for Children (WeeFIM) (System, 1990), Activities Scales for Kids (ASK) (Young, 1996), the Child Health Questionnaire (CHQ) (Landgraf et al., 1996), the Canadian Occupational Performance Measure (COPM) (Law et al., 1998), Vineland Adaptive Behavior Scales (VABS) (Sparrow et al., 1984), and the Adaptive Behavior Assessment System (ABAS) (Harrison & Oakland, 2000). An overview of these assessment tools (domains assessed, age range, environments, administration, time, reliability, validity and measurement method) is provided in Table 10.3.

Table 10.1 Basic activities of daily living (BADL) for children.

Specific BADL tasks	Definition*	Childhood examples
Bathing, showering	Obtaining and using supplies (such as soap, shampoo); washing body parts; maintaining bathing position in tub; transferring to and from bathing positions in tub or shower.	**Toddler:** bath or shower with parental supervision; playing with wet cloth or water toys. **Early school-age:** bath or shower with parental supervision; soaping and rinsing body parts; getting in and out of bath independently; applying shampoo and rinsing hair with parental supervision. **Pre-adolescent:** having daily shower by self; washing with soap; getting in and out of shower independently; drying self with towel.
Bowel and bladder management	Complete, conscious control of bowel and bladder movements.	**Toddler:** wears diaper/nappy to bed over night; tells parent when diaper/nappy is wet or soiled by pointing, vocalizing or pulling at nappy/diaper; tells parent or indicates when they have had a bowel movement; learning voluntary control of bladder and bowel; starting to urinate and defecate using potty or toilet; starting to ask to use toilet. **Early school-age:** is dry over night; has regular bowel movement routine established; will take self to toilet when has urge to urinate or defecate; wipes self, flushes toilet; and washes hands. **Pre-adolescent:** is continent of bowel and bladder; takes self to toilet when has urge to urinate or defecate; wipes self and flushes toilet independently; undoes and fastens clothing as required.
Dressing	Selection of clothes and accessories suitable for time of day, weather and occasion; dressing and undressing; fastening and adjusting clothing; putting on and taking off shoes; washing and drying clothes.	**Toddler:** assists with putting arms and legs through shirts and pants; inserts feet into loose shoes; removes front opening coat, jacket or shirt without assistance; may be able to put on pull-up clothes with elastic waistbands. **Early school-age:** chooses clothing to wear, dresses self; pulls on shoes; may require assistance with buttons, zippers and snaps; puts shoes on correct feet with assistance; may not be able to tie shoe laces. **Pre-adolescent:** dresses independently; chooses what clothes to wear; ties shoe laces; does up buttons and zippers; has well developed sense of clothing preferences and fashion.

(Continued)

Table 10.1 (cont'd)

Specific BADL tasks	Definition*	Childhood Examples
Eating and drinking	Ability to keep and manipulate food and fluids in mouth as well as swallow mouth contents.	**Toddler:** drinks and swallows liquids; drinks from cup unassisted; chews solids and swallows them; drinks through straw. **Early school-age:** drinks and swallows liquids independently; chews and swallows solid foods independently; food likes and dislikes become more established. **Pre-adolescent:** drinks and swallows liquids independently; chews and swallows solid foods independently.
Self feeding	Process of setting up, arranging and bringing food or fluids to mouth from plate or cup.	**Toddler:** drinks from bottle or adapted cup with some spilling; brings pieces of food to mouth and places in mouth with hands; feeds self with spoon with minimal spillage. **Early school-age:** gets cup from cupboard and pours liquid into cup; drinks from cup or uses straw; uses spoon or fork; may need assistance with cutting food with knife. **Pre-adolescent:** drinks from glass or uses straw with ease; uses spoon or fork; uses knife to cut food up.
Functional mobility	Moving from one position to another during the completion of everyday activities such as mobility in bed, transfers (such as bed, car, tub, toilet, chair, floor), functional ambulation and transporting objects.	**Toddler:** rolls over in bed; climbs in and out of low bed or cot; gets from sitting position on floor to standing position; sits in bath; sits in highchair at table; walks as a primary means of mobility; may start climbing up stairs. **Early school-age:** gets in and out of bed with ease; gets into and out of car; stands in shower; sits on toilet independently; walks up and down stairs with alternating feet without assistance; runs smoothly with changes in speed and direction; opens and closes doors using door knobs; sits at table to colour and draw; climbs on and off playground equipment; rides bicycle with/out training wheels. **Pre-adolescent:** gets in and out of bed, car with ease; gets on and off of toilet, stands in shower; sits on chair in front of computer; sits on school bus seat; carries books to and from school.

Term	Definition	Age-specific descriptions
Personal device care	Using, cleaning and maintaining personal care items such as hearing aids, contact lenses, glasses, braces, retainer, or toothbrush.	**Toddler:** does not perform these activities. **Early school-age:** will rinse toothbrush under tap. **Pre-adolescent:** will clean contact lenses or glasses; will rinse toothbrush under tap after use; will clean braces or retainer on teeth.
Personal hygiene and grooming	Washing body; washing, drying and combing hair; nail care (hands and feet); caring for skin, ears, eyes and nose; shaving; applying deodorant; cleansing mouth; brushing and flossing teeth; applying and removing cosmetics.	**Toddler:** rinses hands under tap; needs assistance with body washing, hair and nail care; attempts to brush teeth with supervision. **Early school-age:** washes hands by self; washes body parts, dries body parts with towel with supervision; washes and dries face without assistance; uses tissue to blow nose; puts toothpaste on brush and brushes teeth by self; requires assistance with hair washing and nail care. **Pre-adolescent:** independent in all aspects of personal hygiene and grooming; completes hair care routine; applies deodorant; brushes and flosses teeth; applies moisturiser to skin; girls may start to apply make-up; boys may start to shave face; girls may start shaving legs.
Toilet hygiene	Managing clothing and position on toilet and transferring to and from toilet; using toilet paper to cleanse self; flushing toilet.	**Toddler:** using diapers/nappies; indicates wet or soiled nappies/diapers by pointing, vocalizing or pulling at nappy/diaper; will start to urinate and defecate using potty chair or toilet. **Early school-age:** transfers on and off of toilet; sits on toilet by self; uses toilet paper; flushes toilet; undoes and does up clothing. **Pre-adolescent:** transfers on and off toilet; undoes and does up clothing; wipes self with toilet paper; flushes toilet.
Sleep-rest	A period where one is inactive and may or may not sleep.	**Toddler:** requires nap during day; usually full night's sleep; parents in charge of bedtime routine. **Early school-age:** usually up for full day; requires full night's sleep; parents in charge of bed time routine. **Pre-adolescent:** takes responsibility for sleep cycle and rest periods; able to take responsibility for waking self up in morning for school and other commitments.

* Definitions adapted from: American Occupational Therapy Association (2002). Occupational therapy practice framework: domain and process. *American Journal of Occupational Therapy, 56*, 609–639.

Table 10.2 Instrumental activities of daily living (IADL) for children.

Specific IADL tasks	Definition*	Childhood examples
Care of others	Arranging, supervising, or providing the care of others.	**Toddler:** not applicable. **Early school-age:** not applicable. **Pre-adolescent:** children may be left on their own for periods of time or may take responsibility for looking after others for limited periods (for example baby-sitting; looking after younger sibling).
Care of pets	Arranging, supervising, or providing care for pets.	**Toddler:** not applicable. **Early school-age:** child may assist with feeding and watering family pet under supervision and guidance of adult. **Pre-adolescent:** child may take responsibility for care and feeding of family pets.
Communication device use	Using equipment such as pens, pencils, telephones, pagers, text messaging, videotapes, typewriters, computers, call lights, emergency systems and augmentative communication systems to send and receive information.	**Toddler:** not applicable due to young age of child; child may pretend to use toy telephone or manipulate computer mouse to play game; child may become adept at TV/VCR/DVD player remote control buttons. **Early school-age:** uses telephone, pencils to draw, and computers to play games; child may become adept at using TV/VCR/DVD player remote control buttons. **Pre-adolescent:** uses telephone, pens, pagers, and computers to send and receive information with ease; uses pay-phone independently.
Community mobility	Moving self in and around the community and using public or private transport such as strollers, cars, bicycles, scooters, skateboards, buses, trams, trains, or taxis.	**Toddler:** dependent on parents or care-givers for community mobility. **Early school-age:** dependent on parents for community mobility to a large extent; walks with adult to playground or local library; can be taken in car or on public transport by adults; able to ride bicycle with/out training wheels in yard or on driveway; able to roller-skate or ice-skate. **Pre-adolescent:** walks around neighbourhood; uses public transport by self; can be driven in car to destination by adult; rides bicycle or skateboard; roller-skates or ice-skates.
Financial management	Using financial services such as bank account, bank card, writing cheque, credit card; using cash to pay for expenses and to buy items; planning short and long-term financial goals.	**Toddler:** not applicable. **Early school-age:** uses money to purchase small items; may save money in piggy bank. **Pre-adolescent:** manages own bank account, uses bank card to withdraw funds, uses money to purchase items or saves money; may receive allowance for completion of household tasks; orders meals in restaurant.

Health management and promotion	Formulating, managing and carrying out routines for health promotion such as physical fitness, nutrition and minimizing health risk activities (such as smoking).	**Toddler:** not applicable. **Early school-age:** will be dependent on parental or care-giver guidance for health management and promotion activities. **Pre-adolescent:** takes more responsibility for fitness and exercise routines; sun care, may start experimenting with risky health activities such as smoking.
Home establishment and management	Obtaining and maintaining personal and household possessions and environment (for example bedroom, kitchen, bathroom, yard, home, garden).	**Toddler:** not applicable. **Early school-age:** puts away toys, makes bed and clears dinner dishes from table with parental supervision; puts clean clothes away with assistance when asked. **Pre-adolescent:** takes more responsibility for home maintenance tasks such as yard work, washing dishes, clearing dinner dishes from table, making bed, sweeping floors, tidies own room.
Meal preparation and clean up	Planning, preparing and serving meals as well as cleaning up after meal is finished.	**Toddler:** not applicable. **Early school-age:** assists parents in meal preparation such as stirring cake batter, pouring ingredients into bowl, mixing cookie dough under parental supervision; sets table for meal with assistance; clears dishes after meal completion. **Pre-adolescent:** prepares, serves and cleans up after basic meal (for example making cake, cooking pasta, warming up canned soup); uses microwave and stove correctly for cooking; uses kitchen applies such as toaster, blender, electric fry pan with ease.
Safety procedures and emergency responses	Being aware of and performing actions to maintain safe environment as well as recognizing unexpected dangerous situations and initiating emergency procedures to reduce threat to health and safety (for example contact fire department, police or paramedics).	**Toddler:** not applicable. **Early school-age:** child relies on parents for safety during emergency situations; child can be street proofed to ensure safety when in public venues; child can be educated what to do in case of fire or emergency situation. **Pre-adolescent:** takes more responsibility for safety procedures and emergency responses; could take course in basic first aid procedures; child can be educated what to do in case of fire or emergency situation; takes more responsibility for personal safety such as obeying traffic lights, rules of road as a pedestrian and road signs.
Shopping	Preparing shopping list, selecting and paying for items	**Toddler:** not applicable. **Early school-age:** purchases small items such as candy, toys or other treats. **Pre-adolescent:** makes a list of items to be bought and goes to store to purchase them.

* Definitions adapted from: American Occupational Therapy Association (2002). Occupational therapy practice framework: domain and process. *American Journal of Occupational Therapy*, 56, 609–639.

Table 10.3 BADL & IADL instruments.

	Areas measured	Age range	Environments	Completion time	Reliability	Validity	Measurement methods
Pediatric evaluation of disability inventory (PEDI) Activity and participation level	BADL IADL Cognition (self-care, mobility, social function)	6 months to 7.5 years	Home School Hospital outpatient Clinic	45 to 60 minutes	Inter-rater = .96–.99 Intra-rater = .67–1.00 Internal consistency = .95–.99 Test-retest = .80–.95	**Content:** expert content panel and Rasch modelling used to determine sequence of items. **Criterion:** scores correlate with WeeFIM (.80–.97), Gross motor function measure (.75–.85), Peabody developmental motor scales (.24–.95), and Battelle developmental inventory (.62–.97). **Construct:** hypothesis that PEDI scores increase with age support; functional skills and care-giver assistance supported hypothesis that they are separate constructs.	Interview Observation
Functional independence measure for children (WeeFIM) Activity level	BADL IADL Social Cognition (self-care, sphincter control, mobility, locomotion, communication, and social cognition)	6 months to 7 years	Home School Hospital	15 minutes	Inter-rater = .98 Intra-rater = .98 Internal consistency = NR * Test-retest = .83–.99 ICC = .94–.97 score ICC = .73–.99 for subscales	**Content:** good evidence. **Predictive:** scores predict amount of assistance needed. **Concurrent:** correlates with measures of developmental status. **Construct:** scores correlated to age; Rasch analysis confirmed the motor and cognitive scales; was able to discriminate between normal and impaired children; criterion validity demonstrated.	Interview Observation

Measure	Domains measured	Age	Setting	Time	Reliability	Validity	Report type
Activities scales for kids (ASK) Activity level	BADL IADL Leisure (performance and capacity measures of personal care, dressing, eating and drinking, locomotion, stairs, play, transfers and standing skills)	5 to 15 years of age	Home School Childcare centre	30 minutes for first time completing; 10 minutes on subsequent completion	Inter-rater = .96–.98 Intra-rater = .94–.98 Internal consistency = .99 Test-retest = .97–.98	**Content:** established through expert review and Rasch analysis of item characteristics. **Convergent:** .82–.85 correlation with child health assessment questionnaire. **Divergent:** ASK had correlations of .15 and .09 with measures of emotion and speech. **Criterion:** correlation of .92 between children's self-rating of capability and clinicians' observation of children's performance of ability. **Construct:** ASK ratings were compared to global ratings of severity and disability; significant differences were found on the ASK scores of children with different global ratings.	Self-report or parental report
Child health questionnaire (CHQ) Activity and Participation Level	BADL IADL (physical and psycho-social wellbeing of children)	5 years or older	Home School Clinic Childcare centre	15 to 45 minutes	Inter-rater = NR Intra-rater = NR Internal consistency = .90 Test-retest = NR	**Content:** items generated from literature review, existing measures and use of experts. **Discriminant:** CHQ was able to discriminate between general population and clinical groups. **Construct:** factor analysis confirmed the two-dimensional factor structure of physical and psychosocial dimensions.	Child report and parent report
Canadian occupational performance measure (COPM) Activity level	BADL IADL Productivity Leisure (client's self-perception of occupational performance)	Can be used across the lifespan	Home School Childcare centre	30 to 60 minutes	Inter-rater = NR Intra-rater = NR Internal consistency = .41–.71 Test-retest = .63–.84 ICC = .90 and above	Evidence of content and criterion validity provided. No evidence of construct validity provided.	Interview

(Continued)

Table 10.3 (cont'd)

Instrument/ ICF level	Areas measured	Age range	Environments	Completion time	Reliability	Validity	Measurement methods
Vineland adaptive behaviour scales (VABS) Activity and participation level	BADL IADL Leisure Social participation (ADL, cognition, language, play and social competency)	Birth to 18 years of age	Home School Childcare centre	20 to 90 minutes (depending on version used)	Inter-rater = .96 Intra-rater = NR Internal consistency = .78–.94 Test-retest = .77–.98	**Content:** items identified through literature review and subsequent factor analytic techniques. **Convergent:** moderate correlations with Kaufman assessment battery and high correlations with other measures of adaptive behaviour. **Divergent:** VABS scores had low correlations with intelligence tests. **Construct:** scores of VABS follow developmental progression and are able to differentiate children with and without difficulties in adaptive behaviour.	Interview of parent, health professional, or teacher by rater. Observation.
Adaptive behaviour assessment system (ABAS) Activity and participation level	BADL IADL Productivity Leisure Social participation (communication, functional academics, community use, home living, health and safety, self-care, social, leisure, self-direction and work)	Birth to 89 years of age	Home School Childcare centre	15 to 20 minutes	Internal consistency = .86–.97	**Content:** items identified that were consistent with the 10 AAMR adaptive skill domains. **Construct:** scores of ABAS follow developmental progression and are able to differentiate children and adults with and without difficulties in adaptive behaviour.	Parental or teacher report for ages 5 to 21. Self-report on adult form by individual or a care-giver. Interview Observation

* NR = scores not reported.

Table 10.4 outlines the types of occupational therapy management (direct, indirect, advocacy and health promotion), the occupational therapy role, the service environments, the methods used and the service recipients involved in the delivery of self-care services. Direct management involves hands-on service by the occupational therapist to the client. For example, an occupational therapist might use neurodevelopmental treatment techniques to improve postural tone and alignment in the upper body in preparation for self-feeding. In the case of children, service recipients can also include parents, care-givers, siblings and teachers.

Indirect service refers to any services provided when the client is not actively engaged in the therapy session, such as providing advice to parents, or when consulting with other professionals, accessing funding for adaptive equipment, or consulting with a classroom teacher. Advocacy deals with an occupational therapist lobbying for children with special needs, for example provision of wheelchair accessible bathroom facilities in a school setting. This can occur at many levels, such as local city government, state/provincial government, federal/commonwealth governments and international agencies dealing with children's rights. A final role that occupational therapists can fulfil is that of health promoter. For example, encouraging healthy eating choices may occur alongside developing self-feeding skills in young children. By promoting healthy engagement and participation in occupations, occupational therapists act as consultants, educators and change agents, enabling children's self-care, self-maintenance, health, and wellbeing.

Intervention frameworks targeting impairment and activity limitations may include the biomechanical approach (Trombly & Scott, 1983), sensory processing (Kimball, 1999), and the neurodevelopmental treatment (Schoen & Anderson, 1999). These usually require direct treatment. Intervention frameworks that underpin participation and environmental restrictions may include the Person–Environment–Occupation model (PEO) (Law et al., 1996) and the Model of Human Occupation (Kielhofner, 1997). These will often be operationalized through indirect modes of intervention. When assisting children and their families to manage self-care issues there is a need to draw from frameworks at all levels of the ICF (WHO, 2001) depending on where the child's performance issues arise.

Application of ICF model to paediatric self-care issues

A case study will be used to demonstrate how the ICF model can be applied to the self-care issues of a child diagnosed with cerebral palsy, named Maria. First, the case history is provided, followed by the specifics of the ICF model, including body structure/function, activity limitations in self-care and participation restriction in self-care. In addition, personal factors and environmental issues are outlined (see Figure 10.1). Maria's self-care abilities will be discussed at three developmental stages: toddlerhood (2–3 years), early school-age (5–6 years), and pre-adolescence (12–13 years). At each of these stages, the occupational therapy assessments that could be used, the results of the assessment process and occupational therapy management strategies to enable optimal participation in self-care will be discussed.

Table 10.4 Occupational therapy management of children's self-care challenges.

Levels of management	Occupational therapist service role	Service environments	Methods	Service Recipients
Direct service	Service provision	Home Childcare School Play contexts (for example playgroup) Clinical sites (for example early intervention centre, children's treatment centre, hospital, community health centre)	Hands-on service: NDT, positioning, adaptive equipment, skills teaching, modelling.	Child Parent Other family members Other service providers (such as teachers, assistants, child care staff)
Indirect service	Modification Maintenance Prevention Monitoring Consultation	School Childcare Play contexts (for example playgroup) Clinical sites (for example early intervention centre, children's treatment centre, hospital, community health centre)	Equipment provision Environmental modification Education, demonstration and skill teaching Consultation Contextual interventions (for example create, maintain, modify, prevent).	Parent Teachers Other care-givers Other service providers
Advocacy	Lobbying Advocating Consultation Political activism Change agent	Government (all levels) Industry Community School Global: WHO, international aid agencies.	Education Change agent Children's rights advocacy Lobbyist	Children Parents Educators Law makers Politicians Global community
Health promotion	Modification Maintenance Prevention Monitoring Consultation Lobbying Advocating Change agent	School Childcare Play contexts (for example playgroup) Clinical sites (for example early intervention centre, children's treatment centre, hospital, community health centre) Industry Community Global: WHO, international aid agencies.	Education and skill teaching Demonstration Monitoring Consultation Maintenance Prevention	Children Parents Educators Law makers Politicians Global community

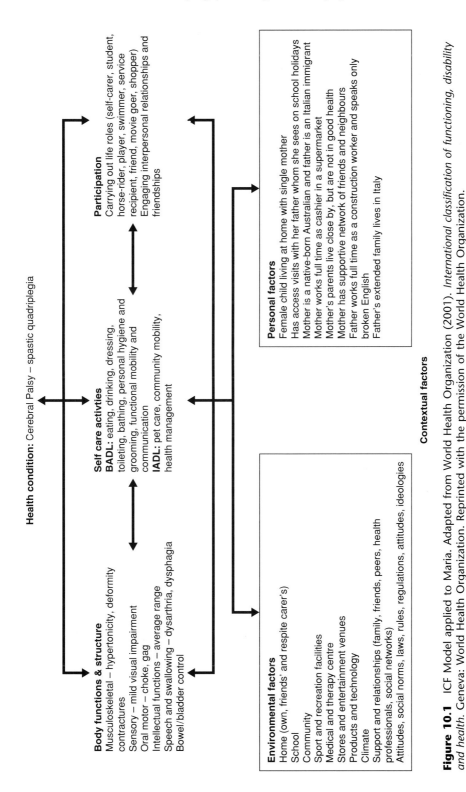

Figure 10.1 ICF Model applied to Maria. Adapted from World Health Organization (2001). *International classification of functioning, disability and health.* Geneva: World Health Organization. Reprinted with the permission of the World Health Organization.

Maria

Personal factors

> Maria is an only child, living with her mother. She has regular access visits to her father on a monthly basis and sees him for a full week on alternate school holidays. Maria's mother works full time as a cashier at a supermarket in a suburban shopping centre. Maria's maternal grandparents are supportive and live close by; however, neither of them is in good health. Maria's mother is Australian and her father is a recent Italian immigrant who works in the construction industry. Maria has no direct contact with her paternal grandparents (other than letters, pictures and gifts) since they live in Italy. Maria attends a cluster school that has a special class for children with physical disabilities. In addition, Maria has regular contact with therapists from a community agency every six months for review as well as more frequent contact with school based therapists (who are contracted to work at the school she attends). For her medical needs, Maria sees an orthopaedic surgeon and paediatric neurologist at a children's hospital outpatient clinic once a year.

Environmental factors

Maria's school is physically accessible. While she attends a special class, Maria also spends a significant period of time in a regular classroom with her age peers. She uses a wheelchair for functional mobility, a communication device and a computer for academic tasks. At home she lives in a ground floor accessible unit in a public housing estate. Once a month, Maria attends out-of-home respite care with a regular carer, to provide her mother with a break. Maria's community environments (which include a shopping centre, movie theatres, a corner shop, restaurants and supermarkets) are generally accessible, as is the pony riding for the disabled complex where she goes riding fortnightly on a Saturday afternoon. She goes swimming at school.

Body structure and function

Maria presents with cerebral palsy, feeding difficulties and incontinence. She was born after a premature delivery at 34 weeks gestation and had an extended hospital stay for two months in a special care nursery. She was initially hypotonic and then developed increased tone in her extremities by three months of age. Early difficulties with feeding were experienced by Maria since she would often choke and gag. Maria has spastic quadriplegia and dysarthria, which becomes more marked when she becomes excited. She has had two surgical interventions to correct developing lower limb deformities and has difficulties with voluntary bowel and bladder control. Hence, in ICF terms her health condition, cerebral palsy, resulted in Maria having a number of body structure and function issues, for example musculoskeletal and movement difficulties (hypertonicity, deformity), swallowing difficulties (dysphagia), speech difficulties (dysarthria), bowel and bladder incontinence, and sensory issues (mild visual impairment) requiring corrective lenses. Her speech is slow but intelligible and she is learning to use a computer for written communication. While unable to be assessed reliably due to her motor and communication impairments, it would appear from her level of awareness and alertness and her understanding of language that Maria is functioning at least within the average range of intellectual ability.

Self-care activity limitations

In terms of activity limitations in the area of self-care, Maria experiences difficulties with all BADL including eating, drinking, toileting, bathing, dressing, grooming and functional mobility. She manages soft textured food and is spoon fed by her mother. She drinks through a cup with a straw and is prone to gagging and choking. Her toileting regime involves regular timed visits to the bathroom. She wears incontinence pads in case of accidents. These limitations will be discussed below at various stages of childhood. In the area of functional mobility, Maria is unable to transfer independently to the toilet either at home or school, and requires her mother or attendant to assist her with removing clothes and wiping. In terms of dressing she is dependent on her mother or carer at school to dress and undress her. She needs assistance transferring to the bath and while Maria can maintain sitting balance, she needs to be bathed by her mother. Maria has long hair that requires washing, combing and braiding by her mother every two days. Teeth care and other grooming tasks also require assistance.

Participation restrictions

In relation to participation, Maria attends school on a full-time basis. She enjoys playing computer games with classmates at lunch-time in the school library. Even though Maria swims with her classmates, she does not fully participate in regular physical education classes due to her mobility restrictions. Once a week, Maria visits her best friend (since her house is wheelchair accessible). Maria has developed a positive relationship with her regular respite carer and enjoys visits to her home and going on outings to the park, restaurants, movie theatre and shops. She enjoys listening to music, watching television, going to the movies, visiting the local zoo and botanical gardens, as well as shopping. In particular, Maria enjoys her fortnightly pony riding lessons which are also attended by three friends from her school class. Maria visits her father once a month for a weekend and sees him for a week on alternate school holidays. Her father lives in a small, less accessible apartment and takes her to children's museums, the local amusement park and indoor bowling. She mobilizes with a wheelchair at home, school and in the community. Maria uses a wheelchair accessible taxi to get to and from school as well as on community outings. Maria's transportation to school is funded by the school and her mother receives a children's disability pension fortnightly which helps to offset the taxi fare costs at other times.

Maria's participation in dressing, mealtime and personal hygiene routines, as well as community mobility will now be explored with respect to how an occupational therapist might support Maria, her family, care-givers and teachers to facilitate her self-care management.

Toddlerhood (2–3 years of age)

Three self-care assessments were used – COPM, PEDI and the VABS with her mother, as well as informal observations of self-care routines. At two years of age, the occupational therapy assessment results indicated that Maria was able to complete the following BADL:

(1) Functional mobility: is able to roll over; unable to sit independently; when supported in sitting, able to reach and grasp larger objects such as toys; able to use switch operated toys; and totally dependent for transporting from one place to another; mother uses a pusher/stroller with a special insert to transport Maria around when she takes her out

(2) Eating: dependent on mother/carer to feed her soft textures with spoon; gags easily; drinks thickened liquids through a straw in cup; unable to hold cup and bring it up to mouth by herself; not finger feeding; drools; needs to be positioned for eating to ensure symmetry; and adequate nutrition and fluid intake are an ongoing problem

(3) Dressing: totally dependent on mother or carer for undressing and dressing needs

(4) Toileting: uses nappies day and night; requires mother or carer to change nappies; and has no awareness of toileting needs

(5) Bathing: totally dependent for transfers, washing and drying

(6) Personal hygiene/grooming: totally dependent for teeth brushing, combing hair, nail care and skin care

(7) Sleep/rest: has a regular bedtime routine and sleeps well through the night

As a toddler, Maria was too young to participate in any IADL. Occupational therapy management strategies took the form of direct service, occurring mainly in Maria's home environment. Strategies involved Maria, her mother, other family members and the respite care-giver. In terms of direct hands-on service strategies, the main focus was on positioning Maria for transfers, feeding and dressing, as well as educating Maria's mother about proper back care and lifting techniques. Another area of focus was adaptive equipment, such as a bath seat support, moulded seating system for Maria's upright play, eating and television viewing. Education and demonstration of self-care routines focused mainly on feeding and transfers.

Young school-age (5–6 years of age)

Maria attended a preparatory year at school. The COPM, PEDI, and ABAS, and clinical observations were used to assess Maria's self-care skills at this age. The COPM and PEDI were completed with Maria's mother via interview. The ABAS was completed with Maria's classroom teacher. Maria was also observed by the occupational therapist in her home environment completing self-care routines, as well as at school in her classroom during lunch and physical education class time with her aide. At five years old, assessment results indicated that Maria was able to complete the following BADL:

(1) Functional mobility: used a wheelchair accessible taxi to get to and from school; and mother had access to use of wheelchair accessible van at the weekends that she used to transport Maria to her social and recreational activities

(2) Eating: at home and school Maria was dependent in eating and drinking (getting cup to mouth); ate in her wheelchair at school and seating system at home; and was able to finger feed some foods such as soft fruit (for example banana)

(3) Dressing: dependent, but Maria could roll over to assist the person dressing her

(4) Toileting: toilet training successful for the most part, but occasional accidents at home or school; and totally dependent for transfers on/off toilet and for wiping

(5) Bathing: dependent for transfers into tub; used sponge to wash face and front of trunk; mother or carer needed to wash back and extremities; mother used hand-held shower to rinse Maria off in tub; and was totally dependent for drying

(6) Personal hygiene/grooming: could bring toothbrush to mouth (electric) and tried to brush, but needed adult for supervision and finishing off; and dependent with hair care, washing, drying and braiding

(7) Sleep/rest: continued to sleep well, but needed assistance of mother/carer for transferring from wheelchair to bed

Based on the assessment results and informal clinical observations, Maria also required assistance with the following IADL:

(1) Looking after a pet budgie in a cage; was unable to care for it, mother fed bird and cleaned cage

(2) Learning to use computer and communication device

(3) Asking for musical toy accessed by a switch and stuffed toy animals at the toy store as well as videos and DVDs at video shop

Occupational therapy management strategies took the form of direct and indirect service, taking place mainly in Maria's home and school environments. Strategies involved Maria, her mother, other family members, respite care-giver, classroom teacher and aide. In terms of direct hands-on service strategies, the focus was on neurodevelopmental treatment and biomechanical techniques to improve active postural alignment and control in sitting, to develop appropriate supported seating and positioning in preparation for activity engagement. Indirect areas of service included environmental modification; equipment recommendations and purchase (such as self-care assistive devices and wheelchair); education regarding Maria's positioning, transfers and self-feeding; and modification of self-care tasks.

Late childhood (12 years of age)

Maria attended grade 6 at school. The COPM, ASK, ABAS and informal clinical observations were used to assess Maria's self-care skills at 12 years. The COPM was completed with Maria's mother and Maria via interview by the occupational therapist. The ABAS was completed by the occupational therapist interviewing Maria's classroom teacher. The ASK was completed with Maria using her communication device. Maria was also observed by the occupational therapist in her home environment completing self-care routines, as well as at school with her aide.

At 12 years of age, the assessment results indicated that Maria was able to complete the following BADL:

(1) Functional mobility: used electric wheelchair now in home, school, recreation and community environments; used wheelchair accessible taxi to get to and from school; and mother had access to use of wheelchair accessible van at the weekends
(2) Eating: able to tolerate more textures and soft solids; ate in her wheelchair pushed under the kitchen table; ate some foods with spoon; still drank from cup with straw; needed food to be cut up; and mother still fed Maria since she was a very slow eater and fatigued easily
(3) Dressing: dependent for undressing and dressing; assisted with pulling pants down to knees; sat up for upper limb dressing on bed or in wheelchair; needed help with lower limb dressing; and was dependent with donning/doffing socks, shoes and underwear
(4) Toileting: continent of bowel and bladder; bowel and bladder was regime regulated, but still required assistance of one person with toilet transfers and wiping self
(5) Personal hygiene and grooming: able to brush own teeth with electric brush once paste was placed on brush by another person; needed assistance with hair care, nail care and deodorant application
(6) Sleep: no problems except for supervision and assistance with transfers

In terms of participation issues regarding mobility, communication, and personal self-maintenance, and based on the assessment results and clinical observations, Maria required assistance with the following IADL: learning to cross road with supervision in electric chair when dropped at school, use of automatic dial on phone and speaker phone for general use to facilitate functional communication. She took responsibility for making sure her budgie was fed and cleaned by reminding others. She was a buddy/mentor to a six-year-old girl with physical disabilities at school.

Occupational therapy management strategies primarily took the form of direct and indirect service mainly in Maria's school environment. Direct intervention with Maria in terms of transfers, self-feeding and self-maintenance occured at home and school. School based strategies primarily involved Maria, classroom teacher and aide. Indirect areas of service involved monitoring and consultation. Methods of intervention included environmental modifications, education, equipment recommendations, and strategies related to positioning, transfers, feeding and other self-care tasks. Indirect methods also included advocacy in the form of including self-care as part of her curriculum (for example, teacher's aide to provide one-to-one assistance for self-care), community advocacy regarding wheelchair access in shopping malls, and government advocacy for funding for teacher's aides, access to adequate transportation methods, wheelchairs and other adaptive devices. Information gained from the COPM on reassessment at 12 years of age, indicated that Maria was generally pleased with her performance in relation to self-care goals. Her mother was also satisfied with her level of independence. The importance of developing personal identity and self-efficacy related to self-care management can not be underestimated.

The importance of self-care skills

Self-care skills are important to all people at all stages of their lives (Perr, 2004). Infants and toddlers are largely dependent on their parents/care-givers to meet their self-care needs. By the time a child starts school, they are fairly independent in completing their basic daily living tasks. School-age children are still dependent on their parents, however, for safety, supervision, provision of meals and washing of clothes. By adolescence, young people are able to look after themselves completely in terms of bathing, toileting, grooming, dressing and eating (Davis & Polatajko, 2004).

The development of self-care skill independence is therefore fundamentally important for the optimization of personal identity and self-esteem. Self-management of self-care needs is linked to the development of autonomy, self-efficacy, self-awareness and life satisfaction (Barnes & Case-Smith, 2004). For many children with significant physical disabilities, like Maria, there is also a need to develop the ability to inform and direct personal care attendants about how to best assist with personal self-care tasks. Many young people with physical disabilities such as cerebral palsy may never be fully independent in self-care. During their later childhood and adolescent years, they need to decide which tasks they can realistically master and those for which they will need ongoing assistance. These decisions require consideration of safety issues, as well as the physical exertion and time requirements. Parents and health professionals need to assist young people with these decisions and accept that there will be tasks where assistance may always be required. Being able to make these decisions and learning to employ, roster, manage and instruct personal care staff with respect to one's own self-care needs is an important developmental self-care task for many young people with physical disabilities. Health professionals need to assist these young people to develop the skills to positively manage this important aspect of their lives so as to ensure self-dignity and personal autonomy.

Summary

The ability to manage self-care needs is an essential requirement of adulthood. For some children, however, full independence is not possible. In this chapter, we described self-care skills (both BADL and IADL) throughout various stages of childhood. A number of assessments that can be used by clinicians to evaluate children's self-care skills were briefly reviewed. The ICF was used to provide a framework for understanding children's self-care activities and participation. Occupational therapy assessment and management of self-care challenges faced by Maria as a toddler, school-age child and pre-adolescent were then outlined. Finally, the importance of self-care management for the development of psychological and emotional wellbeing in children and adolescents was discussed. The term self-care management was used rather than independence, as it is recognized that some young people will never be fully independent in self-care. As health care providers and children's advocates, occupational therapists are concerned with the optimal development of self-care skills in children and adolescents. Recognizing the difference between 'I can do it' and 'I can do it myself' is essential, if occupational therapists are to assist young people in managing their own self-care, with or without the help of others. This will minimize the activity limitations and participation restrictions that children with disabilities may experience as a result of not being able to manage their self-care needs.

References

American Occupational Therapy Association (2002). Occupational therapy practice framework: domain and process. *American Journal of Occupational Therapy*, 56, 609–639.

Barnes, K. J. & Case-Smith, J. (2004). Adaptive strategies for children with developmental disabilities. In: C. H. Christiansen & K. M. Matuska (Eds.), *Ways of living: adaptive strategies for special needs* (2nd ed.) (pp. 109–147). Bethesda, MD: AOTA Press.

Canadian Association of Occupational Therapists (1997). *Enabling occupation: an occupational therapy perspective*. Ottawa, Ont.: CAOT Publications.

Case-Smith, J. (2002). *Occupational therapy for children*. St Louis, MO: C.V Mosby.

Christiansen, C. H. & Matuska, K. M. (2004). *Ways of living: adaptive strategies for special needs*. Bethesda, MD: AOTA Press.

Davis, J. A. & Polatajko, H. J. (2004). Occupational development. In: C. H. Christiansen & E. A. Townsend (Eds.), *Introduction to occupation: the art and science of living* (pp. 91–119). Upper Saddle River, NJ: Prentice Hall.

Furuno, S., O'Reilly, K. A., Hosaka, C. M., Inatsuka, T. T., Allman, T. L. & Zeisloft, B. (1985). *Hawaii early learning profile (HELP)*. Palo Alto, CA: VORT Corporation.

Haley, S., Coster, W., Ludlow, L. H., Haltiwanger, J. T. & Andrellos, P. J. (1992). *Pediatric evaluation of disability inventory (PEDI). Version 1.0: development, standardization and administration manual*. Boston, MA: PEDI Research Group.

Harrison, P. & Oakland, T. (2000). *Adaptive behavior assessment system (ABAS)*. Marickville, NSW: The Psychological Corporation.

Harvey, A. S. & Pentland, W. (2004). What do people do? In: C. H. Christiansen & E. A Townsend (Eds.), *Introduction to occupation: the art and science of living* (pp. 63–90). Upper Saddle River, NJ: Prentice Hall.

Hong, C. S. & Howard, L. (2002). *Occupational therapy in childhood*. London: Whurr Publishers.

Kielhofner, G. (1997). *Conceptual foundations of occupational therapy*. Philadelphia: F. A. Davis.

Kimball, J. G. (1999). Sensory integration frame of reference: theoretical base, function/dysfunction continua, and guide to evaluation. In: P. Kramer & J. Hinojosa (Eds.), *Frames of reference for pediatric occupational therapy* (pp. 119–168). Philadelphia: Lippincott, Williams & Wilkins.

Landgraf, J. M., Abetz, L. & Ware, J. E. (1996). *The child health questionnaire (CHQ) User's Manual*. Boston, MA: The Health Institute, New England Medical Centre.

Law, M., Cooper, B., Strong, S., Stewart, D., Rigby, P. & Letts, L. (1996). The person–environment–occupation model: a transactive approach to occupational performance. *Canadian Journal Occupational Therapy*, *63* (1), 9–23.

Law, M., Baptiste, S., Carswell, A., McColl, M., Polatajko, H. & Pollock, N. (1998). *Canadian occupational performance measure (COPM) Manual*. Ottawa, Ont.: CAOT Publications.

Law, M., Baum, C. & Dunn, W. (2001). *Measuring occupational performance: supporting best practice in occupational therapy*. Thorofare, NJ: Slack Incorporated.

Newborg, J., Stock, J. R. & Wnek, L. (1984). *Battelle developmental inventory examiner's manual*. Allen, TX: DLM Teaching Resources.

Perr, A. (2004). Range of human activity: self-care. In: J. Hinojosa & M. L. Blount (Eds.), *The texture of life: purposeful activities in occupational therapy* (pp. 397–413). Bethesda, MD: AOTA Press.

Porr, S. M. & Rainville, E. B. (1999). *Pediatric therapy: a systems approach*. Philadelphia: F. A. Davis Company.

Schoen, S. A. & Anderson, J. (1999). Neurodevelopmental treatment frame of reference. In: P. Kramer & J. Hinojosa (Eds.), *Frames of reference for pediatric occupational therapy* (pp. 83–118). Philadelphia: Lippincott, Williams & Wilkins.

Sparrow, S. S., Balla, D. A. & Cicchetti, D. V. (1984). *Vineland adaptive behavior scales*. Circle Pines, MN: American Guidance Service.

System, U. D. (1990). *Guide for the Use of the Pediatric Functional Independence Measure*. Buffalo, NY: Research Foundation, State University of New York.

Trombly, C. & Scott, D. (1983). *Occupational therapy for physical dysfunction* (2nd Ed.). Baltimore, MD: Williams & Wilkins.

World Health Organization (WHO) (2001). *International classification of functioning, disability and health: ICF* (Short version ed.). Geneva: World Health Organization.

Young, N. L. (1996). *The activities scale for kids (ASK) manual*. Toronto, Ont.: The Hospital for Sick Children.

Chapter 11

THE TRANSITION TO SCHOOL

Cathy McBryde, Jenny Ziviani and Monica Cuskelly

Children undergo many transitions throughout their journey into adulthood. Some are small, such as moving from inside play in home corner to group time on the mat at kindergarten. Some are more profound, such as negotiating various developmental stages (crawling to walking), or moving from one educational environment to another (commencing primary or secondary school). Each transition can be accompanied by a change in occupational role, some of which will be more challenging than others. Transitions can therefore be conceptualized in terms of a necessary phase that occurs as children move from one occupational role to another. There is not a great deal of research into early childhood transitions, possibly because there is no accepted model on which to base or conceptualize transition practices. Transitions have been described, however, as significant recurrent processes involving an element of change that occur periodically throughout life. They are an inevitable part of our existence and can be stressful (Wolery, 1999).

One childhood transition that has attracted increasing attention within many western countries is the transition to year one. This particular transition is a potentially difficult one for children to make, owing to the many differences that can exist between the early childhood environment from which they are coming, and the school environment to which they are heading. The physical environment of the latter will be much larger and perhaps initially more challenging in terms of negotiating playgrounds; becoming accustomed to a bigger class size, with only one teacher as opposed to a teacher and a teacher's aide in early childhood settings; self-care such as toileting which may be more difficult owing to facilities being located outside the classroom and children being uncertain about whether they must wait for a break; tasks usually needing to be completed within a time limit and being more structured; and children needing to be able to respond to directions from their teacher regardless of whether or not they feel like complying at the time (Sweet & Percival, 1996).

This chapter examines the concept of transition in the context of commencing primary school and highlights the importance of transitions in terms of children's success in fulfilling their occupational roles as school students. Differing conceptualizations of transitions will be discussed, incorporating an examination of school readiness. The importance of the 'goodness-of-fit' between children and the context in which they must function will be highlighted, in conjunction with a consideration of the function of the occupational therapist in preparing children for their role as a school student within a multidisciplinary team approach. It is acknowledged that children in some countries do not attend formal educational environments, and consequently are not required to make transitions to schools. The focus of this chapter, however, will be on the inclusive education practices within most western countries.

The aims of this chapter are to:

(1) Explore the importance of a successful transition to school with respect to the child's ability to function optimally in the role of student, and participate in the classroom environment
(2) Examine the concept of school readiness and the perceived link between readiness and subsequent school adjustment
(3) Discuss the factors that influence beliefs about the concept of school readiness and how a child's readiness for school is currently determined
(4) Highlight the importance of an optimal *fit* between the personal character-istics of the child, previous environmental influences and the context in which the child is expected to function in the role of student
(5) Acknowledge the roles undertaken by families, communities and health professionals in preparing children for their roles as school students

Occupational therapy and preparing children for school

Little has been documented about the role of the occupational therapist in sup-porting children and their families to make a successful transition to school (Prigg, 2002). There has, however, been a considerable amount of occupational therapy literature addressing how children in early childhood settings are assessed and treated for perceived delays or difficulties in the attainment of a range of developmental, self-care and play skills (see for example Dubois, 1996). There has also been considerable attention paid to the development of skills regarded as prerequisites for functional performance, for example fine motor skills as a prerequisite for handwriting (see for example Amundson & Weil, 1996).

More recently, however, occupation based models of practice, emphasizing optimal occupational performance as the desired outcome, have assumed greater prominence (Law et al., 2001). Enabling occupation and occupational performance is achieved by considering the dynamic relationship between individuals, their environment and their occupation (Townsend, 1998); 'Optimal occupational per-formance is achieved when the fit between the child, environment and occupation is maximized' (Primeau & Ferguson, 1999, p. 509). This type of practice aligns well with the International Classification of Functioning, Disability and Health (ICF) (World Health Organization, 2001) model, which postulates that the ability of children to achieve required activities (in this case, to function in the role of school student and participate to an optimal level in the classroom), is contingent on a combination of children's personal characteristics (for example, developmental level, temperament, behaviour, sensory processing ability, gender), as well as the context in which children must operate (that is, the expectations of the school environment and classroom teacher, as well as home environment influences) (Simeonsson et al., 2003).

Despite this change of perspective, the task of *readying* children for school remains popular. Programmes continue to be developed by occupational therapists and administered to groups of children with the aim of addressing skill deficits that are considered to be affecting a child's readiness to progress to school (see for example Roberts & Carter, 2003). Prigg (2002) interviewed six occupational therapists about their roles and experiences with children with special learning needs during the period of transition to school. One of the most common roles described was preparing the child for the school experience, which involved assisting the child to develop the abilities considered to be required for successful participation. This included pencil and scissor skills, and achieving independence with self-help skills. Written programmes for specific skill development were also frequently provided to parents and teachers once school had commenced.

There is no question that possessing certain skills and abilities assists children to make smoother transitions to school (Dockett & Perry, 2001). Assisting children to acquire specific skills is a useful and valid occupational therapy intervention. The difficulty with the use of an exclusively child-centred approach, however, is that research has demonstrated little direct relationship between skill components and actual functional abilities (Badley, 1995). La Paro & Pianta (2000) demonstrated that less than 25% of the variability in children's academic school performance could be explained by the actual skills of the child as demonstrated in their preschool year. McBryde (2001) found a significant predictive relationship between preschool teacher perceptions of school readiness and year one teacher perceptions of adjustment to school. However, the relationship was moderate, implying that factors in addition to their characteristics were contributing to children's school adjustment. Caution must therefore be exercised in adopting an occupational therapy approach involving intervention strategies (such as the remediation of skills and school readiness groups) in isolation. Factors other than the characteristics of the child are obviously influential.

Understanding childhood transitions

Wolery (1999) described three types of transitions pertinent to young children. First, are those transitions that involve movement from one setting to another such as occurs when children move from early childhood settings to primary school environments, from primary to secondary school, or are referred from one educational programme or therapy setting to another. This has also been spoken of as a vertical transition in terms of the continuity of experiences children have between different phases of their lives, moving up or down into a completely different environment (Kagan & Neuman, 1998).

Second, are the daily transitions that occur when children must leave parental care, move to care provided by another adult, and subsequently change back to parental care. This kind of transition can be very difficult for some children in early childhood settings where children can often be observed clinging to their parents when being dropped off, but not wanting to go home when parents return at pick-up time. Within primary school environments too, daily transitions may occur between the regular classroom, special subject classes such as physical education, music and library, and learning support classes.

Third, 'in-class' or 'in-home' transitions occur within settings. In-class transitions might involve moving from group time on the mat to small group work at desks, to morning tea. In-home transitions might include moving from playing with siblings, to taking a bath, to having dinner, to going to bed (Wolery, 1999). These last two types of transitions are also referred to as horizontal, indicating movement within or between the same or parallel environments (Kagan & Neuman, 1998). Wolery (1999) argued that transitions are likely to be difficult to a certain extent for all children and their families, and are potentially even harder for children with disabilities. This chapter focuses on the vertical transition children experience when moving from the early childhood environment to school.

Making the transition to primary school

Starting school involves a 'significant ecological shift', with children having to negotiate increased academic and social demands, and physical changes to learning environments, as they progress from preschool to school (Law et al., 2001). Entwisle & Alexander (1998) noted that the *internal* or cognitive world of the school-aged child is developing and changing rapidly during the first few years at school (5–8 years), marked by the progression, in Piagetian terms, from pre-operational to operational stages of development. Acquisition of academic abilities, particularly literacy and numeracy skills, become paramount. At the same time, the *external* worlds of these children, consisting of the classroom environment in which they are expected to function, and the nature of their social experiences, have also undergone dramatic change (Entwisle & Alexander, 1998). The goals and demands of the school environment are very different from that of the early childhood environment from which children have come. Social networks change from a primary interaction with adults and family members, to same age peers. Interactions with teachers change, as a result of increased child-to-teacher ratios and shift in focus from developmentally or play based programmes oriented towards social development, to more cognitive and structured academically oriented approaches (Rimm-Kaufman & Pianta, 2000) (see Figure 11.1).

Measures of success also alter with children's transition to school. School is compulsory, and children generally have no choice about which school they attend, who their teacher is and what they will do in the classroom. At school, children's performance is compared to a group of their peers, not only academically, but also socially and behaviourally. Children who may be successful in their own home environment where they are able to choose the play activities that interest them, may not experience the same level of achievement in the classroom where they must participate in all assigned tasks regardless of their level of expertise or inclination.

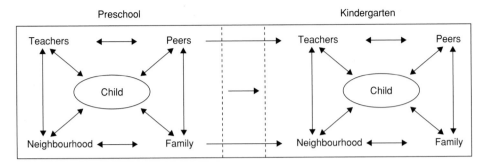

Figure 11.1 An ecological model of transition. Adapted from R. C. Pianta & M. Kraft Sayre. (2003). *Successful kindergarten transition: your guide to connecting children, families, and schools.* Baltimore: Paul H. Brookes Publishing Co. Reprinted with the permission of Paul H. Brookes Publishing Co.

Children are also, for the first time, compared to a large group of their peers. The ability of children to experience success will therefore be relative to the talents of the rest of the class group, as the peer group with which children must function will influence teachers' perceptions of an individual child's success (Entwisle & Alexander, 1998).

The transition to school has been identified as a 'critical or sensitive period' for children's academic and social development, 'a life stage of *limited duration* where an unusual response potential of an organism is coupled with particular kinds of environmental stimulation' (Entwisle & Alexander, 1998, p. 352). A good example of a critical period is the imprinting stage in newborn chicks and ducklings, whereby, for a period of 24 hours after birth, they instinctively follow and become attached to any large animal (including humans) in their immediate environment. While Entwisle & Alexander identified that there is no actual evidence for such a neurologically based critical period in children as is observed in baby chicks or ducks, they argue that the imagery of a critical period is worth considering for children starting school, given that they are making significant transitions into new academic and social roles.

Transitions to school are therefore considered to have important and far-reaching consequences for future school achievement. 'Because a sensitive period is one in which considerable fluidity occurs, both positive and negative consequences can be strongly influenced' (Pianta & Cox, 1999, p. 367). Early school success and positive transitions tend to translate to higher levels of social competence and academic achievement that remain stable over time (Pianta & Cox, 1999). Self-image, particularly in terms of being a learner, is also directly determined by the experiences children have in their early school years (Dockett et al., 1999). Conversely, children who do not experience early school success are far more likely to drop out of school later on.

'Drop out is not an isolated event that occurs in high school. Rather, it is the culmination of a process of disengagement from school that stretches back over many years . . . very likely to children's earliest encounters with the school.' (Entwisle & Alexander, 1993, p. 411)

The obvious course of action would appear to be ensuring that children experience a successful transition to year one, and certainly many suggestions have been made and programmes implemented with this aim in mind. The reality is, however, that children enter school demonstrating marked diversity in skills as a consequence of normal differences in development at school entrance age (National Association for the Education of Young Children [NAEYC], 1995). Some children will be reading fluently, and others will not yet recognize all the letters of the alphabet or their sounds. Children also come from diverse home environments and varied life experiences, including the amount of television viewing permitted, opportunities for social interactions with others, and the degree to which children are read to and taken on trips to parks or museums. Consequently, children will experience the transition to school in very different ways (Dockett et al., 1999), with some being more successful in negotiating the journey than others.

Models of transition

Pianta & Kraft-Sayre (2003) proposed four models to describe transition into school: the skills only model, which views transition as a factor of the child's personal characteristics; the environmental input model, which asserts that a child's experiences within certain environments influence transition; the linked environments model, which emphasizes not only the environmental impact but the importance of the connections between various settings and communities in the life of the child; and the developmental model, which incorporates aspects of the previous three models but stresses that these interactions occur over time.

Given that occupational therapists regularly focus on developing children's skills and abilities in preparing them for school transitions (Prigg, 2002), the skills only model of transition will be addressed in considerable depth, incorporating a discussion regarding school readiness. Also highlighted will be the developmental model of transition and the importance of this model as an alternative for underpinning occupational therapy practice.

The skills only model of transition

In the skills only model, transition to school is conceptualized in relation to child characteristics, including factors such as school readiness and level of maturity. The focus of school readiness as the key to ensuring children make successful transitions to school has traditionally centred around children's ability to demonstrate particular skills and characteristics thought to be required for a successful school adjustment. The limitation in adopting this approach to school transitions is the associated inference that *readiness* is unidimensional and the responsibility of the child. In reality, however, the factors that influence a child's performance and personal characteristics are multidimensional, extremely variable across individuals, and influenced by the culture and context in which the child functions (Meisels, 1999).

'If readiness consists of a mastery of simpler skills that permit a person to reach higher or more complex skills, one child's readiness may be another child's long-ago accomplishment or another child's yet-to-be achieved success.' (Meisels, 1999, pp. 43–44)

This view of transition remains popular and has perpetuated a focus on the skills and abilities individual children bring with them to the classroom. Contemporary literature continues to present discussion of school readiness in these terms. Many child centred readiness checklists have been compiled, and are widely accepted by parents and teachers alike.

In his book *Thriving at school*, John Irvine presented an extensive *readiness checklist* itemizing educational characteristics, social characteristics and self-help characteristics (Irvine, 2000). Other books written for parents and teachers list skills under headings such as physical skills, intellectual skills, social skills and emotional skills (Sweet & Percival, 1996), level of independence, ability to function in a group, concentration level and physical factors such as whether they are unusually big or small for their age (Hill, 1991). Rief (2001) argued that the children most prepared for school are those who can demonstrate or have nearly acquired 60 *readiness skills* listed under self-care/self-help/self-awareness; verbal/language; perceptual; motor; cognitive and academic; and social/adaptive/behavioural sections.

Generally, in Australia assessment prior to school is only undertaken for children suspected of giftedness or as having special learning needs, for the purpose of determining areas of strength and limitation, and individualizing the curriculum to ensure optimal success for the individual. Some privately run schools, however, screen potential students on the basis of IQ assessments (see for example Doherty, 2003) and criterion based readiness checklists based on different aspects of children's skills, such as social-emotional, motor and language development.

Basing educational or therapeutic services around a framework of school readiness, in which school transition is the child's responsibility, however, is fraught with danger. Adopting a school readiness model of transition, requires that certain assumptions about readiness are able to be met, namely: that the concept of readiness can be adequately defined; that school readiness can be measured; and that the results of such measurement can predict how a child will cope at school (Meisels, 1999). These assumptions are not easy to validate, as the following discussion will illustrate.

Defining readiness

School readiness is a very difficult concept to define, owing to its basis in early psychological, developmental and learning theories regarding a child's skill acquisition. Conceptualizations differ markedly, with a primary point of contention being the degree to which school readiness is influenced by biology or environment.

Gesell's *maturation theory* provided the basis for the first model of school readiness, and has remained the most influential for educational philosophy and practice (Watson, 1996). Maturation theory asserts that development is biological or genetically predetermined: something that proceeds from within (Gredler,

1992). Growth is viewed solely as a function of maturation, with environmental influences on the child having minimal impact or influence. Children are believed to develop according to individual time clocks at individual rates and will therefore not all be ready for the same thing at the same time (Meisels, 1999). Maturationists advocate delaying entry to school if the requisite developmental abilities have not emerged (Gredler, 1992; Powell, 1995).

The contrasting school readiness perspective is the *environmentalist approach* originating in behaviourism, and based on the work of learning theorists Thorndike and Skinner (Weber, 1984). This approach emphasizes the importance of early environmental experiences and early stimulation for intellectual and affective development. The influence of heredity is not discounted; however, it is believed to exert a proportionately small influence over learning compared to environment. Assessing readiness for school is not a consideration for supporters of this view, as children are always deemed ready to learn. This perspective resulted in strong advocacy for early intervention, and provided the basis for many of the programmes aimed at at-risk or environmentally disadvantaged children such as Headstart in America (De Cos, 1997).

Both the maturationist and environmentalist approaches have been criticized for their tendency to define readiness in the extreme: either as a child centred characteristic or an environmental characteristic (De Cos, 1997). Attempts to resolve the heredity–environment dilemma resulted in the evolution of the *interactionist approaches*, which are significantly influenced by Piaget's cognitive theory. In these approaches, readiness is considered to be a cognitive entity, dependent on the interaction between two principal factors: a child's intellectual maturity and specific learning experiences.

The most recent conceptualization of school readiness adopts a dynamic social and cultural orientation, in which school readiness is believed to be constructed through social interaction (Pianta & Walsh, 1996). Graue (1992) proposed the *social constructionist model* of readiness, postulating that meanings about school readiness were constructed within a social and cultural context: '. . . readiness means different things in different situations, and children could be "ready" for one type of school experience, but not another' (Dockett & Perry, 2002, p. 71).

Proponents of this conceptualization of school readiness believe that it is a relative entity influenced by a teacher's personal beliefs about growth and development; the expectations of the school the child will attend; the level of parent involvement in the child's education; and the characteristics of the group of children to which an individual child's performance will be compared. The relationship between the child and the school is considered pivotal in ensuring a smooth transition (Dockett & Perry, 2002). Obtaining information from many different types of assessment and from many different perspectives is advocated, and includes assessment of children's development and personal characteristics, interview and questionnaire information from teachers and parents, and observations of children in group settings such as the classroom (Meisels, 1999).

Diversity about what constitutes readiness has been illustrated in the preceding discussion and makes reaching consensus about a definition of school readiness very difficult. Consequently, the more simplistic maturationist and environmentalist approaches remain widely held and influence the way in which parents, and health and education professionals approach the issue of school transitions. It is likely, for example, that teachers having maturationist beliefs will advise parents uncertain about whether to send their children to school to give them another year at home. Conversely, teachers adhering more to an environmentalist philosophy will be inclined to recommend that children commence school, in the belief that their skills will develop from being in a stimulating early childhood environment.

It is suggested that occupational therapists tend to assume a maturationist approach to children's transition owing to the importance of development and maturation as one of the underlying tenets of occupational therapy practice. Adopting this perspective will undoubtedly, and perhaps subconsciously, influence recommendations made to parents about children's ability to start school. With maturationist beliefs, occupational therapists are more likely to recommend another year at preschool if doubts exist about children's ability to cope with school. This may well be at odds with parents and early childhood teachers who hold differing perspectives, and it is important for occupational therapists to be mindful of these potential and very real differences in viewpoints when discussing school transitions with families and schools.

Measuring school readiness

The inability to define or quantify school readiness, has generated many problems with its measurement (Meisels, 1999). Currently in Australia, eligibility for school entry is determined by chronological age: when children reach a designated age within a particular time period, they are legally required to commence school. Consequently, but perhaps not appropriately, chronological age has been utilized as an indicator of school readiness.

Dissatisfaction with age as a criterion has resulted in numerous attempts by those in education to determine readiness in a more meaningful way, with a consequent increase in the development and use of assessments designed to measure characteristics considered to reflect a child's readiness for school (Pianta & La Paro, 2003). Measurement of children's skills by occupational therapists and other educational personnel has been, and remains, extremely useful for providing information about a child's strengths and skills, and facilitating individualization of the curriculum. What increasingly occurred, however, was that a child's skill deficits were identified for the purposes of making placement decisions (American Academy of Pediatrics, 1995). The use of these assessments to make judgements about whether or not children could progress to school has received widespread condemnation for several reasons.

First, skill development is so inconsistent and varied at the age at which children start school that an isolated assessment administered several months prior to school entry may not be indicative of future school performance (Gredler, 1997). Second, most available assessments do not capture the influence of context on a child's peformance (Powell, 1995). Lastly, test results were being used inappropriately to make decisions about a child's readiness for school, in the absence of acceptable psychometric properties such as adequate reliability and validity (May & Kundert, 1997). Lack of predictive validity is the most commonly cited problem of school readiness measures. Many of the assessments are not able to predict future academic functioning or social adjustment, and yet they were being used to make decisions about where children should be placed within the education system (Bredekamp & Shepard, 1989). Research regarding the precision of these assessments in predicting later school performance has consistently revealed low correlations between the two, indicating only a small degree of accuracy in correctly identifying *ready* and *unready* children (Gredler, 1992; Meisels, 1992).

Assessments to measure readiness have consequently fallen from favour and chronological age remains the sole criterion for school entry in many countries (Narahara & Lass, 1998). Unfortunately, this age related criterion for school admission continues to be confused as a measure of children's ability to make a successful transition to school. Consequently, policy makers persist in pushing for an increase in the age of entry of children to school by bringing the cut-off dates for entry forward, in the mistaken belief that this will somehow increase the readiness of children to begin (Graue, 1999). The reality is that there will always be a child who is the youngest in the intake year and a wide range of normal developmental differences at school entry age. This is not a factor of chronological age but typical differences in development, and it is important for schools to employ teachers who understand these differences (namely those with early childhood backgrounds or specialist training) in the first few years of school.

In practice, judgements about children's ability to progress to school are made by parents and early childhood teachers, based on their perceptions of individual abilities and their ideas about the skills required for a successful transition (Lewit & Baker, 1995). Consequently, a child believed to be *unready* by a parent, or teacher, or both, may be withheld from school, despite being chronologically eligible.

Research indicates that parents and teachers hold definite beliefs about children and their development (Smith & Shepard, 1988). Factors considered by parents and teachers in their deliberations specifically regarding school readiness tend to be quite uniform, and include developmental, behavioural, and temperamental characteristics, plus chronological age (Dockett et al., 1997; McBryde et al., 2004). Perceptions held by parents and teachers are strongly influenced and, in many respects, constructed by their cultural and social environment. Ideas and beliefs formulated in response to cultural and social influences are known as naïve theories (Goodnow, 1988) and tend to be intuitive rather than based on any sort of scientific evidence (Lightfoot & Valsiner, 1992).

Naïve theories can be, and are, *reproduced* (passed from one generation to another). An example of a reproduced naïve theory is the belief espoused by our parents and grandparents that flat lemonade is good when we are sick. Naïve theories can also be *produced* by community interactions, in which a community creates a shared subjective understanding and belief system about certain things (Holloway et al., 1995). An example of a recently produced naïve theory is that the older children are the more ready they are for school. Despite any definitive evidence, this perception is strongly held by both parents and teachers. Research has also demonstrated that parent and teacher beliefs, in turn, influence their behaviours (Miller, 1988). For example, if adults believe that younger children will not cope as well in the school environment, observations will tend to reinforce these perceptions.

Developmental model of transition

In the developmental model, transition to school is understood by examining the influence of contexts, and draws on Bronfenbrenner's bio-ecological model (Bronfenbrenner & Morris, 1998), and Pianta & Walsh's (1996) contextual systems model (Pianta & Kraft-Sayre, 2003). This model proposes that any consideration of readiness with a view to enabling a successful transition to school needs to take account of the broader picture: that a child's skills are relative to the context in which they are demonstrated, and are significantly influenced by the contribution of family and early childhood environments. This includes the school environment, teacher expectations, family attitudes and level of support provided at home. This is a broad view of transition in which it is recognized that there are many contributors to the transition experience, and that the perspectives and expectations of contributors all shape children's experiences in some way (Dockett & Perry, 2001).

Assisting children to make optimal transitions does not simply involve teaching specific pre-academic or readiness skills, but includes assisting children to engage within the classroom and with the teacher with whom they will be working. Ideally, this would involve an ecological assessment of the classroom well before the transition occurs (Wolery, 1999). Believing that the qualities children require to start school can be quantified and improved implies that it is a finite entity: something that must be completed by the first day they enter the classroom. In reality, starting school is a process that occurs over time rather than a single event in time (Pianta & Kraft-Sayre, 1999). The transition period has been defined as a period of 18–21 months duration, beginning 6–9 months before a child starts school, and ending 12 months after commencing (New South Wales Department of School Education, 1997). 'Fundamentally, transition is a process that involves four facets: ready schools, community participation and support, family knowledge and involvement, and preschool and childcare settings committed to preparing children' (Pianta & Kraft-Sayre, 2003, p. 9).

Assisting children to make optimal transitions

Occupational therapists cannot assist children to make any sort of transition, let alone the transition to school, in isolation. Any service provided to children undergoing the transition to school needs to incorporate multiple types of information from sources such as parents, early childhood teachers, the primary school environment and philosophy, and the child themselves. Information from health and educational professionals such as occupational therapists, speech pathologists, physiotherapists, psychologists and audiologists is also vital.

Parents provide important perceptions and knowledge pertaining to their child's capabilities and characteristics and their expectations about their child's school experience. Early childhood teachers also know the children whom they teach intimately and it has been demonstrated that early childhood teacher perceptions of a child's ability to cope with the demands of year one, are able to predict that child's adjustment to school as measured by the year one teacher (McBryde, 2001). Results of studies, however, comparing early childhood teacher and parent perceptions of children have consistently demonstrated either no correlation (see for example Porwancher & De Lisi, 1993), or low correlation between different raters (Margetts, 1994). It has been hypothesized that such a low level of agreement relates to the fact that observations are being made in entirely different environments (Achenbach et al., 1987). It is therefore imperative that multiple views across different contexts are incorporated into any consideration of the transition to school.

Information about the primary school environment and philosophy will include issues such as school and class size, accessibility, the degree of support provided for students with additional needs, and the willingness of staff to adapt both educational practices and environment to maximize the likelihood of a successful transition. The children themselves will provide important information about their particular skills and characteristics, including developmental abilities, behaviour, attention, temperament characteristics such as persistence and adaptability, sensory processing style, social and communication skills, and proficiency in play.

Other health and educational professionals will have additional information on individual children. The behaviours and skills witnessed in a one-to-one occupational therapy assessment conducted in a quiet environment, for example, may well be quite different from the same child's behaviour and skill level in the busier educational setting. Collaborative teamwork is generally considered the accepted model of service provision for children undergoing transition, and is particularly ideal because planning and coordination of services needs to be comprehensive and inclusive (Prigg, 2002).

Goodness of fit

It has been illustrated repeatedly in this chapter that focusing on children's characteristics in isolation by completing readiness checklists or skills based assessments is inadequate. Similarly limiting are definitive checklists providing criteria to assist with choosing a school (see for example Irvine, 2000). Obviously, school resources, physical facilities such as classroom and playground equipment, reputation and happy students are important considerations. However, in isolation they will be meaningless if the skills and needs of particular children are not considered simultaneously. It is imperative that the school and the child *fit* together optimally if transition is to be successful. The local school may have an excellent reputation, be well resourced, have very dedicated teaching staff and 1400 students. A child who is very shy, finds social interactions difficult and is easily overwhelmed by a lot of sensory stimulation (noise and movement), however, may not *fit* very well into an environment with this many students and hence make a very poor transition, despite the school scoring well on a school checklist.

The degree or *goodness* of fit between children, their occupation as students and the school environment is a paramount consideration. Children's individual characteristics are not viewed as *good* or *bad* in this kind of approach. Rather the fit between children's individual characteristics and the environment in which they function is the key to understanding adjustment and successful transitions (Feagans et al., 1991). The issue of goodness of fit is not an isolated consideration when children first commence year one. Each vertical transition between year groups raises new deliberations for parents and educational staff about how well children will fit into the new classroom and respond to the expectations of a different teacher. While not often documented in policy manuals, some schools attempt to maximize the goodness of fit for their students by altering the composition of the groups of children in classrooms every year to ensure that individual children are placed in a teaching environment that suits them best. Deliberations such as these require considerable flexibility of approach and a genuine desire to provide children with the best learning experience possible. Judgements are based on wide consultation with the child's teacher from the previous year group, the learning support and gifted and talented support teachers, parents and the principal, with primary consideration given to keeping key friendship groups together and ensuring an optimal fit between the individual child and the proposed teacher's teaching style and classroom learning environment (see Figure 11.2).

Occupational therapy assessment

Assessment of children when uncertainty exists about their ability to make a successful transition to school is a very important occupational therapy role. Occupational therapists cannot use assessment results, however, in order to make judgements or recommendations about a child's school readiness, or their ability to make a successful transition to school. This does not mean that occupational therapy assessment is not useful, but it does recognize that assessments should only be used for the purpose for which they have been developed. For example, they may indicate the level of skill a child has attained at a certain age. Ideally, assessment should also be based on multiple sources of information, in recognition that the issues impacting on children's ability to make successful transitions to school are multifaceted. There is a very real need for parents, teachers, and other health and educational personnel to work collaboratively to obtain a full complement of information prior to making decisions.

Occupational therapy intervention

Assisting children to develop certain skills and abilities remains an important and valid part of any occupational therapy intervention, and will certainly assist children to make smoother transitions to school (Dockett & Perry, 2001). It is important to bear in mind, however, that lasting improvements in achievement are least

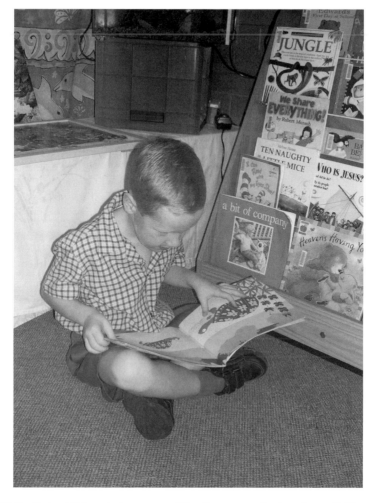

Figure 11.2 Early childhood classrooms utilize floor space for learning activities, as well as desks and more formal classroom spaces.

noted when children are *remediated* by trying to teach them isolated skills. If skills are learned in meaningful contexts they are more likely to be generalized to other contexts (National Association for the Education of Young Children [NAEYC], 1995). The occupational therapy perspective must therefore be broader than simple skill acquisition.

Prigg (2002) identified several additional roles identified by six occupational therapists interviewed about their experiences with children with special learning needs during the period of transition to school. In addition to addressing skill acquisition, occupational therapists also worked with and made recommendations to school personnel regarding the degree of teacher aide time required, made modifications to equipment or the school environment, used adaptive and compensatory treatment approaches such as altering classroom or playground environments, and adapted classroom activities. Provision of parent support in terms of assisting parents to make decisions about the type of school or classroom environment that would be suited to a particular child was also identified.

Occupational therapists are well placed to empower parents to investigate thoroughly all available educational options for their children in order to maximize the goodness of fit. Encouraging parents to interview school principals to obtain a sense of the ethos of the school in which their children will be functioning will assist greatly with decision making. What support does the school offer to children with special needs? What kinds of social programmes and anti-bullying measures are in place? Does the school place children with teachers each year based on an informed and deliberate consideration of which classroom environment and teaching style would best suit them? What roles are parents encouraged to play by the school in order to facilitate an optimal transition for their children?

Summary

Transitions can be conceptualized in terms of a phase that occurs between occupational roles. Some transitions will be negotiated with ease, and others will prove more problematic. One particular transition occurring in many children's lives is that which occurs when children start school. Transition to school is a complex process with many influences. The context in which transition occurs appears to have a strong impact on the outcome of transitions, but it is still not well understood. Traditionally, those considering transitions to school for young children have focused on a skills only model of transition, which emphasizes the importance of child characteristics such as school readiness. More recently, perspectives have broadened and a developmental model of school transition has been proposed, which centres on the broader interactions between children, families and school factors (Lloyd et al., 1999). In reality, however, it appears that our expanding knowledge and broadening understanding of the interactive nature of school transition remains primarily academic. In practice, school transitions continue to be predominantly conceptualized in terms of school readiness models. With increasing emphasis placed on performance criteria and assessment of students as a means of making schools accountable for children's progress, the attention placed on children's abilities and deficiencies has escalated even further (La Paro & Pianta, 2000).

Occupational therapists assisting children to make optimal transitions to their new roles as school students will need to work closely within a multidisciplinary team in order to achieve a full complement of information from whoever is involved in the transition process. Assisting in transition may involve working with the child to develop certain skills. It may also involve assisting parents to assess, advocate and make choices about the environment in which their child will best fit. It may also mean speaking to the teacher about how best to support the child in that particular classroom.

Ramey & Ramey (1999) considered that successful school transitions involved five key elements:

(1) Children have positive feelings about school, teachers and peers.
(2) Children make good progress in all aspects of their development (physical, social, emotional and intellectual).
(3) Parents express positive attitudes towards the school and encourage their children's learning.
(4) Teachers provide developmentally appropriate experiences in a supportive and nurturing classroom environment.
(5) Relationships between families and school environments are mutually supportive

It can be seen from these elements that successful school transition is not purely dependent on the developmental capabilities of children, but involves a complex interplay of the child, their family, school, social and physical environment.

References

Achenbach, T. M., McConaughy, S. H. & Howell, C. T. (1987). Child/adolescent behavioural and emotional problems: implications of cross-informant correlations for situational specificity. *Psychological Bulletin, 101*, 213–232.

American Academy of Pediatrics (1995). The inappropriate use of school 'readiness' tests. *Pediatrics, 95*, 437–438.

Amundson, S. J. & Weil, M. (1996). Prewriting and handwriting skills. In: J. Case-Smith, A. S. Allen & P. N. Pratt (Eds.), *Occupational therapy for children* (pp. 524–561). St Louis, MO: Mosby.

Badley, E. M. (1995). The genesis of handicap: definition, models of disablement and role of external factors. *Disability and Rehabilitation, 17*, 53–62.

Bredekamp, S. & Shepard, L. (1989). How best to protect children from inappropriate school expectations, practices and policies. *Young Children, 44* (3), 14–24.

Bronfenbrenner, U. & Morris, P. A. (1998). The ecology of developmental processes. In: W. Damon & R. M. Lerner (Eds.), *Handbook of child psychology: theoretical models of human development* (pp. 993–1029). New York: John Wiley & Sons.

De Cos, P. L. (1997). *Readiness for kindergarten: what does it mean?* (No. ERIC Document Reproduction Service No. ED 415 969). Sacramento, CA: California Research Bureau, California State Library.

Dockett, S., Perry, B. & Tracey, D. (1997). *Getting ready for school.* Paper presented at the Annual Conference of the Australian Association for Research in Education, Brisbane, Australia. (ERIC Document Reproduction Service No. ED 421 248).

Dockett, S., Perry, B., Howard, P. & Meckley, A. (1999). *What do early childhood educators and parents think is important about children's transition to school? A comparison between data from the city and the bush.* Paper presented at the Australian Association for Research in Education, Melbourne. Retrieved 25 June 2004 from http://www.aare.edu.au/99pap/per99541.htm

Dockett, S. & Perry, B. (2001). Starting school: effective transitions. *Early Childhood Research and Practice, 3* (2). Retrieved from http://ecrp.uiuc.edu/r3n2/dockett.html

Dockett, S. & Perry, B. (2002). Who's ready for what? Young children starting school. *Contemporary Issues in Early Childhood, 3*, 67–89.

Doherty, L. (2003). Making the grade. *The Sydney Morning Herald* (1–2 November p. 33).

Dubois, S. A. (1996). Preschool services. In: J. Case-Smith, A. S. Allen & P. N. Pratt (Eds.), *Occupational therapy for children* (pp. 671–692). St Louis, MO: Mosby.

Entwisle, D. R. & Alexander, K. L. (1993). Entry into school: the beginning school transition and educational stratification in the United States. *Annual Review of Sociology*, *19*, 401–423.

Entwisle, D. R. & Alexander, K. L. (1998). Facilitating the transition to first grade: the nature of transition and research on factors affecting it. *The Elementary School Journal*, *98*, 351–364.

Feagans, L. V., Merriwether, A. M. & Haldane, D. (1991). Goodness of fit in the home: its relationship to school behaviour and achievement in children with learning disabilities. *Journal of Learning Disabilities*, *24*, 413–420.

Goodnow, J. J. (1988). Parents' ideas, actions and feelings: models and methods from developmental and social psychology. *Child Development*, *59*, 286–320.

Graue, M. E. (1992). Readiness, instruction and learning to be a kindergartener. *Early Education and Development*, *3*, 92–114.

Graue, M. E. (1999). Diverse perspectives on kindergarten contexts and practices. In R. C. Pianta & M. J. Cox (Eds.), *The transition to kindergarten* (pp. 109–142). Baltimore, MD: Paul H. Brookes Publishing Co.

Gredler, G. R. (1992). *School readiness: assessment and educational issues*. Brandon, Vt: Clinical Psychology Publishing Company.

Gredler, G. R. (1997). Issues in early childhood screening and assessment. *Psychology in the Schools*, *34*, 99–105.

Hill, J. (1991). *Ready, set, school. A guide to the primary years*. Bacchus Marsh, Vic.: Jeanette Hill.

Holloway, S. D., Rambaud, M. F., Fuller, B. & Eggers-Pierola, C. (1995). What is 'appropriate practice' at home and in childcare? Low-income mothers' views on preparing their children for school. *Early Childhood Research Quarterly*, *10*, 451–473.

Irvine, J. (2000). *Thriving at school*. East Roseville, New South Wales: Simon & Schuster.

Kagan, S. L. & Neuman, M. J. (1998). Lessons from three decades of transition research. *The Elementary School Journal*, *98*, 365–379.

La Paro, K. M. & Pianta, R. C. (2000). Predicting children's competence in the early school years: a meta-analytic review. *Review of Educational Research*, *70*, 443–484.

Law, M., Missiuna, C., Pollock, N. & Stewart, D. (2001). Foundations for occupational therapy practice with children. In: J. Case-Smith (Ed.), *Occupational therapy for children* (pp. 39–70). St Louis, MO: Mosby.

Lewit, E. M. & Baker, L. S. (1995). School readiness. *The future of children*, *5*, 128–139.

Lightfoot, C. & Valsiner, J. (1992). Parental belief systems under the influence: social guidance of the construction of personal cultures. In: I. E. Sigel, A. V. McGillicuddy-De Lisi & J. J. Goodnow (Eds.), *Parental belief systems. The psychological consequences for children*. (pp. 393–414). Hillsdale, NJ: Lawrence Erlbaum Associates.

Lloyd, J. W., Steinberg, D. R. & Wilhelm-Chapin, M. K. (1999). Research on the transition to kindergarten. In: R. C. Pianta & M. J. Cox (Eds.), *The transition to kindergarten* (pp. 305–316). Baltimore, MD: Paul H. Brookes Publishing Co.

McBryde, C. L. (2001). *Factors influencing parent and preschool teacher perceptions of readiness for, and adjustment to, school*. Unpublished Doctoral thesis, University of Queensland, Brisbane, Australia.

McBryde, C. L., Ziviani, J. & Cuskelly, M. (2004). School readiness and factors that influence decision making. *Occupational Therapy International*, *11*, 193–208.

Margetts, K. (1994). *Children's adjustment to the first year of school.* Unpublished Masters thesis, the University of Melbourne, Melbourne, Australia.

May, D. C. & Kundert, D. K. (1997). School readiness practices and children at-risk: examining the issues. *Psychology in the Schools, 34,* 73–83.

Meisels, S. J. (1992). Doing harm by doing good: iatrogenic effects of early childhood enrolment and promotion policies. *Early Childhood Research Quarterly, 7,* 155–174.

Meisels, S. J. (1999). Assessing readiness. In: R. C. Pianta & M. J. Cox (Eds.), *The transition to kindergarten* (pp. 39–66). Baltimore, MD: Paul H. Brookes Publishing Co.

Miller, S. A. (1988). Parents' beliefs about children's cognitive development. *Child Development, 59,* 259–285.

Narahara, M. & Lass, M. J. (1998). *Kindergarten entrance age and academic achievement* (ERIC Document Reproduction Service No. 421 218). Long Beach, CA: California State University.

National Association for the Education of Young Children (NAEYC) (1995). *NAEYC position statement on school readiness.* Retrieved 2 November 2003 from http://naeyc.org/resources/position_statements/psredy98.htm

New South Wales Department of School Education (1997). *Transition to school for young children with special learning needs.* Sydney: New South Wales Department of Education.

Pianta, R. C. & Walsh, D. J. (1996). *High-risk children in schools. Constructing sustaining relationships.* New York: Routledge.

Pianta, R. C. & Cox, M. J. (1999). The changing nature of the transition to school: trends for the next decade. In: R. C. Pianta & M. J. Cox (Eds.), *The transition to kindergarten* (pp. 363–379). Baltimore, MD: Paul H. Brookes Publishing Co.

Pianta, R. C. & Kraft-Sayre, M. (1999). Parents' observations about their children's transitions to kindergarten. *Young Children, May,* 47–52.

Pianta, R. C. & Kraft-Sayre, M. (2003). *Successful kindergarten transition.* Baltimore, MD: Paul H. Brookes Publishing Co.

Pianta, R. C. & La Paro, K. (2003). Improving early school success. *Educational Leadership, April,* 24–29.

Porwancher, D. & De Lisi, R. (1993). Developmental placement of kindergarten children based on the Gesell school readiness test. *Early Childhood Research Quarterly, 8,* 149–166.

Powell, D. R. (1995). *Enabling young children to succeed in school.* Washington DC: American Educational Research Association.

Prigg, A. (2002). Experiences and perceived roles of occupational therapists working with children with special learning needs during the transition to school: a pilot study. *Australian Occupational Therapy Journal, 49,* 100–111.

Primeau, L. A. & Ferguson, J. M. (1999). Occupational frame of reference. In: P. Kramer & J. Hinojasa (Eds.), *Frames of reference for pediatric occupational therapy* (pp. 469–516). Philadelphia: Williams & Wilkins.

Ramey, C. T. & Ramey, S. L. (1999). Beginning school for children at-risk. In: R. C. Pianta & M. J. Cox (Eds.), *The transition to kindergarten* (pp. 217–252). Baltimore, MD: Paul H. Brookes Publishing Co.

Rief, S. F. (2001). *Ready start school.* Paramus, NJ: Prentice Hall Press.

Rimm-Kaufman, S. E. & Pianta, R. C. (2000). An ecological perspective on the transition to kindergarten: a theoretical framework to guide empirical research. *Journal of Applied Developmental Psychology, 21,* 491–511.

Roberts, J. & Carter, A. (2003). *Hi ho, hi ho, it's off to school we go! School readiness group programs: an innovative approach*. Paper presented at the OT Australia (Qld) 2nd Paediatric Conference – What works with kids., Brisbane.

Simeonsson, R. J., Leonardi, M., Lollars, D., Bjorck-Akesson, E., Hollenweger, J. & Martinuzzi, A. (2003). Applying the international classification of functioning, disability and health (ICF) to measure childhood disability. *Disability and Rehabilitation*, 25 (11–12), 602–610.

Smith, M. L. & Shepard, L. A. (1988). Kindergarten readiness and retention: a qualitative study of teachers' beliefs and practices. *American Educational Research Journal*, 25, 307–333.

Sweet, L. & Percival, F. (1996). *Start school smiling*. Glen Luce, Vic.: Prentagast Publishers.

Townsend, E. (1998). Using Canada's 1997 guidelines for enabling occupation. *Australian Occupational Therapy Journal*, 45, 1–6.

Watson, R. (1996). Rethinking readiness for learning. In: D. R. Olsen & N. Torrance (Eds.), *The handbook of education and human development. New models of learning, teaching and schooling* (pp. 148–172). Cambridge, MA: Blackwell.

Weber, E. (1984). *Ideas influencing early childhood education: a theoretical analysis*. New York: Oxford University Press.

Wolery, M. (1999). Children with disabilities in early elementary school. In: R. C. Pianta & M. J. Cox (Eds.), *The transition to kindergarten* (pp. 253–280). Baltimore, MD: Paul H. Brookes Publishing Co.

World Health Organization (WHO) (2001). *International classification of functioning, disability and health: ICF* (Short Version ed.). Geneva: World Health Organization.

Chapter 12

STUDENT PARTICIPATION IN THE CLASSROOM

Jenny Ziviani and Mary Muhlenhaupt

Being part of a school community is an important aspect of children's development. Participating in school enables children to undertake their primary role as student, while at the same time developing aspects of their roles as player and friend. Research has identified positive outcomes for families, school personnel and for *all* students when children with disabilities are educated along with their peers within inclusive environments (Cole et al., 2004; Fisher & Meyer, 2002). Yet there are countries in which children, particularly those with disabilities, are denied their right to education (Brohier, 2001) as presented in the World Declaration on Education for All (United Nations General Assembly, 1989). For those fortunate enough to have this right enacted in legislation, the process by which it is achieved can still present a number of challenges.

For all children the management of self-care, mobility, communication, learning and play activities forms an integral part of their school experience. It has been estimated that 12% of children have a disability which impacts on their abilities in these areas (Msall et al., 2003). It is these children who commonly come in contact with occupational therapy. Understanding the nature of a student's difficulties and how to best facilitate the fit between the child's skills and abilities, the demands of the curriculum and classroom activities, the expectations of teachers, as well as the school's physical, social and cultural environments forms the basis for occupational therapy interventions. Children who have difficulties, and their teachers, often have a long-term and changing interaction with occupational therapists. This affiliation becomes a partnership in participation. The relationship between occupational therapist, student and teacher is often most active at times of transition between grades and schools.

In this chapter we explore the process through which a student's participation in the school environment is enhanced. The chapter objectives are to:

(1) Identify student roles and occupations, and the activities and tasks which underpin school participation: in this process the child as a student, player and friend will be examined
(2) Examine the dynamic relationships between the student, the environment, and the activities and routines of school, which contribute to effective student participation

(3) Discuss ecological and occupation based evaluation approaches that lead to interventions that support student participation in school experiences
(4) Present a framework for designing occupational therapy services that enable children to participate in activities, routines and experiences in the classroom and across the school.

Occupational role of student

The primary role of a child at school is that of student. School provides the structure whereby formal education is delivered and children start on a trajectory that leads them towards deciding on a career or employment path. School has also been described as a child's first workplace (Chapparo & Hooper, 2002). Children as young as six years clearly distinguish between activities as work or play even when learning experiences are playful. When activities involve instruction, writing, thinking, sitting still or listening, then the activity is classified as work.

A secondary role that students adopt at school is that of player. The role of player has particular significance in the early school years. Often it is difficult to distinguish what is play and what is learning for children. Through play children learn concepts, develop social skills, cooperative behaviours and work skills. Their learning may be further optimized by appropriate physical settings, equipment and materials, as well as through exchanges with peer and adult playmates (Rigby & Huggins, 2003). Preschool and beginning school-age programmes feature curricula that emphasize discovery and learning through play activities and small group experiences (Dodge et al., 2002). These classrooms are often set up with open areas for floor activity and small group engagement. Toys and materials for imaginative play are readily accessible on open shelves or in containers, encouraging independence.

The role of friend develops as children become more skilled with the social and behavioural aspects of communication, negotiation, self-awareness and humour. School provides the opportunity for children to meet a wide range of children with a variety of backgrounds and experiences. Learning how to accommodate diversity and manage interpersonal challenges is just as important an aspect of school as the academic requirements. Establishing some close networks of children with whom they can share life experiences is an important buffer for children when faced with adversity.

As children progress through primary grades to intermediate and secondary levels, the roles they assume change. These transitions occur in reaction to expanded school and community expectations, and also as a result of their own maturation. As learners they are expected to become more independent and self-directed as they reach their final years of schooling (Spencer et al., 2003). As players their behaviour becomes more subtle in the confines of school. Instead of running out into the playground as would be the case in the early years, children in middle and high school tend to congregate and share jokes or plan out of school social gatherings. This can represent a merger between the roles of player and friend.

■ **Performance in areas of occupation**
Activities of daily living (ADL)*
Instrumental activities of daily living (IADL)
Education
Work
Play
Leisure
Social participation

■ **Performance skills**
Motor skills
Process skills
Communication/interaction skills

■ **Performance patterns**
Habits
Routines
Roles

■ **Context**
Cultural
Physical
Social
Personal
Spiritual
Temporal
Virtual

■ **Activity demands**
Objects used and their properties
Space demands
Social demands
Sequencing and timing
Required actions
Required body functions
Required body structures

■ **Client factors**
Body functions
Body structures

Figure 12.1 Engagement in occupation to support participation in context or contexts. Adapted from American Occupational Therapy Association. (2002). Occupational therapy practice framework: domain and process. *American Journal of Occupational Therapy, 56* (6), 611. Reprinted with the permission of the American Occupational Therapy Association.
* Also referred to as basic activities of daily living (BADL) or personal activities of daily living (PADL).

The student

To become effective students, children depend upon multiple inherent characteristics, including a range of cognitive, psychological, sensory and motor skills, and the capacity to self-regulate behaviour. The occupational therapy practice framework (AOTA, 2002) defines these *body functions* and *body structures*, as *client factors* that influence a person's participation in a context (see Figure 12.1). These client factors, together with other student attributes and external influences, shape a student's performance for learning, play and friendship roles. Readers are referred to AOTA (2002) for full details. A number of detailed descriptions concerning the foundation and development of specific sensory, motor, cognitive and psychosocial functions are also available, along with schedules of milestones accomplished by children who are developing typically, as well as those with disabilities (see for example the American Academy of Pediatrics http://www.aap.org/topics.html).

In addition to the contribution of client factors, the student also develops skills, and relies on habits and routines in order to support performance in everyday occupational pursuits. Performance skills, habits and routines are distinct from the underlying capacities and functions (client factors) that influence them (AOTA, 2002). While client factors relate to what the student *has*, performance skills, habits and routines relate to what he or she *does*. AOTA's practice framework defines motor, process and communication/interaction skills as 'observable elements of action that have implicit functional purposes' (AOTA, 2002, p. 612). Holding and picking up a glass to drink milk or coordinating both hands together while manipulating jacket closures are examples of *motor skills*. Attending to one's own assignment while other classmates engage in a small group activity, or arranging cups that hold different rock specimens and placing tools in the workspace during a science lab experiment exemplify important *process skills* related to self-control and organization. Making and keeping eye contact with a teacher or classmate during conversation and taking turns while playing a game at recess reflect *communication* and *interaction skills* that contribute to social engagement.

The habitual or routine behaviours that a student uses in the course of daily performance are the final aspect of the student included in this discussion. Habits are the automatic behaviours that develop over time and support an individual as they carry out activities (AOTA, 2002). An effective repertoire of performance patterns depends upon a variety of useful habits that are consistently expressed. An example of a *habit* that contributes to successful school participation is always checking that one's homework notebook is packed in one's schoolbag before leaving school. Some habits, however, are not useful, and maladaptive behaviour can result when they predominate and interfere with function (such as a compulsion to pile any available papers into a neat and organized stack). Habits that are not well developed or not well established also limit a student's participation (such as when a student only sometimes remembers to include their name on each assignment submitted).

Routines are 'established sequences of occupations or activities that provide a structure for daily life' (AOTA, 2002, p. 612). Routines can apply to both groups and to individuals. For example, daily school routines may include arrival, morning class work, lunch, recess, afternoon class work and dismissal. Within the classroom, especially in the younger grades, teachers support routines that reflect the class of students as a group. For example, upon arrival, students may complete a period of independent morning work, followed by a sequence of teacher instruction for the whole group. Classroom routines may include lessons that alternate between sedentary and movement oriented activity. As they mature, develop reliable work habits and are capable of choice making, individual students adopt routines that reflect increased diversity and uniqueness. For example, students pack materials to go home at the end of the school day independently.

In concluding this section, it is important to understand that while general developmental patterns and trends provide a guide, children possess and develop their own unique combinations of inherent attributes, skills, habits and routines as they engage in daily occupations. These variables are a significant influence on each child's performance, but by themselves they do not determine student participation. In order to understand and support a student's engagement in a variety of occupations, the relationship of their personal traits and abilities with features and characteristics in the multiple environments surrounding them needs to be considered.

The learning environment

The importance of environmental prerequisites to school participation by students with disabilities is receiving increased recognition (Baker & Donelly, 2001;

Hemmingson & Borell, 2002; Mihaylov et al., 2004). The interface of the learner's attributes with features that characterize the educational, social and physical environments experienced at school is often indicative of how successfully the student negotiates this period of life (Rigby & Letts, 2003). Occupational therapists consider these associations in order to identify and address supportive, neutral or limiting relationships that influence student participation (Muhlenhaupt, 2003).

The types of tools and materials that are available for a student's use, the physical arrangement of furniture within the classroom, its sights, sounds and scents are some obvious examples of environmental factors that influence student participation. Beyond immediate surroundings, the environment in a broader sense also influences participation. School rules, the way adults encourage interactions between children and a teacher's understanding about how instructional approaches may be modified for a student with a disability are examples of some of these factors.

Physical domain
Building design and architecture varies dramatically across regions and climates, between rural and urban locations and when newly built schools are considered in relation to mature or ageing designs. A unique combination of building style and size, floor plan, spatial elements, designated areas and contents characterizes each individual school and affords different opportunities and challenges for students during the school day.

The classroom spaces in which students spend their time are a focal point when considering the immediate environment for children's school experiences. Low tables and chairs for small groups of students and a designated floor area for teacher led instruction are typical in classrooms for younger students. For older students, individual desks and chairs may be arranged in pairs, clusters, or in rows. Classrooms may include learning centres, specific areas in which students can learn and practise skills or receive individualized instruction (Salend, 2005). The physical arrangement of furniture, work areas, supplies and materials in the classroom is generally teacher directed. Some teachers discourage movement of desks and chairs from their preferred arrangement, while others solicit student ideas or recommendations when planning or rearranging the classroom (Sanoff, 1993).

Aspects of the physical environment are important concerns for occupational therapists as they conduct evaluations and devise strategies to increase student participation in desired activities throughout the school campus. A correct fit between the size of the student and their desk/table and chair affords comfortable and efficient body positioning in relation to work tasks (Smith-Zuzovsky & Exner, 2004). Further, attributes of the physical furnishings and issues surrounding ergonomics have been correlated with student satisfaction related to learning (Zandvliet & Straker, 2001).

Instructional materials such as text books, workbooks, paper, classroom tools and other supplies may be stored on shelves, in containers, cupboards or drawers in the classroom or in outside lockers. Students may also be responsible for the maintenance of their own supply of often used items, such as personal notebooks, paper, pens, pencils, ruler, a calculator and crayons. The physical attributes as well as the ways these materials are presented and used by an individual during instruction are important considerations related to student participation. Each situation is unique, and different experiences are evident among students. It may be difficult for one student to contain letters within the same narrow lined paper that supports another student's handwriting legibility. A tie closure on a notebook may prevent one student from accessing its contents, but for another student, may be a way to provide practice opportunities to master a needed skill.

The sounds available within the classroom include voice, music, phone signals, computers, noise from students moving themselves or their materials, or noise from activity going on outside an open window. Small groups of children may be assigned to learning stations to complete assignments simultaneously, with or without a supervising adult in each group. Concerns have been expressed about the increased noise level in modern classrooms as a result of interactive learning strategies. Children younger than 13 years are less able to hear an oral instruction in the presence of background noise than adults, as a result of immature auditory figure ground perception (Anderson, 2001). High noise levels can compromise the learning of children with hearing impairment, autistic spectrum disorder, visual impairment, attention deficit disorder and for children for whom the spoken language is their second language.

In addition to the sensory stimuli that are naturally present when groups of children assemble together in a learning context, the environment in many classrooms is enriched in order to augment instruction. Teachers use visual aids as a background or as a focal point for instruction. Many classrooms are decorated with photographs, posters, charts or graphs that pertain to current instructional topics. While in progress, and once they are complete, the results of student projects are exhibited in many classrooms. These materials add to the intensity of the students' visual environment. The same stimuli that are unnoticed or offer beneficial elements of interest for some students, may present a distraction or source of distress to others. For example, sensory overstimulation has been identified as a factor that has the potential to impede learning in students with Asperger's syndrome (Myles et al., 2000).

Students participate in activities within secondary learning environments at school, such as the library, gymnasium, cafeteria, computer, art or science labs, and these areas are another focus of the occupational therapist's attention. As part of their education, students may also experience environments beyond the school grounds. Community based work assignments that provide opportunities for students with disabilities to learn skills and routines in the context in which they will be used are an important part of many students' secondary education programmes (Bates et al., 2001; Kluth, 2000). The altered physical context inherent in these experiences is, however, difficult to anticipate until teachers or therapists visit the specific field site.

Social domain
Social aspects of the school environment include students' relationships and interactions with their classmates and playmates, with other students in the school, and

with teachers and other adults who provide instruction and support. Social relationships are complex and interactive, with exchanges between students and their peers, or between students and teachers, or other adults in the school environment, representing variables that influence the subsequent response and performance of each person involved. Research has identified different social behaviour repertoires between students with and without disabilities (Hughes et al., 2002; Lee et al., 2003) and has also shown that the social environment may influence school participation by students with disabilities (Hemmingson & Borell, 2002).

The social environment is carefully considered by teachers in the classroom or in other school experiences. Particular children may be separated with the aim of enhancing the learning environment, while others are *buddied* with a partner to support their learning or positively influence their participation. Establishing positive social relationships between adults and students with special needs is another important factor in supporting constructive student behaviour and social inclusion (Robertson et al., 2003). To this end, an occupational therapist may offer a teacher useful and practical information about a student's medical diagnosis and allay fears related to safety concerns when the student participates in school experiences. Strategies to enhance teacher student interaction may include identifying specific daily arrival routines that the teacher can implement and facilitating interaction between students and their peers.

Many curricula reinforce opportunities to support a positive social environment through instructional approaches that integrate the teaching of both academic and social skills (Winterman & Sapona, 2002). These programmes are advocated to benefit *all* students. Teachers may include a variety of different opportunities for cooperative learning groups (York & Stanford, 2002) in which students work together with less direct instruction and teacher supervision. Benefits in learning and social behaviour have been reported when students play an active role in their learning and take responsibility for evaluating and documenting their performance (Gilberts et al., 2001; Gunter et al., 2002).

Recognizing the importance of the social environment in relation to student participation and learning, occupational therapists devise strategies that support positive interactions between the student with a disability, his/her peers and adults in the education environment. The focus of intervention may be to make the social environment more inclusive, rather than on developing the social skills of the student with a disability.

Temporal domain

When temporal aspects of everyday life are considered, we generally think about clock time and the duration of events within a given period. What is an individual student scheduled, or required, to do during the hours of the schoolday? How long does each task extend or how long should the performance be sustained? Depending upon how scheduling is managed, a student's daily routine may vary with regard to flexibility and predictability. The length of lessons generally increases as students advance through the grades, with increasing expectations that students learn to structure their own time and develop independent work skills within the lesson. Teachers may sequence or alternate prescribed tasks within an instructional period, or encourage students to be responsible for their own time management.

By themselves, these temporal concerns are neither inherently positive nor negative. For example, knowing that a student typically requires fifteen minutes to copy homework assignments from the board does not indicate whether or not that accomplishment represents a desirable level of performance. When other variables are considered, the relevance and usefulness of this student's level of performance becomes clear. Once we know that the teacher writes the nightly homework on the board just before the ten-minute dismissal period, during which students are expected to record or verify their homework assignments, pack their books, retrieve other personal belongings and move to the bus loading zone, we have a more complete picture. Knowing that this student's bus is one of the early buses adds more information that helps us consider how to enable his/her participation.

Beyond the immediate experience of traditional time concepts just discussed, we can consider an individual's *perception of time* and *the meaning of time*, and how these factors contribute to the multidimensional temporal environment that influences his/her participation in everyday activities (Zemke, 2004). A teacher's own perspective regarding time influences the choices made about how daily routines are sequenced and the time allotted for their completion. The teacher's expectations for how individual students manage their work and the importance the teacher gives to timely completion of students' tasks are additional relevant environmental variables.

Cultural and institutional domains

Children with disabilities may be enrolled in neighbourhood schools or they may attend separate schools that are designated to serve only students with disabilities. These school options include programmes that are government funded as well as privately supported programmes with particular secular or non-secular affiliations. All of these different types of schools emphasize values and develop goals and plans that reinforce their particular mission. Occupational therapists working in schools should be familiar with the mission and vision statements that guide programmes and services. The principal's leadership is also important in promoting a culture of inclusion for students with disabilities (Praisner, 2003).

School and classroom rules are designed to shape positive behaviour by individuals and the group as a whole. They are also enlisted to support an environment that is conducive to the specific activities and tasks in which students are engaged. Rules may be explicit or implicit. Teachers often post their priority rules in their classroom, such as 'Raise your hand to ask a question,' 'Do your own work,' 'Be a good friend'. In addition, many unwritten rules exist, such as 'No running in the classroom,' and 'Come to class prepared, with last night's homework completed'. Both adults and students need a clear understanding of both explicit and implicit rules. A classroom teacher may have unique expectations regarding an individual student's compliance with rules and this may be a factor that either supports or limits the child's participation. For example, a teacher who expects that children with Down's Syndrome have reduced attention abilities may continue reading aloud when the student leaves the book corner during the middle of story time. As there is no consequence for leaving the group, nor an effort to bring the student back, the desired behaviour is not reinforced and participation is not facilitated. Holding students accountable to follow school rules and consistent reinforcement of these expectations are strategies used to support positive behaviour and student success.

The curriculum

Curriculum refers to a set course of study. The learning curriculum relates to the structures and processes which are part of a school programme for the delivery of the curriculum. When considering curricula it is not possible to divorce this from the political and institutional structures which are in place to determine its implementation. Inclusive education (where children with special learning requirements are accommodated in regular schools) is now firmly established as a policy imperative in many countries (Lindsay, 2003; UNESCO, 2000). In practice, inclusion may incorporate a range of options, including full-time integration into mainstream classrooms, *pull-out* for extra support, or co-location of special units in school grounds with the sharing of limited class opportunities. Alternative programmes may be provided for students with severe disabilities (for example, students with very limited mobility and communication and/or multiple impairments). The literature reports a divide between the attitudes of special education and regular teachers with respect to inclusion, with the former being more positive than the latter (Avramidis & Norwich, 2002). The reasons are usually related to practical matters and not to the concept, per se. There is also a disparity between what happens in developing and post-industrial countries, with the latter relying more heavily on segregated educational models for children with disabilities (Sakari & Hannu, 2003).

Multiple educational theories (such as Rogoff et al., 1996) support diverse teaching philosophies, techniques and methods that characterize instructional approaches in the classroom. Teachers are influenced by these perspectives during their pre-service preparation, through on-the-job experiences and from continuing professional development pursuits. In the absence of particular evidence regarding pedagogical practices that facilitate the inclusion of learners with different abilities in general education classrooms (Katz et al., 2002), students with disabilities experience a variety of different instructional approaches. Student participation in learning activities is facilitated when the instructional approach used is compatible with the individual's unique strengths and needs. For example, teaching reading to a child with autism using a visual learning approach may be preferred over the phonetic linguistic methodology that is typical in many classrooms (Broun, 2004).

For children with special needs in a regular educational environment the curricula may need to be adjusted to meet their individual learning needs. In the same way that accessibility issues have influenced the design and building of physical space, the need to afford students with disabilities access to learning and to instructional materials has influenced curriculum design. Universal Design for

Table 12.1 Universal design for learning resources.

- ERIC clearinghouse on disabilities and gifted education (1998, Fall). *A curriculum every student can use: design principles for student access* (ERIC/OSEP Topical Brief). Rockville, Md.: ERIC clearinghouse on disabilities and gifted education. http://www.cec.sped.org/osep/ud-sec1.html
- Goodrich, B. (2004, March). Universal design for learning and occupational therapy. *School System Special Interest Section Quarterly, 11* (1), 1–4.
- CAST: Universal Design for Learning. 'CAST is a research and development organization that uses technology to make education more flexible and accessible for all students, especially those with disabilities.' www.cast.org

Learning (UDL) (Rose & Meyer, 2002) is one approach that has gained momentum in recent years. The goal of UDL is to create flexible instructional methods and materials that meet individualized needs and enable learning by all students (see Table 12.1 for additional resources). The most effective modifications to curriculum are designed to provide both social and instructional participation for children with special learning needs (Janney & Snell, 2000). The adaptations are also only as *special* as is necessary to enable participation (Giangreco, 2000) and, ideally, are not intrusive. Where possible, the sensitivities of students with regard to appearing *different* from their peers, should be respected.

The curriculum influences priorities within the classroom, what is valued by the classroom teacher, and the way course material is structured and presented. Standards are used to measure student learning and accomplishment, both incrementally as the student progresses through the grades, and in the longer term to define student graduation from the programme. The development of an understanding of the curriculum will assist occupational therapists to work collaboratively with other school personnel in meeting the specific learning needs of children (Nochajski, 2001).

Occupational therapy to support children's education

A primary goal of occupational therapy services that are provided in the school environment is to enable participation by students in the play, learning and social experiences that are a part of that context. Occupational therapy's focus on performance has application across the academic, social, personal management and extra-curricular activities in which all students engage. The profession's concern over how an individual derives meaning and achieves mastery from participation in activity within a context is relevant when considering the school experiences of a particular student, as well as those of groups of students. The evaluation process underlies decisions regarding how and when occupational therapy services are provided to enable participation by individuals or groups of students, and provides essential information that is needed by the therapist to design an effective programme plan.

Occupational therapy evaluation in the schools

The key functions of evaluation for occupational therapists working in school settings are to:

(1) Determine the nature of the concerns regarding the student's school participation
(2) Identify what types of interventions may support the student's participation
(3) Determine the success of intervention strategies

If, as we have indicated above, the performance of children with special needs is context specific then obviously practitioners should adopt assessments of functional ability which are specific to student participation within the school setting's routines and activities. Furthermore, occupational therapists need to relate evaluation to the educational goals of children. As the focus of occupational therapy involvement with children in school contexts is on educational outcomes (Whallen, 2003), it is necessary to adopt evaluation methods that assist in the development of educationally relevant interventions and the documentation of educationally relevant outcomes.

In keeping with the approach adopted by the World Health Organization (2001) we can apply the ICF model to demonstrate how evaluation starts at the level of participation and then unfolds to take into account activity, environmental and personal considerations. Following an evaluation of the student's performance on school tasks, the impact of underlying skills relating to specific body functions and structures may be assessed to determine if impairment or dysfunction at this level has an impact on performance. The analogy of only 'drilling down as far as necessary' is useful if the outcome is functional performance and participation. Certainly the top-down evaluation approach advocated in occupational therapy literature (Coster, 1998) is an application of this interpretation of the ICF model.

Children are commonly referred to school based occupational therapists because of handwriting difficulties (Case-Smith, 2002; Lockhart & Law, 1994). Using the top-down evaluation approach, the therapist first determines what the student's participation looks like. For example, the student is having difficulty in taking class notes within a reasonable time and hence is not able to complete task requirements. Further, any change to the speed of note taking results in handwriting becoming illegible. Having determined the nature of the participation difficulty, the therapist may evaluate the activity by using an assessment of handwriting speed and legibility. In addition, during an observation of the student taking notes in the classroom, the therapist may attend to the environment and note the physical features (seating, lighting, implement) as well as the social factors (expectations, interactions, distractions) impacting on participation. The therapist gathers perspectives from others through discussion with school personnel, family and the student. At this time the therapist reflects on the personal characteristics that influence participation, identifying those that may operate as facilitators (such as the child may be highly motivated, the family may be very supportive) or barriers (such as the child may have a cognitive limitation, or this aspect of school participation is not valued by the family). Only when this information is available to the therapist might it be necessary to determine if there are particular structures and function issues which might be impacting performance (such as low muscle tone, motor planning difficulties, visual perceptual problems).

With this backdrop let us look at what ecologically based evaluation methods are available to therapists working in schools to evaluate student participation. Ideally, evaluation needs to consider the dynamic relationships among a student's inherent characteristics, the activities and task demands of a curriculum and the supports necessary for student performance. Skilled observation by an occupational therapist encompasses much more than noticing how a student approaches, engages in and completes a task. The unique variables that exist within an environment and ultimately support or limit student performance are important concerns that are noted by the occupational therapist. As there are currently relatively few formal measures which support occupational therapists in this process, clinical reasoning and judgement are widely used (Bryte, 1996; Hanft & Place, 1996). There are, however, some promising developments in the area of formal evaluation.

The School Function Assessment (SFA) (Coster et al., 1998) was developed specifically to measure children's function within a school environment. It was designed and normed in schools in the USA. Nevertheless, there is now support for the use of the SFA assessment both in the USA and also in other countries. The SFA is a detailed instrument which can be used to establish base-line performance, structure intervention and also determine outcomes. The need for a time efficient method of determining school based outcomes has also been identified (McEwen et al., 2003). There is currently developmental work being undertaken on the School Outcome Measure (McEwen et al., 2003). This measure looks at school based performance in self-care, mobility, student role, expression of learning and behaviour. With further refinement this instrument may offer the potential to provide a minimal data set for determining therapy outcomes in schools.

Finally, the School Assessment of Motor and Processing Skills (SCAMPS) (Fisher et al., 2002) is a naturalistic observation based assessment conducted in the child's classroom during their typical routine, where the student performs teacher assigned tasks. Writing, drawing, colouring, cutting and pasting, computer and other manipulative tasks are addressed.

Occupational therapy intervention in the schools

A range of occupational therapy service approaches currently exist within schools. Service provision models that categorize the different ways therapists may direct their time as they intervene to support individuals have included *direct services*, *integrated or supervised therapy* and *consultation* (Dunn, 2000). While these differentiations offer a helpful way to define a continuum of service options, the intervention process is dynamic (AOTA, 2002) and it is not accurate to depict a well-planned intervention programme as fitting within any one particular service model. Contemporary discussions about school system practice (Swinth, 2003) acknowledge a need for therapists to include a variety of service delivery approaches within their intervention plans in order to meet students' needs across situations and settings. In practice, this means that what the therapist does as part of a student's school based therapy service varies over time. For example, during one week the therapist may work in the classroom to help the student learn to use adapted writing tools and an alternate set-up of materials designed to increase participation during written assignments. In the following week the service for this same student may be delivered through a meeting with the classroom teacher to plan new strategies to increase the student's independent work behaviours in the science curriculum.

The elements of the intervention programme that is ultimately implemented depend upon the particular variables that are targeted for change in each student's unique situation. For example, evaluation results may indicate that a student needs to develop a specific skill, ability or performance pattern that is absent, delayed or dysfunctional. When principles of 'least restrictive environment' (Rueda et al., 2000), 'cascade of services' (Wolfe & Hall, 2003) and integrated programming (Dieker, 2001; Giangreco, 2000) are applied, a sequence of options emerges and provides a framework for occupational therapist's clinical reasoning about appropriate intervention plans (see Table 12.2). As a first alternative, the therapist considers whether or not the needed skill or pattern can be developed through the student's continued participation in the already available classroom and special subject programmes. For many students, their current levels of participation in aspects of the curriculum are an appropriate means for them to increase skills and master desired behaviours.

The occupational therapist may identify and recommend that the team consider the use of specific adaptive equipment or environmental modifications as a means to develop skills, optimize performance and support learning. Classroom furniture may be replaced with alternatives that provide needed support for independent seatwork. Furniture arrangements may be reconfigured to increase a child's function in tasks requiring positioning and mobility. Adapted handles may be added to the student's locker, or classroom storage bins, in order for a student to access and store materials independently. Sometimes, simply changing the kinds of cues that are available in the environment makes a significant difference and increases a student's function. For example, the teacher may encourage peer models during clean-up time to facilitate participation by the student who doesn't initiate activity in response to verbal instructions. Specific environmental supports, such as graphic organizers or other visual aids to help a student learn prosocial behaviour, self-regulation or effective work habits may be developed in collaboration with other team members for classroom use (Daly & Ranalli, 2003; Rock, 2004).

As a next step, modifications in the existing curriculum (changes within the activity or materials) are considered, so that the naturally occurring opportunities available to students are tailored to their unique needs. For example, raised line drawings, the availability of three-dimensional props through story boxes or book

Table 12.2 Continuum of intervention options to support children's education programmes.

Begin with the first option and add only as many interventions as necessary to enable student participation

Option	Indications for implementation
• Use natural environment and routines already available in student's current school context.	• Activities and tasks within curriculum afford opportunities for continued practice and experience to develop targeted behaviour. • Therapist highlights beneficial opportunities that are already available, to ensure student's participation.
• Embedding additional strategies into natural environment and routines.	• Alterations that increase opportunities for participation and practice are compatible with current context and routines (examples: use of adapted equipment, alternate tools and materials, placement of student's desk and chair in classroom, use of written instructions, specified work set-up or schedule). • Additional cues from peers and others in environment result in increased student participation (examples: gestures to accompany verbal interaction, cooperative learning, peer-tutoring).
• Alternate curriculum or instructional methods.	• Changes in the teacher's instructional method and/or student's means of response enables access to learning opportunities (examples: incorporate student preview of lesson, break task directions into specific steps, use pictures or concrete materials, student answers questions aloud rather than in writing). • Adjustment to the content and/or conceptual level of material enables student's participation (examples: student answers multiple choice questions rather than write essay, student listens to story as classmates read sections aloud, student paints abstract picture while classmates learn still-life drawing).
• Separate intervention by specialist, in small group or individually with student in classroom.	• Intensive, individualized instruction between student and adult is necessary in order to develop targeted performance (examples: pre-teaching lesson, developing requisite concepts).
• Intervention outside classroom context.	• Only when all other options do not result in increased participation. • Temporary, time-limited approach. • Must include plan for generalization of behaviour into classroom routine.

bags, and self-made books with representational objects stored in pockets, or attached to pages, are some strategies that may be used to help students with visual impairments access primer level story books (Lewis & Tolla, 2003).

The literature includes numerous reports of successful learning when individualized approaches are implemented within routines in their natural context (Fisher & Meyer, 2002; Wehmeyer et al., 2003; Xin & Holmdal, 2003). Studies have also documented increased classroom participation when unique therapeutic knowledge is applied to create strategies that are easily embedded into existing school routines. As an example, occupational therapists may recommend that a student wear a vest containing weights as a means to provide specific organizing and calming sensory input (touch pressure and proprioception) and help the student attend (Olson & Moulton, 2004). Researchers have documented increased focused attention and on-task behaviour by some students when this strategy was implemented during classroom instructional time (Fertel-Daly et al., 2001; VandenBerg, 2001). Increased productivity was correlated with periods during which selected students sat on ball chairs, rather than on their regular firm seats during deskwork in the classroom (Schilling et al., 2003).

In these examples, the situations that were created considered the individual student's needs and the specific context – classroom environment, peer grouping, instructional demands and the desired learning targets and mastery levels. The therapist's expertise was used to design strategies that enabled student performance and, at the same time, were compatible with teacher's goals and plans for how the lesson unfolded. These types of intervention may be thought of as 'behind the scenes' ways to facilitate student participation in the natural routines of the day. This approach to intervention enriches the student's experiences in social and learning situations encountered with peers throughout the school day. Further, when therapists identify ways to support children in the classroom context, they ultimately provide more opportunities for skills practice, thus meeting a primary intent of service provision (Hanft & Pilkington, 2000).

The need for therapists to continue to look for ways to support children within available daily routines and everyday life situations rather than implement specialized interventions and activities is receiving increasing attention in the literature (Campbell, 2004; Dunn, in press; Rush et al., 2003). This concern is particularly relevant for school based therapy practice, when the purpose of education and its unique contextual variables are considered. When therapists find ways to utilize natural routines as a means to support students' goal attainment, their practice represents the essence of occupational therapy. At the same time, these approaches help to make inclusive educational experiences available to all students.

Students are only withdrawn for individual occupational therapy programmes, when natural opportunities embedded in school routines do not provide sufficient exposure and experience to develop the necessary skills to enhance participation. This occupational therapy programme may involve direct intervention to ameliorate, restore or maintain the skills required for the student to overcome the performance challenge, participate and learn in school activities. These sessions may be delivered to small groups of students who have similar or complementary needs that can be addressed within the activity context. Enabling students to access opportunities and experiences together with their peers in the classroom and other school environments is always a priority. As a result, this type of segregated and separate intervention programme is continued only for the duration that it is necessary.

Summary

This chapter has examined the role of student as children engage in the experience of schooling. This is an important developmental period for children and one which can provide numerous challenges, especially for those with disabilities. Occupational therapy services aim to identify and implement strategies that maximize or promote the variables that have a positive influence on the student, task and environment fit; and minimize or eliminate the variables that negatively influence this fit.

References

American Occupational Therapy Association (AOTA) (2002). Occupational therapy practice framework: domain and process. *American Journal of Occupational Therapy*, 56, 609–639.

Anderson, K. L. (2001). Voicing concern about noisy classrooms. *Educational Leadership*, April, 77–79.

Atchison, B. T., Fisher, A. B. & Bryze, K. (1998). Rater reliability and internal scale and person response validity of the school assessment of motor and process skills. *American Journal of Occupational Therapy*, 52, 843–850.

Avramidis, E. & Norwich, B. (2002). Teachers' attitudes towards integration/inclusion: a review of the literature. *European Journal of Special Needs Education*, 17, 2, 129–147.

Baker, K. & Donelly, M. (2001). The social experiences of children with disability and the influence of environment: a framework for intervention. *Disability and Society*, 16, 71–85.

Bates, P., Cuvo, T., Miner, C. & Korabek, C. (2001). Simulated and community-based instruction involving persons with mild and moderate mental retardation. *Research in Developmental Disabilities*, 22, 95–115.

Brohier, W. G. (2001). Breaking the barriers to social integration of disabled persons: 'education for all'? What next? *Asia Pacific Disability Rehabilitation Journal*, 12, 2, 149–154.

Broun, L. (2004). Teaching students with autistic spectrum disorders to read: a visual approach. *Teaching Exceptional Children*, 36, 36–40.

Bryte, K. (1996). *Classroom intervention for the school based therapist*. San Antonio, Tex.: Therapy Skill Builders.

Campbell, P. (2004). Participation-based services: promoting children's participation in natural settings, *Young Exceptional Children*, 8, 20–29.

Case-Smith, J. (2002). Effectiveness of school based occupational therapy intervention on handwriting. *American Journal of Occupational Therapy*, 56, 17–25.

Chapparo, C. J. & Hooper, E. (2002). When is it work? Perceptions of six-year-old children. *Work*, *19*, 291–302.

Cole, C., Waldron, N. & Majd, M. (2004). Academic progress of students across inclusive and traditional settings. *Mental Retardation*, *42*, 136–144.

Coster, W. (1998). Occupation-centered assessment of children. *American Journal of Occupational Therapy*, *52*, 337–344.

Coster, W., Deeney, T., Haliwanger, J. & Haley, S. (1998). *School function assessment*. San Antonio, TX: the Psychological Corporation.

Craig, S., Haggart, A. & Hull, A. (1998). Integrating therapies into the educational setting: strategies for supporting children with severe disabilities. *Physical Disabilities: Education and Related Services*, *17* (2), 91–109.

Daly, P. & Ranalli, P. (2003). Using countoons to teach self-monitoring skills. *Teaching Exceptional Children*, *35* (5), 30–35.

Dieker, L. (2001). Collaboration as a tool to resolve the issue of disjointed service delivery. *Journal of Educational and Psychological Consultation*, *12*, 268–271.

Dodge, D., Colker, T. & Heroman, C. (2002). *The creative curriculum for preschool* (4th ed.). Washington DC: Teaching Strategies, Inc.

Dunn, W. (2000). Designing best practice services for children and families. In: W. Dunn, (Ed.), *Best practice occupational therapy: in community service with children and families* (pp. 109–134). Thorofare, NJ: Slack Incorporated.

Dunn, W. (in press). Supporting children to participate successfully in everyday life by using sensory processing knowledge. *Infants and Young Children*.

Fertel-Daly, D., Bedell, G. & Hinojosa, J. (2001). Effects of a weighted vest on attention to task and self stimulatory behaviors in preschoolers with pervasive developmental disorders. *American Journal of Occupational Therapy*, *55*, 629–640.

Fisher, A. G., Bryze, K. & Hume, V. (2002). *School AMPS: school version of the assessment of motor and process skills*. Fort Collins, CO: Three Star Press.

Fisher, M. & Meyer, L. (2002). Development and social competence after two years, for students enrolled in inclusive and self-contained educational programmes. *Research and Practice for Persons with Severe Disabilities*, *27*, 165–74.

Giangreco, M. (2000). Related services research for students with low incidence disabilities: implications for speech language pathologists in inclusive classrooms. *Language, Speech and Hearing Services in the Schools*, *31*, 230–239.

Gilberts, G., Agran, M., Hughes, C. & Wehmeyer, M. (2001). The effects of peer delivered self-monitoring strategies on the participation of students with severe disabilities in general education classrooms. *Journal of the Association for Persons with Severe Handicaps*, *26*, 25–36.

Gunter, P., Miller, K., Venn, M., Thomas, K. & House, S. (2002). Self-graphing to success: computerized data management. *Teaching Exceptional Children*, *35* (2), 30–34.

Hanft, B. E. & Place, P. A. (1996). *The consulting therapist: a guide for OTs and PTs in schools*. San Antonio: TX, Therapy Skill Builders.

Hanft, B. & Pilkington, O. (2000). Therapy in natural environments: the means or end goal for early intervention? *Infants and Young Children*, *12* (4), 1–13.

Hemmingson, H. & Borell, L. (2002). Environmental barriers in mainstream schools. *Child Care Health and Development*, *28*, 57–63.

Hughes, C., Copeland. S., Wehmeyer, M., Agran, M., Cai, X. & Hwang, B. (2002). Increasing social interaction between general education high school students and their peers with mental retardation. *Journal of Developmental and Physical Disabilities*, *14*, 387–402.

Janney, R. & Snell, M. E. (2000). *Modifying schoolwork*. Baltimore, MD: Paul H. Brookes Publishing Co.

Katz, J., Mirenda, P. & Auerbach, S. (2002). Instructional strategies and educational outcomes for students with developmental disabilities in inclusive 'multiple intelligences' and typical inclusive classrooms. *Research and Practice for Persons with Severe Disabilities*, 27, 227–238.

Kluth, P. (2000). Community referenced learning and the inclusive classroom. *Remedial and Special Education*, 21, 19–26.

Lee, S., Yoo, S. & Bak, S. (2003). Characteristics of friendships between children with and without mild disabilities. *Education and Training in Developmental Disabilities*, 38, 157–166.

Lewis, S. & Tolla, J. (2003). Creating and using tactile experience books for young children with visual impairments. *Teaching Exceptional Children*, 35, 22–28.

Lindsay, G. (2003). Inclusive education: a critical perspective. *British Journal of Special Education*, 30, 1, 3–12.

Lockhart, J. & Law, M. (1994). The effectiveness of a multisensory writing program for improving cursive writing ability in children with sensorimotor difficulties. *Canadian Journal of Occupational Therapy*, 61, 4, 206–214.

McEwen, I., Arnold, S., Hansen, L. & Johnson, D. (2003). Content validity and interrater reliability of a minimal data set to measure outcomes for students receiving school based occupational therapy and physical therapy. *Physical and Occupational Therapy in Pediatrics*, 23, 77–95.

Mihaylov, S., Jarvis, S., Colver, A. & Beresford, B. (2004). Identification and description of environmental factors that influence participation of children with cerebral palsy. *Developmental Medicine and Child Neurology*, 46, 299–304.

Msall, M., Avery, R., Tremont, M., Lima, J., Rogers, M. & Hogan, D. (2003). Functional disability and school activity limitations in 41 300 school-age children: relationship to medical impairments. *Pediatrics*, 111, 548–553.

Muhlenhaupt, M. (2003). Enabling student participation through occupational therapy services in the schools. In: L. Letts, P. Rigby & D. Stewart (Eds.), *Using environments to enable occupational performance* (pp. 177–196). Thorofare, NJ: Slack, Incorporated.

Myles, B., Cook, K., Miller, N., Rinner, L. & Robbins, L. (2000). *Asperger's syndrome and sensory issues: practical solutions for making sense of the world*. Shawnee Mission, KS: Autism Asperger's Publishing Co.

Nochajski, S. M. (2001). Collaboration between team members in inclusive educational settings. *Occupational Therapy in Health Care*, 15, 101–12.

Olson, L. & Moulton, H. (2004). Use of weighted vests in pediatric occupational therapy practice. *Physical and Occupational Therapy in Pediatrics*, 24, 45–60.

Praisner, C. (2003). Attitudes of elementary school principals toward the inclusion of students with disabilities. *Exceptional Children*, 69, 135–145.

Rigby, P. & Huggins, L. (2003). Enabling young children to play by creating supportive environments. In: L. Letts, P. Rigby & D. Stewart (Eds.), *Using environments to enable occupational performance* (pp. 155–176). Thorofare, NJ: Slack, Incorporated.

Rigby, P. & Letts, L. (2003). Environment and occupational performance: theoretical considerations. In: L. Letts, P. Rigby & D. Stewart (Eds.), *Using environments to enable occupational performance* (pp. 17–32). Thorofare, NJ: Slack, Incorporated.

Robertson, K., Chamberlain, B. & Kasari, C. (2003). General education teachers' relationships with included students with autism. *Journal of Autism and Developmental Disabilities*, 33, 123–30.

Rock, M. (2004). Graphic organizers: tools to build behavioral literacy and foster emotional competency. *Intervention in School and Clinic, 40*, 10–37.

Rogoff, B., Matusov, E. & White, C. (1996). Models of teaching and learning: participation in a community of learners. In: D. Olson & N. Torrance (Eds.), *The handbook of education and human development: new models of learning, teaching and schooling* (pp. 388–414). Oxford: Blackwell Publishers, Ltd.

Rose, D. & Meyer, A. (2002). *Teaching every student in the digital age: universal design for learning.* Alexandria, Vic.: Association for Supervision and Curriculum Development.

Rueda, R., Gallego, M. & Moll, L. (2000). The least restrictive environment: a place or a context? *Remedial and Special Education, 21*, 70–78.

Rush, D., Shelden, M. & Hanft, B. (2003). Coaching families and colleagues: a process for collaboration in natural settings. *Infants and Young Children, 16*, 33–47.

Sakari, M. & Hannu, S. (2003). Struggling for inclusive education in the North and South: educators' perceptions on inclusive education in Finland and Zambia. *International Journal of Rehabilitation Research, 26* (1), 21–31.

Salend, S. (2005). *Creating inclusive classrooms: effective and reflective practices* (5th ed.) Upper Saddle River, NJ: Prentice Hall.

Sanoff, H. (1993). Designing a responsive school environment. *Children's Environments, 10* (2), 140–154.

Schilling, D., Washington, K., Billingsley, F. & Deitz, J. (2003). Classroom seating for children with attention deficit hyperactivity disorder: therapy balls versus chairs. *American Journal of Occupational Therapy, 57*, 534–541.

Smith-Zuzovsky, N. & Exner, C. E. (2004). The effect of seated positioning quality on typical six- and seven-year-old children's object manipulation skills. *American Journal of Occupational Therapy, 58* (4), 380–388.

Spencer, J. E., Emery, L. J. & Schneck, C. M. (2003). Occupational therapy in transitioning adolescents to post-secondary activities. *American Journal of Occupational Therapy, 57*, 435–441.

Swinth, Y. (2003). Interventions to promote participation: section II. Education. In: E. Crepeau, E. Cohen & B. Schell (Eds.), *Willard and Spackman's occupational therapy* (10th ed.) (pp. 561–567), Philadelphia: Lippincott Publishing Co.

UNESCO (2000). *Dakar framework for action. education for all: meeting our collective commitments.* Paris: United Nations Educational, Scientific and Cultural Organization.

United Nations General Assembly, Convention on the Rights of the Child, Resolution 44/25, adopted 20 November 1989.

VandenBerg, N. (2001). The use of a weighted vest to increase on-task behavior in children with attention difficulties. *American Journal of Occupational Therapy, 55*, 621–628.

Wehmeyer, M., Yeager, D., Bolding, N., Agran, M. & Hughes, C. (2003). The effects of self-regulation strategies on goal attainment for students with developmental disabilities in general education classrooms. *Journal of Developmental and Physical Disabilities, 15*, 79–91.

Whallen, S. S. (2003). Effectiveness of occupational therapy in the school environment. CanChild Centre for Childhood Disability Research. Retrieved 16 August 2004 from www.fhs.mcmaster.ca/canchild

Winterman, K. & Sapona, R. (2002). Everyone's included: supporting young children with autism spectrum disorders in a responsive classroom learning environment. *Teaching Exceptional Children, 35* (1), 30–35.

Wolfe, P. & Hall, T. (2003). Making inclusion a reality for students with severe disabilities. *Teaching Exceptional Children, 35* (4), 56–61.

World Health Organization (WHO) (2001). *International classification of functioning, disability and health* (ICF). Geneva, Switzerland: World Health Organization.

Xin, J. & Holmdal, P. (2003). Snacks and skills: teaching children functional counting skills. *Teaching Exceptional Children, 35* (5), 46–51.

York, C. & Stanford, C. (2002). Learning to cooperate: a teacher's perspective. *Teaching Exceptional Children, 34* (6), 40–44.

Zandvliet, D. & Straker, L. (2001). Physical and psychosocial aspects of the learning environment in technology rich classrooms. *Ergonomics, 44*, 838–857.

Zemke, R. (2004). The 2004 Eleanor Clarke Slagle lecture: time, space and the kaleidoscopes of occupation. *American Journal of Occupational Therapy, 58*, 608–620.

Chapter 13

CHILDREN'S PARTICIPATION IN PHYSICAL ACTIVITY AT SCHOOL

Doune Macdonald, Jenny Ziviani and Rebecca Abbott

This chapter introduces physical activity and examines why it is important for children, before examining contemporary patterns of physical activity engagement. The context for this discussion is school oriented physical activity: curricular, extra-curricular, and remedial. The aims of the chapter are therefore to:

(1) Locate physical activity in the various roles which children undertake as students
(2) Clarify the place and purposes of physical activity within the school environment
(3) Suggest principles for creating sustainable and engaging physical activity in and beyond schools

Physical activity: definitions, benefits and determinants

Definitions

Physical activity is any bodily movement produced by skeletal muscles resulting in energy expenditure. This definition reminds us to think about physical activity as occurring in daily occupations and manifesting in transport, play and household chores. Any attempts to increase physical activity levels in children should therefore account for these varied opportunities. Studies suggest that children have a narrow understanding of what constitutes physical activity and wrongly equate physical activity with physical fitness and low body weight (Burrows et al., 2002; Trost et al., 2000). Body size and shape are determined genetically, and by what children eat and how active they are. It is essential that children understand that being active is more important than their body size, that being thin does not equate with being fit, and that being overweight and active is healthier than being thin and inactive. On this basis, along with negative effects sometimes observed when children focus on weight measurement, schools are advised to invest in the promotion of physical activity.

Benefits

Within the epidemiological literature, the development of positive attitudes towards physical activity and adoption of a physically active lifestyle are considered to be major components of preventive medicine that should begin in childhood (Royal College of Physicians, 1991). Part of the rationale for this is that the level of engagement in physical activity tracks from childhood through to adulthood (Anderssen et al., 1996; Raitakari et al., 1994) and that physical inactivity in adulthood is correlated with an increased incidence of chronic diseases (Katzmarzyk et al., 2000). Furthermore, there is clear evidence demonstrating that:

- Children who engage in weight bearing activities have better bone density and skeletal health, both in the short and long term (Bailey et al., 1999)
- Learning by doing at an early age is fundamental to the quality of skill acquisition (Behets, 1997) and the optimal *age of readiness* is 5–6 years of age (Blanksby et al., 1995)
- Children who are more physically active are less likely to be overweight (Berkey et al., 2003; Moore et al., 1995)
- Children who are physically active are more likely to have higher self-esteem, positive body image and less stress and anxiety than less active children (Alfermann & Stoll, 2000)

Determinants

The physiologic, environmental, psychosocial and socio-demographic factors that influence children's choices to participate in physical activity have been widely studied. The most consistently documented influences are age and gender; with physical activity declining with age, and at all ages boys being more active than girls (Hovell et al., 1999; Trost et al., 2002). The role of the family as a major influence upon children's physical activity is undisputed, and relates to beliefs and expectations held by parents, interacting with gender and socio-economic status (Brustad, 1993; Raudsepp & Viira, 2000). In Brustad's study (1996) of eight to eleven-year-old children, boys' attraction to physical activity was most strongly related to parental encouragement, whereas in girls, the most important parental socialization variable was perceived parental enjoyment of physical activity. Peers also have a strong influence on attitude to, and participation in, physical activity (Raudsepp & Viira, 2000; Zeijl et al., 2000). In the study by Zeijl et al., peer influence became more dominant as children got older, with ten to twelve-year-old children spending a substantial part of their leisure time with parents and siblings but after fourteen years of age, children's leisure interests were more aligned with those of their peer groups.

Clearly, the factors influencing physical activity do not work in isolation, but interact with each other alongside socio-economic status, race, ethnicity and geographical location. For example, the Australian Bureau of Statistics' figures from 2000 indicated that 59% of Australian children aged between five and fourteen years old were involved in organized sport outside school hours and that 29% participated in one or more *cultural* activities (Australian Bureau of Statistics, 2000). However, when such data sets are examined in terms of income, location and ethnicity, children from low socio-economic, minority and rural backgrounds have less participation, due to limitations such as money, parental encouragement and transport (Brown et al., 2001; Woodfield et al., 2002; Wright et al., 2003).

The majority of psychosocial studies that have sought to determine children's motivations for physical activity have employed structured questionnaires. This line of research has shown that *fun, fitness* and *competence* are important reasons for children to participate in sport and that fun is more important for younger children, whilst physical motives are more important for older children (Buonamano, 1995; Kolt & Capaldi, 2001; Wang & Wiese-Bjornstal, 1996; Weinberg et al., 2000). Furthermore, a recent Australian study with seven and eight-year-olds also suggested that while fun and companionship were important even at this early age, there was a sense of the imperative for children to care for their bodies (Macdonald et al., 2005).

Current dilemmas surrounding children and physical activity

Children's physical activity, obesity, screen based activities and diet have become front page news. While for those working in the physical activity field these issues have been of growing concern for a number of years, it is only relatively recently that they have been taken up by politicians and the media. The response to this has included the blaming and shaming of individual young people, a plethora of testing (both fitness and weight), and a return to the 'old days when everyone played sport'.

Through the education system, children and young people are now expected to become healthy citizens who are informed about risks to their health, self-regulating with regard to their own health practices, and critically reflective of health practices in general (Tinning & Glasby, 2002). The individual is required to constantly monitor diet, exercise and consumption of such unhealthy products as tobacco, alcohol and fast foods (Petersen, 1997). Consequently, 'public health knowledge and practices play a central role in regulating the body by prescribing bodily practices through which health should be accomplished and illness avoided' (Lupton, 1998, p. 122). Alongside these health messages, advertising, TV soap operas and lifestyle magazines have become new regulatory techniques for the shaping of the self, thereby replacing much of the traditional authority of education (Bunton & Burrows, 1995; Rose, 2000). These messages are largely based upon the assumption that the individual has the ability to make healthy choices, a supposition that is contested by statistics, which indicate the limiting effects of social structures such as income, ethnicity, or even gender.

In the current rush to curtail what is being called a *crisis* in young people's health, the misuse of *popular knowledge* rather than that informed by research can prove to be not only ineffective but potentially detrimental to student learning and growth. For example, in Australia and elsewhere, we are seeing an increase in fitness testing and weight measurement practices. Armstrong & Biddle (1992), amongst others, argue against compulsory fitness testing as they maintain there are no tests that are suitable for use in the school environment or that provide valid and objective measures of fitness. Research also suggests that fitness testing can be a major contributor to negative attitudes towards physical education (Armstrong & Biddle, 1992; Luke & Sinclair, 1991).

Most scholars in the field of physical activity and health would agree, however, that a major challenge for schools is to provide enough time for children to be physically active and also offer children a range of physical activities in which they are interested and that can be sustained, perhaps across the lifespan (Armstrong & Welsman, 1997; Baranowski et al., 1992; Cavill et al., 2001). This should cause schools to question the place of compulsory, traditional, competitive physical activity and sport in their curricula. In many western contexts there is evidence of increasing interest in non-traditional and recreational physical activities and sports (such as surfing, skate boarding, martial arts), and that children and young people want opportunities to *snack* on activities across shorter time spans, making less commitment to equipment purchases, club fees and seasonal competitions.

Finally, it is curious that at a time when there are calls for increased participation in physical activity and sport, physical education still holds a somewhat marginal status in many schools. There remains a common-sense view that schooling is about educating the mind while at the same time taming the body. This is reflected in the promotion of academic subjects (such as science and maths) over practical subjects (such as physical education and art), in superiority of cognitive word based communication (such as reading and writing) over other forms of communication (such as visual and movement), and in the coupling of serious learning with stationary, individual deskwork in classroom settings rather than physically active work. This mind/body dualism is partly responsible for discourses which on the one hand may serve to devalue physical activity in schools, yet on the other hand may rebuke students who may be overweight and thereby demonstrating irresponsibility (Young, 1998).

Physical activity within the school curriculum

Physical education is the subject within the formal curriculum which explicitly focuses upon physical activity. Physical education is that part of a child's education which uses physical activity as the primary medium for education. In some countries, physical education is a stand alone subject with its own syllabus (such as USA and France), while in other countries it is part of a key learning area (such as health and physical education in Australia and New Zealand). Definitions and purposes of physical education vary in their scope and philosophies, as indicated below.

Physical education is any process which increases a child's ability and desire to participate, in a socially responsible way, in physical activity in the form of games, sport, dance, adventure activities and other leisure pursuits. The USA National

Association for Sport and Physical Recreation (NASPR) (1995, p. 1) has described a physically educated person as one who:

(1) Demonstrates competency in many movement forms and proficiency in a few
(2) Applies movement concepts and principles to the learning and development of motor skills
(3) Exhibits a physically active lifestyle
(4) Achieves and maintains a health enhancing level of physical fitness
(5) Demonstrates responsible personal and social behaviour in physical activity settings
(6) Demonstrates understanding and respect for differences among people in physical activity settings
(7) Understands that physical activity provides opportunities for enjoyment, self-expression, and social interaction

As part of a key learning area rather than a stand alone subject, physical education often sits alongside health education, personal development, outdoor education, aspects of home economics and religious education, to name a few. As a broader field of study it aims to: 'develop the knowledge, skills, attitudes and motivation to make informed decisions and to act in ways that contribute to personal wellbeing, the wellbeing of other people and that of society as a whole' (New Zealand Ministry of Education, 1999, p. 6).

Place and structure of school sport

Best practice in physical education reflects contemporary research in learning that draws on several constructivist principles, such as engagement with real problems, inclusion and negotiation (Wright et al., 2004). In physical education settings, two pedagogies, teaching games for understanding (TGfU) and sport education highlight student centred, context based approaches to teaching and learning. By starting with the tactical dimensions of the game rather than learning a set of discrete, game related skills and drills, TGfU has been shown to increase students' learning and rigor in a range of game-like physical activities (Grehaigne & Godbout, 1995). Sport education seeks to engage children and young people as players, coaches, managers, scorers and trainers in units of work that involve student managed competition, with a view to better aligning physical education to the sporting community (Kirk & Macdonald, 1998). Other pedagogical approaches in physical education, such as cooperative learning (Dyson, 2002), negotiated curricula (Glasby & Macdonald, 2004), problem based pedagogies and integrated curricula (Macdonald et al., 2004) also seek to engage children and young people with personal, social and environmental issues that are meaningful to them (Carlson, 1995; Macdonald, 2004).

What is understood and practised as school sport varies worldwide and it is claimed that 'the relationship between sport and physical education in the school context has often been uncertain and unclear' (Evans, 1990, p. 6). Sport can be understood as games or pastimes involving gross bodily movement, for regular competitive physical activity, governed by constituted rules. Sport ranges between informal game-like play (with rules, fixed time and space) to highly institutionalized activities (for example dedicated coached programmes, such as rowing and tennis). In some contexts, a semi-regular afternoon of sport constitutes the school's physical education programme. In other contexts, such as fee paying schools in Australia, New Zealand or the UK, school sport comprises regular, highly structured intra- and inter-school competition that is central to the school's image and ethos. Despite these different configurations, the idea, or indeed the ideal, of school sport is valued by many parents and young people. Indeed, research suggests that many parents consider that sport participation engenders personality traits such as teamwork, effort and responsibility.

We have previously argued the potential benefits of school based physical activity, of which one form is sport. If carried out safely (both physically and emotionally), proponents of sport would argue that it is a powerful cultural practice in which the majority of young people should become literate (Siedentop, 1994). The extensive use of modified sports (that is those which use child friendly equipment and spaces, in addition to simplified and inclusive rules) has done a great deal to attract and maintain the interest of a broader range of children. Others have criticized sport for becoming increasingly commodified, and overly stressing a 'performance ethic' in which young people are 'encouraged to evaluate their experiences in terms of developing technical skills and progressing to higher personal levels of achievement in one or more sports' (Coakley, 2001, p. 113).

Research also suggests that many young people reject sport when there is an over-emphasis on winning, and an under-emphasis on fun (Brustad et al., 2001). Various alienating factors, alongside aspects of youth and risk cultures, have led to increased participation in non-traditional, alternate, often unstructured sports such as skate boarding, in line skating and 'x' sports (extreme sports such as BMX bike-jumping and snowboarding) (Wright et al., 2003). With the concern that many children have too much pressure on them to develop sporting expertise at an early age, Cote (1999) developed a model to map appropriate participation pathways. Cote described the ages of six to thirteen years as the *sampling* years, which are dominated by deliberate play, enjoyment and immediate rewards; a period in which children develop interest and become involved in various sports. This is followed by the *specializing* years, between 13 and 15 years, when children tend to focus on one or two specific sporting activities. Whilst fun and excitement remain central to the sporting experience, the key feature of this phase is the development of sport specific skills.

Physical activity: making friends and enemies within the curriculum

While acknowledging that some young people have positive experiences in physical education and sport, and healthy attitudes to physical activity and their bodies, many young people still leave school oppressed by the tyrannies of elitism, sport and cult of the body. Practices resulting in the marginalization of young people from physical education and sport have included a lack of personal meaning, lack of control and isolation (Carlson, 1995), and a lack of opportunity for some groups such as students with disabilities (Hutzler, 2003). Other reasons why young people can become alienated relate to discrimination on the basis of gender (Reay, 2001), sexuality (Portman & Carlson, 1991), social class (Lee et al., in press), geographic isolation (Lee et al., in press), race (Daiman, 1995), age (Hunter, 2002; Tinning & Fitzclarence, 1992), physicality (Shilling, 1993) and religion (Zaman, 1997). Much of this research indicates that the understanding of equity and inclusion is still poor in some contexts and that the teaching of, and with, difference within a class is at best difficult, and at worst ignored. Ironically, it is those children who may be marginalized from participation in mainstream physical activity in the playground or community who are most in need of an inclusive curriculum.

Addressing the needs of those students for whom physical activity participation does not come easily is complex. It is important to recognize differences within a group such as girls, or young people with disabilities, or those who are geographically isolated. Yet, in taking a blanket approach to meeting the needs of these groups, teachers or therapists can overlook important individual differences and the ability individuals may have to move beyond their marginality. The implications of this for those working with children and young people are that they need to be simultaneously aware of the structural, societal and physical limitations on some groups' access to physical activity (such as working in a low socio-economic school), while at the same time seeing the differences amongst those children.

This perspective provides signposts for how therapists and teachers might approach physical activity in the curriculum. Here we take the example of physical activity provision in a low socio-economic school. The student population may have less equipment at home, less space in which to play, less money to buy uniforms and for club fees, reduced access to transport, less control over leisure time and options, and thereby possibly less opportunity to develop motor skills. In these contexts, the provision of school based physical activity is particularly important and, as such, the programmes should pay particular attention to:

- Motor skill development in a playful, game-like, non-competitive atmosphere
- Linking physical education to intra-school opportunities for constructive play and sport related celebrations
- Recruiting members of the community to assist with the provision of physical education
- Educating and encouraging generalist teachers to value and enjoy teaching physical education and including movement across the curriculum
- Assisting children to access low-cost community activity options

Those working with school based physical activity need to be reflective of not only *what* is being taught (is it contemporary, relevant, health-promoting?) and *how* it is being taught (is the context and pedagogy safe, inclusive, respectful, fun?), but also how it is being assessed (what is being rewarded?).

Physical activity beyond the school curriculum

Although physical education within the curriculum and school sport are considered to be the time in the school day when children engage in physical activity, there are many other areas of school life that provide activity opportunities.

Recess

Recess or breaktime provides a recreational break for children within the school day, and in most schools lunch-time also has a component of recess. It is a time for children to escape from the classroom, to get outside, let off steam and play with friends. The amount of time devoted to recess or breaktimes during a school-day varies, but estimates range from between 15 and up to 25% of the schoolday (Blatchford & Sumpner, 1998; Zask et al., 2001). Recess can therefore play a significant role in enabling children to be physically active.

Research shows that recess is seen by children as an enjoyable time when they can play, meet friends, have freedom from adult control and develop social skills and competence (Blatchford, 1998). Recess also has important developmental and educational implications, in particular in its facilitation of peer relations and friendships (Pellegrini & Smith, 1993). In the study by Blatchford & Sumpner (1998), one of the major reasons primary schoolchildren cited for liking recess, was the 'opportunity to play games'. It can facilitate the art of simple play. Play is most generally defined in terms of serving no immediate purpose, and yet in many ways it is the quintessential developmental activity of childhood (Pellegrini & Blatchford, 2000). Through active free play and peer interaction, children can develop a respect for rules, gain self-discipline and construct an appreciation for other children's cultures and beliefs (National Association of Early Childhood Specialists/State Departments of Education, 2001). Through active play, children can also learn about their bodies' capabilities, through practise of physical skills such as running, climbing, jumping, chasing, batting and kicking.

Although recess provides the opportunity to be active, it does not necessarily follow that children will be active. Studies from America (Kraft, 1989; McKenzie et al., 1997) suggest that children are becoming less active, with the most recent surveys suggesting that children spend less than 50% of their recess time in moderate to vigorous physical activity (MVPA). Similar findings have been reported for Australia (Zask et al., 2001), though a study of English children found that as little as 15% of their recess was spent in moderate to vigorous physical activity (Stratton, 1999).

Evidence is emerging which indicates that recess in schools worldwide is undergoing a significant change. In many Australian schools, there is no afternoon recess, and the traditional lunch-hour has been reduced to 45–50 minutes (Evans, 2003).

In the UK, between 1991 and 1996, more than 38% of primary schools and 26% of infant schools reduced the length of the lunch-break, and more than one in four schools abolished the afternoon break (Blatchford & Sumpner, 1998). These changes came despite an increase in the length of the schoolday over the same time period. The reasons cited are manifold, and include: concerns about pupil health and safety, and pressures on staff to increase academic learning time to improve numeracy and literacy standards.

One of the major concerns regarding declining recess times is the effect this may have on children's physical activity levels. Research suggests that children who have less opportunity to be active during the day, do not compensate after school (Dale et al., 2000). Reduction in time dedicated to recess is not the only concern. As Evans (2003, p. 56) detailed in a recent commentary on the changes in Australian school recess, the following sign, actually witnessed, is typical of what might be seen in primary school playgrounds today:

'In this school there is to be:
 NO running on or jumping off playground equipment
 NO running in or around the school buildings
 NO fighting or playing games that involve tackling
 NO climbing trees or playing in or under them
 NO ball games played near the school buildings.'

This sign depicts the rising concern for safety and risk in the school context. However, as schools adopt more sanitized play environments, with *safer* equipment and more rules governing its use, the risk is simply altered. This supposed *safer* environment, may be in itself less stimulating for the engagement of physical activity, which carries its own risk to health.

Attempts to increase physical activity in school break periods have demonstrated that physical activity can be increased by 17–60% with simple low-cost interventions (Jago & Baranowski, 2004). The painting of school playgrounds, and provision of extra equipment and space in which to play, have both been demonstrated to increase engagement in physical activity (Stratton & Leonard, 2002). In today's society, where many children may not have access to either a safe area near home to play or their own equipment, provision of such facilities within the school setting becomes more important.

Transport to and from school

The journey to and from school is a potentially important opportunity for children to engage in physical activity, as well as socialize (Figure 13.1). Although there are no published studies on the health benefits of *actively commuting* to school, by its very nature, *active commuting* contributes to daily activity levels, and has other potential benefits, such as promoting social development, when active commuting takes place with friends or in a group (Tudor-Locke et al., 2001). It is apparent, however, from studies in Australia, the UK and the USA, that actively

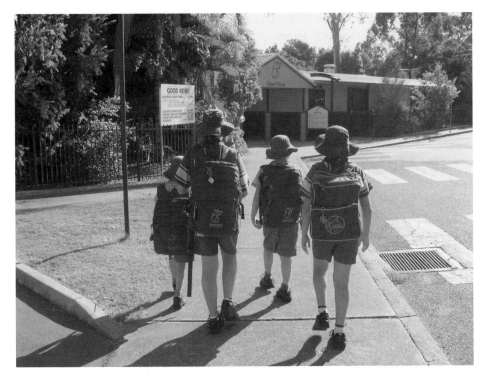

Figure 13.1 Walking to school provides physical activity, as well as opportunity for socialization.

commuting to school by children is in decline. In the UK, the prevalence of children walking to school dropped by 20% from 1970 to 1991 (Hillman, 1993). In the USA, there has been a 37% decline in the number of trips made by children on foot or bicycle from 1977 to 1995 (McCann & Delille, 2000). In fact, the majority of children in the USA do not walk or bike to school, with approximately half being driven, one third riding a school bus and less than one trip in seven made by walking or cycling (US Department of Transportation, 1997). In a recent Australian study, the active transport levels of children were found to be very low, with children walking or cycling on average about 600 metres per day, with only a third of all trips being made by walking or cycling (Harten & Olds, 2004).

Increasing car usage, busy roads, concerns for child safety, perceived crime danger and greater distances between homes and schools all contribute to the falling levels of children walking to school (Centers for Disease Control, 2002; Ziviani et al., 2004). This decline has both an immediate effect on children's opportunity to attain physical activity recommendations, and can carry over into less physical activity after school (Cooper et al., 2003; Sjolie & Thuen, 2002). With this is in mind, many schemes have been introduced at local and national levels in different countries to promote active transport to school (Boarnet et al., 2005; Staunton et al., 2003).

The walking school bus (WSB), is one approach that has been trialled internationally. The WSB is a walking group that is led by a minimum of two parents or teachers and picks up children on a planned route to school. It is safe and convenient, promotes social support and friendship, and enables children to be active at the start and end of each school day. Schools that have introduced a WSB scheme have seen a reduction in the number of children being driven to school. Indeed, in the state of Victoria, Australia, more than 2000 primary schoolchildren from 192 schools, now walk to school as part of a WSB programme (VICHEALTH, 2005). Despite the success of such programmes, persistent concerns regarding traffic congestion, child safety and insufficient safe walking and cycling routes have meant that there has been little investment to date in promoting active transport. Provision of safe cycle friendly and pedestrian routes, and well lit sidewalks and cycle paths, is needed if children are to engage in and benefit from active transport to and from school.

Remedial activity and occupational therapy

Largely driven by a medical model of remediation, perceptual motor programmes were introduced into schools in the early twentieth century. Identifying perceptual motor parameters to learning, some researchers (Kavale & Mattson, 1983) posited that adequate perceptual motor skills formed the basis for cognitive functioning. Based on this premise it was assumed that children with deficiencies in motor and perceptual functioning would manifest learning problems. Supporting this notion was the finding that many children with learning problems were indeed noted to have problems with motor learning (Campbell, 1997). Hence, numerous structured programmes of skill development were introduced, many of which continue to operate in schools to this day. These programmes occur primarily in the early years of schooling and can replace or supplement physical education curricula.

Perceptual motor programmes take the form of activities designed to improve balance, body image, spatial awareness, directionality, laterality and motor memory. These programmes usually require specialized equipment and are organized in such a way that children rotate through a range of tasks. Teaching staff and sometimes parent assistants oversee particular tasks and support students in their performance. Since 1960, considerable research has been conducted to assess the effectiveness of perceptual motor programmes to remediate academic learning problems (Goodman & Hammill, 1973; Kavale & Mattson, 1983; Salvia & Ysseldyke, 1981). Research has concluded that these are not an effective intervention for academic achievement (Gallahue, 1993). This being the case, how are these programmes to be differentiated from mainstream physical education curricula? As argued by Tinning et al. (1993), all physical education activities, by their nature, are perceptual motor in origin. If the benefit of these programmes is the development of movement skills then this is how they should be evaluated and not on the basis of academic outcomes.

How do perceptual motor programmes perform with respect to physical activity and skill development? Some of the complaints levelled at these programmes are that children spend a lot of time waiting their turn to undertake particular tasks. Given that these programmes often only run for half an hour, the overall amount of physical activity and skill development in which children are involved is potentially very limited. Further criticism has been levelled at the degree of visibility to which children with difficulties are subjected when they cannot perform specific tasks. Unless activity is able to accommodate individual needs, interests and abilities, it is not likely to encourage participation (Campbell, 1997). Especially in early schooling years, associating physical activity with fun is important to the encouragement of ongoing participation.

Occupational therapists usually become involved in the physical activities of children at school when motor difficulties manifest in the performance of occupational tasks such as handwriting and self-care. While physical activity is by no means the total focus of occupational therapy intervention when it comes to school participation (see Chapter 12), limitations imposed by physical disabilities, as well as performance limitations, can restrict participation in physical education, sport and recess. In these circumstances alternative, modified or adapted activities need to be considered. It is well documented that children with physical disabilities are at greater risk of reduced physical activity than their non-disabled peers (King et al., 2003) and, hence, at risk of missing out on the benefits which accrue from participation. Involvement with teaching staff can help to identify ways in which children with disabilities may still participate in school based activity. For example, a child who requires a wheelchair for mobility may not be able to participate in a scheduled game of football, but they may be able to take on scoring or support duties which are integral to the team's functioning. This helps to meet the participation goal, but care needs to be taken not to overlook the need for physical activity as well. More individualized (out of school) time might be needed to help develop other lifelong activity interests such as wheelchair racing or basketball, where more active participation by the young person with a disability may be possible.

For children with mild motor difficulties such as developmental coordination disorder (DCD), the barriers to participation in physical activity are less obvious but equally as real (Poulsen & Ziviani, 2004). DCD has been associated with low levels of physical activity and a reduced level of physical fitness (O'Brien et al., 2004). In the school environment, children with DCD are more likely to take on the role of onlooker, and engage in physically passive activities during recess (Smyth & Anderson, 2000). Physical environments which support physically active play in unstructured, non-competitive situations can be advocated by occupational therapists working in schools, for the benefit of many children. Reducing the emphasis on competitive sports and increasing resources to health related fitness activity has been strongly advocated since the early 1990s; however, schools have not always embraced these recommendations (Sallis & Mackenzie, 1991).

Summary

We have argued throughout this chapter that physical activity, within the school setting, should be seen as a health promoting behaviour in the lives of children. This view of health is reflected in the World Health Organization's charter for promoting health through schools (World Health Organization, 1996). Consistent with this broad approach, a review of school based physical activity interventions indicates that school-wide approaches to the promotion of physical activity that include curriculum, policy and environmental strategies appear to be more effective (Timperio et al., 2004).

Responsibility for how to increase children's opportunities to be physically active must move beyond the individual young person. A social view of health seeks to create contexts in which children's opportunities to be physically active within the school context are optimized. Positive, school based, physical activity experiences are particularly important for young people from lower socio-economic, minority and rural backgrounds who have reduced access to community based physical activity, due to limitations such as financial pressures, less parental encouragement and restricted access to transport, as well as for young people with disability. Increasing the time spent in physical activity within the school day could be attained by modest increases in activity at times that may not normally be thought of as activity opportunities. The following are presented as guidelines.

- *Active curricula*
  Ensure that enough time is allocated to physical education to provide the optimal length and intensity of physical activity to give the *daily allowance*. Physical education is a primary site in which changes to physical activity engagement can be achieved and sustained (Timperio et al., 2004). To reach this goal, within a physical education lesson teachers need to introduce activities which are of interest to students and employ pedagogies that allow all students to fully participate and have high time on task. Further, physical activity can be incorporated in measurement in maths or outdoor excursions in science.

- *Active recess*
  School breaktimes are ideal opportunities for increasing daily physical activity. An increase in breaktimes and in teacher instruction in playful games and activities, prior to and during breaks, has provided promising results, motivating and encouraging children to be active (Kraft, 1989).

- *Active playgrounds*
  The playground environment can be enticing for physical activity if it is clean, safe and stimulating. Freshly painted equipment and surfaces, additional play equipment, and teacher encouragement of activity have been found to increase self-reported physical activity in both genders (Stratton & Leonard, 2002).

- *Active transport*
  Walking or cycling to and from school in groups is safe, convenient, promotes social support and friendship, and promotes physical activity.

- *Clubs, classes and competitions*
  Dance classes, come 'n try clubs, festivals, displays, inter-class tournaments, or sporting fixture training sessions and competitions may together provide a variety of options to interest all students. Sustained attendance is the challenge, as is transport home, for after school clubs or classes. This means that time before school, as well as lunch-breaks, is potentially important time for fun recreational physical activity and sport opportunities.

- *Involving parents, carers and the community*
  It may be that parents, grandparents, or members of the local community can help teachers to lead a variety of activities or to assist with access to equipment and facilities. Finding ways for family members to learn about physical activities in the school and attend special events associated with them (whether it be parents' briefings, newsletters, or spectatorship opportunities) is also important in motivating children to be active.

References

Alfermann, D. & Stoll, O. (2000). Effects of physical exercise on self-concept and well-being. *International Journal of Sport Psychology*, *31*, 47–65.

Anderssen, N., Jacobs, D. R. J., Sidney, S., Bild, D. E., Sternfeld, B., Slattery, M. L., et al. (1996). Change and secular trends in physical activity patterns in young adults: a seven year longitudinal follow-up in the coronary artery risk development in young adults study (CARDIA). *American Journal of Epidemiology*, *143* (4), 351–362.

Armstrong, N. & Biddle, S. (Eds.) (1992). *Health-related physical activity in the national curriculum* (Vol. 2). Champaign, IL: Human Kinetics.

Armstrong, N. & Welsman, J. (1997). *Young people and physical activity*. Oxford: Oxford University Press.

Australian Bureau of Statistics (2000). *Children's participation in cultural and leisure activities*. Canberra: Australian Federal Government.

Bailey, D., McKay, H. A., Mirwald, R. L., Crocker, P. R. & Faulkner, R. A. (1999). A six-year longitudinal study of the relationship of physical activity to bone mineral accrual in growing children: the University of Saskatchewan bone mineral accrual study. *Journal of Bone and Mineral Research*, *14*, 1672–1679.

Baranowski, T., Bouchard, C., Bar-or, O., Bricker, T., Heath, G., Kimm, S. Y., et al. (1992). Assessment, prevalence and cardiovascular health benefits of physical activity and fitness in youth. *Medicine and Science in Sports and Exercise*, *24* (s237–s247).

Behets, D. (1997). Comparison of more and less effective teaching behaviors in secondary physical education. *Teacher and Teacher Education*, *13* (2), 215–224.

Berkey, C. S., Rockett, H. R., Gillman, M. W. & Colditz, G. A. (2003). One-year changes in activity and in inactivity among 10 to 15-year-old boys and girls: relationship to change in body mass index. *Pediatrics*, *111*, 836–843.

Blanksby, B., Parker, H., Bradley, S. & Ong, V. (1995). Children's readiness for learning front crawl swimming. *The Australian Journal of Science and Medicine in Sport*, 27 (2), 34–37.

Blatchford, P. (1998). *Social life in school: pupils experience of breaktime and recess from 7 to 16 years.* London: Falmer Press.

Blatchford, P. & Sumpner, C. (1998). What do we know about breaktime? Results from a national survey of breaktime and lunch-time in primary and secondary schools. *British Educational Research Journal*, 24 (1), 79–94.

Boarnet, M. G., Andersen, C. L., McMillan, T. & Alfonzo, M. (2005). Evaluation of the Californian safe routes to school legislation: urban changes and children's active transportation to school. *American Journal of Preventive Medicine*, 28 (2S2), 134–140.

Brown, W., Macdonald, D., Trost, S., Miller, Y., Braiuka, S. & Hornsey, A. (2001). *Final report to the Australian Sports Commission: young people's participation in physical activity.* Brisbane: the University of Queensland.

Brustad, R. J. (1993). Who will go out and play? Parental and psychological influences on children's attraction to physical activity. *Pediatric Exercise Science*, 5, 210–233.

Brustad, R. J. (1996). Attraction to physical activity in urban schoolchildren: parental socialization and gender influences. *Research Quarterly for Exercise and Sport*, 67, 316–323.

Brustad, R. J., Babkes, M. L. & Smith, A. L. (Eds.) (2001). *Youth in sport: psychological considerations.* New York: John Wiley & Sons.

Bunton, R. & Burrows, R. (Eds.) (1995). *Consumption and health in the 'epidemiological' clinic of late modern medicine.* London: Routledge.

Buonamano, R., Cei, A. & Mussino, A. (1995). Participation motivation in Italian youth sport. *The Sport Psychologist*, 9, 265–281.

Burrows, L., Wright, J. & Jungersen-Smith, J. (2002). 'Measure your belly': New Zealand children's constructions of health and fitness. *Journal of Teaching in Physical Education*, 22, 39–48.

Campbell, L. (1997). Perceptual-motor programs, movement and young children's needs: some challenges for teachers. *Australian Journal of Early Childhood*, 22 (1), 37–42.

Carlson, T. (1995). We hate gym: student alienation from physical education. *Journal of Teaching in Physical Education*, 14 (4), 467–477.

Cavill, N., Biddle, S. & Sallis, J. F. (2001). Health enhancing physical activity for young people: statement of consensus of the United Kingdom expert consensus conference. *Pediatric Exercise Science*, 13, 20–25.

Centers for Disease Control (2002). Barrier to children walking and biking to school – United States 1999. *Morbidity and Mortality Weekly Report*, 51 (32), 701–704.

Coakley, J. (2001). *Sport in society: issues and controversies.* New York: McGraw-Hill.

Cooper, A. R., Page, A. S., Foster, L. J. & Qahwaji, D. (2003). Commuting to school: are children who walk to school more physically active? *American Journal of Preventive Medicine*, 25 (4), 273–276.

Cote, J. (1999). The influence of the family in the development of talent in sports. *The Sport Psychologist*, 13 (395–417).

Daiman, S. (1995). Women in sport in Islam. *Journal of the International Council for Health, Physical Education, Recreation, Sport and Dance*, 32, 18–21.

Dale, D., Corbin, C. & Dale, K. (2000). Restricting opportunities to be active during schooltime: do children compensate by increasing physical activity levels after school? *Research Quarterly for Exercise and Sport*, 71 (3), 240–248.

Dyson, B. (2002). The implementation of cooperative learning in an elementary physical education program. *Journal of Teaching in Physical Education, 22* (1), 69–85.

Evans, J. (1990). *Sport in schools*. Geelong: Deakin University Press.

Evans, J. (2003). Changes to primary school recess and their effect on children's physical activity: an Australian perspective. *Journal of Physical Education New Zealand, 36* (1), 53–62.

Gallahue, D. (1993). *Developmental physical education for today's children* (2nd ed.). Dubuque: I.A. Brown & Benchmark.

Glasby, P. & Macdonald, D. (2004). Negotiating the curriculum: challenging the social relationships in teaching. In: J. Wright, D. Macdonald & L. Burrows (Eds.), *Critical inquiry in health and physical education* (pp. 133–144). Sydney: Routledge Falmer.

Goodman, L. & Hammill, D. (1973). The effectiveness of the Kephart-Getman activities in developing perceptual-motor and cognitive skills. *Focus on Exceptional Children, 4,* 121–126.

Grehaigne, J. F. & Godbout, P. (1995). Tactical knowledge in team sports from a constructivist and cognitivist perspective. *Quest, 47,* 490–505.

Harten, N. & Olds, T. (2004). Patterns of active transport in 11–12-year-old Australian children. *Australian and New Zealand Journal of Public Health, 28* (2), 167–172.

Hillman, M. (Ed.) (1993). *Children, transport and the quality of life*. London: Policies Studies Institute.

Hovell, M. F., Sallis, J. F., Kolody, B. & McKenzie, T. L. (1999). Children's physical activity choices: a developmental analysis of gender, intensity levels and time. *Pediatric Exercise Science, 11,* 158–168.

Hunter, L. (2002). *Young people, physical education and transition: understanding practices in the middle years of schooling* (unpublished). The University of Queensland, Brisbane.

Hutzler, Y. (2003). Attitudes toward the participation of individuals with disabilities in physical activity. *Quest, 55* (4), 347–373.

Jago, R. & Baranowski, T. (2004). Non-curricular approaches for increasing physical activity in youth: a review. *Preventive Medicine, 39* (1), 157–163.

Katzmarzyk, P. T., Gledhill, N. & Shephard, R. J. (2000). The economic burden of physical activity in Canada. *Canadian Medical Association Journal, 163* (11), 1435–1340.

Kavale, K. & Mattson, D. (1983). 'One jumped off the balance beam': meta-analysis of perceptual motor training. *Journal of Learning Disabilities, 16* (3), 165–173.

King, G., Law, M., King, S., Rosenbaum, P., Kertoy, M. K. & Young, N. L. (2003). A conceptual model of the factors affecting the recreation and leisure participation of children with disabilities. *Physical and Occupational Therapy in Pediatrics, 23* (1), 63–90.

Kirk, D. & Macdonald, D. (1998). Situated learning in physical education. *Journal of Teaching in Physical Education, 17* (3), 376–387.

Kolt, G. S. & Capaldi, R. (2001). Why do children participate in tennis? *The ACHPER Healthy Lifestyle Journal, 48* (2), 9–13.

Kraft, R. (1989). Behaviour of children at recess. *Journal of Physical Education Recreation and Dance, 60* (4), 21–24.

Lee, J., Macdonald, D. & Wright, J. (in press). Young men's physical activity choices: the impact of capital, masculinities and location. *Journal of Sport and Social Issues*.

Luke, M. & Sinclair, G. (1991). Gender differences in adolescents' attitudes toward school education. *Journal of Teaching in Physical Education, 11,* 31–46.

Lupton, D. (1998). The body, medicine and society. In: J. Germov (Ed.), *Second opinion: an introduction to health sociology*. Melbourne: Oxford University Press.

Macdonald, D. (2004). Rich tasks, rich learning. In: J. Wright, D. Macdonald & L. Burrows (Eds.), *Critical inquiry in health and physical education* (pp. 120–132). Sydney: Routledge Falmer.

Macdonald, D., Rodger, S., Ziviani, J., Jenkins, D., Batch, J. & Jones, J. (2004). Physical activity as a dimension of family life for lower primary school children. *Sport, Education and Society, 9* (3), 307–326.

Macdonald, D., Rodger, S., Abbott, R., Ziviani, J. & Jones, J. (2005). 'I could do with a pair of wings': perspectives on physical activity, bodies and health from young Australian children. *Sport, Education and Society, 10* (2), 195–209.

McCann, B. & Delille, B. (2000). *Mean streets 2000: pedestrian safety, health and federal transportation spending.* Columbia, SC: Centers for Disease Control and Prevention.

McKenzie, T., Sallis, J., Elder, J., Berry, C., Hoy, P., Nader, P., et al. (1997). Physical activity levels and prompts in young children at recess: a two-year study of a bi-ethnic sample. *Research Quarterly for Exercise and Sport, 68* (3), 195–202.

Moore, L. L., Nguyen, U. D. T., Rothman, K. J., Cupples, L. A. & Ellison, R. C. (1995). Preschool physical activity level and change in body fatness in young children. *Journal of Pediatrics, 118,* 215–219.

National Association for Sport and Physical Recreation (NASPR) (1995). *Moving into the future: national standards for physical education.* St Louis, MO: Mosby.

National Association of Early Childhood Specialists in State Departments of Education (2001). *Recess and the importance of play: a position statement on young children and recess.* Retrieved from http://naecs.crc.uiuc.edu/position/recessplay.html

New Zealand Ministry of Education (1999). *Health and physical education in the New Zealand curriculum.* Wellington: Ministry of Education.

O'Brien, C., Larkin, D. & Cable, T. (2004). Coordination problems and anaerobic performance in children. *Adapted Physical Activity Quarterly, 11,* 141–149.

Pellegrini, A. D. & Smith, P. K. (1993). School recess: implications for education and development. *Review of Educational Research, 63* (1), 51–67.

Pellegrini, A. D. & Blatchford, P. (2000). *The child at school: interactions with peers and teachers.* London: Arnold.

Petersen, A. (1997). Risk, governance and the new public health. In: A. Petersen & R. Bunton (Eds.), *Foucault, health and medicine.* London: Routledge.

Portman, P. & Carlson, T. (1991). Speaking out against silence: Pat Griffin. *Teaching Education, 4* (1), 183–187.

Poulsen, A. & Ziviani, J. (2004). Can I play too? Physical activity engagement patterns of children with developmental coordination disorders. *Canadian Journal of Occupational Therapy, 71* (2), 100–107.

Raitakari, O., Porkka, K., Taimela, S., Telama, R., Rasanen, L. & Viikari, J. (1994). Effects of persistent physical activity and inactivity on coronary risk factors in children and young adults. The cardiovascular risk in young Finns study. *American Journal of Epidemiology, 140* (3), 195–205.

Raudsepp, L. & Viira, R. (2000). Socio-cultural correlates of physical activity in adolescents. *Pediatric Exercise Science, 12,* 51–60.

Reay, D. (2001). 'Spice girls', 'nice girls', 'girlies' and 'tomboys': gender discourses, girls' cultures and femininities in the primary classroom. *Gender and Education, 13* (2), 153–166.

Rose, N. (2000). Community, citizenship and the third way. *American Behavioral Scientist, 43* (9), 1395–1411.

Royal College of Physicians (1991). Medical aspects of exercise: benefits and risks. Summary of a report of the Royal College of Physicians. *Journal of the Royal College of Physicians of London*, 25 (3), 195.

Sallis, J. E. & Mackenzie, T. I. (1991). Physical education's role in public health. *Research Quarterly for Exercise and Sport*, 62, 124–137.

Salvia, J. & Ysseldyke, J. (1981). *Assessment in special and remedial education*. Boston: Houghton Mifflin.

Shilling, C. (1993). *The body and social theory*. London: Sage Publications.

Siedentop, D. (1994). *Sport education: quality physical education through positive sport experiences*. Champaign, IL: Human Kinetics.

Sjolie, A. N. & Thuen, F. (2002). School journeys and leisure activities in rural and urban adolescents in Norway. *Health Promotion International*, 17 (1), 21–28.

Smyth, M. M. & Anderson, H. I. (2000). Coping with clumsiness in the school playground: social and physical play in children with coordination impairments. *British Journal of Developmental Psychology*, 18, 389–413.

Staunton, C. E., Hubsmith, D. & Kallins, W. (2003). Promoting safe walking and biking to school: the Marin County success story. *American Journal of Public Health*, 93 (9), 1431–1434.

Stratton, G. A. (1999). A preliminary study of children's physical activity in one urban primary school playground: differences by sex and season. *Journal of Sport Pedagogy*, 2, 71–82.

Stratton, G. A. & Leonard, J. (2002). The effects of playground markings on energy expenditure of 5–7-year-old children. *Pediatric Exercise Science*, 14, 170–180.

Timperio, A., Salmon, J. & Ball, K. (2004). Evidence based strategies to promote physical activity among children, adolescents and young adults: review and update. *Journal of Science and Medicine in Sport*, 791, 20–29.

Tinning, R. & Fitzclarence, L. (1992). Post-modern youth culture and the crisis in Australian secondary school in physical education. *Quest*, 44, 287–303.

Tinning, R., Kirk, D. & Evans, J. (1993). *Learning to teach physical education*. Sydney: Prentice Hall.

Tinning, R. & Glasby, P. (2002). Pedagogical work and the 'cult of the body': considering the role of HPE in the context of the 'new public health'. *Sport, Education and Society*, 7 (2), 109–119.

Trost, S., Morgan, A., Saunders, R., Felton, G., Ward, D. & Pate, R. (2000). Children's understanding of the concept of physical activity. *Pediatric Exercise Science*, 12, 293–299.

Trost, S., Pate, R., Sallis, J., Freedson, P., Taylor, W., Dowda, M., et al. (2002). Age and gender differences in objectively measured physical activity in youth. *Medicine and Science in Sports and Exercise*, 34 (2), 350–355.

Tudor-Locke, C., Aimsworth, B. E. & Popkin, B. M. (2001). Active commuting to school: an overlooked source of children's physical activity? *Sports Medicine*, 31 (5), 309–313.

US Department of Transportation (1997). *Proceedings from the nationwide personal transportation survey symposium*, Bethseda, Md: US Department of Transportation.

VICHEALTH (2005). Where's this bus going? *VicHealth Letter*, 24, 20–22.

Wang, J. & Wiese-Bjornstal, D. M. (1996). The relationship of school type and gender to motives for sport participation among youth in the People's Republic of China. *International Journal of Sport Psychology*, 28, 13–24.

Weinberg, R., Tenenbaum, G., McKenzie, A., Jackson, S., Anshel, M., Grove, R., et al. (2000). Motivation for youth participation in sport and physical activity: relationships to culture, self-reported activity levels and gender. *International Journal of Sport Psychology, 31*, 321–346.

Woodfield, L., Duncan, M., Al-Nakeen, Y., Nevill, A. & Jenkins, C. (2002). Sex, ethnic and socio-economic differences in children's physical activity. *Pediatric Exercise Science, 14*, 277–285.

World Health Organization (1996). *Promoting health through schools: the World Health Organization's global school health initiative.* Geneva: World Health Organization.

Wright, J., Macdonald, D. & Groom, L. (2003). Physical activity and young people: beyond participation. *Sport, Education and Society, 8* (1), 17–33.

Wright, J., Macdonald, D. & Burrows, L. (Eds.) (2004). *Critical inquiry and problem solving in physical education.* London: Routledge.

Young, M. F. D. (1998). *The curriculum of the future: from the 'new sociology of education' to a critical theory of learning.* London: Falmer Press.

Zaman, H. (1997). Islam, wellbeing and physical activity: perceptions of Muslim young women. In: G. Clarke & B. Humberstone (Eds.), *Researching women and sport* (pp. 50–68). London: Macmillan.

Zask, A., van Buerden, E., Barnett, L., Brooks, L. O. & Dietrich, U. C. (2001). Active school playgrounds – myth or reality? Results of the 'Move it, groove it' project. *Preventive Medicine, 33*, 402–408.

Zeijl, E., te Poel, Y., du Bois-Reymond, M., Ravesloot, J. & Meulman, J. J. (2000). The role of parents and peers in the leisure activities of young adolescents. *Journal of Leisure Research, 32*, 281–302.

Ziviani, J., Scott, J. & Wadley, D. (2004). Walking to school: incidental physical activity in the daily occupations of Australian children. *Occupational Therapy International, 11* (1), 1–11.

Chapter 14

CHILDREN'S PARTICIPATION BEYOND THE SCHOOL GROUNDS

Anne Poulsen and Jenny Ziviani

A significant amount of a child's life belongs to that time when the school doors close and the world beyond the school grounds opens wide. A child's participation in activities beyond school can provide opportunities for skill development and role exploration. Ensuring that all children have equal opportunities for meaningful and satisfying experiences in enjoyable leisure pursuits is an important health and wellbeing concern.

Pursuits beyond the school grounds are frequently chosen by children and their families, rather than being determined by the school curriculum. Ideally, children have greater freedom in pursuing extra-curricular goals and interests out of school. For this reason, leisure time may have more impact on quality of life than any other experience (Kelly, 1996).

Exploring children's out of school time use can offer insights into the feelings, beliefs and values of children and their families (Mannel & Kleiber, 1997). While out of school activities include pursuits such as homework, chores, self-care and transportation, this chapter will focus on the rich world of leisure. To fully understand leisure benefits, an overview of the core issues underpinning the study of leisure time participation is a necessary prerequisite.

The objectives of this chapter are to:

(1) Overview the diverse array and distribution of activities in which children participate beyond the school grounds: classification of out of school time use will be discussed
(2) Understand the child (and environment) level variables that contribute to temporal and occupational role balance: internal and external motivating forces influencing participation will be explored
(3) Apply a model of time use: Synthesis of Child Occupational Performance and Environment – In Time (SCOPE-IT) to help understand the leisure ecosystems of children's lives
(4) Review the positive and negative outcomes of out of school activity engagements and factors that contribute to child physical and mental health

Defining participation beyond the school grounds

Understanding children's out of school time use requires both an appreciation of the wide range of activities included under this umbrella and a consistent approach to classifying and describing these pursuits.

The complex task of classifying out of school activities has been problematic and challenging. Consistent classification has been hampered by the lack of a theory driven structure for systematically describing time use. Examples of classification schemes are listed in Table 14.1. A quick perusal of the categories listed in Table 14.1 highlights differences in terminology used to describe clusters of activity participation. Also apparent are inconsistencies in the grouping of activities, with overlapping attributes used to categorize activities such as physical and/or social contextual features. The variability in classification systems has contributed to difficulties replicating and comparing findings across different settings, populations and cultures. In Table 14.1 out of school time use classification clusters are grouped using the taxonomical division of work, play and self-care, that have philosophically and historically underpinned occupational therapy practice (Poulsen & Ziviani, 2004).

Distribution of out of school time

Information about how children spend their out of school hours has been collected largely through time use surveys in which leisure activities may have been only one part of a wider examination of family life. In 1997, the Child Development Supplement to the Panel Study of Income Dynamics examined time diary data obtained on a random schoolday and a random weekend day from 3600 US children aged from nought to twelve years and compared it with time use in 1981 (Hofferth & Sandberg, 2001). Children spent more time in 1997 in structured environments such as organized sport and less time in outdoor play, household work, eating and watching television than in 1981. Since the 1980s greater attention has been focused specifically on out of school time use during middle childhood (Carpenter et al., 1989; Harrell et al., 1997; Meeks & Mauldin, 1990). A week long diary study of activity distribution after school for US children aged from seven to eleven years showed approximately 48% of time was spent in sleep, 34% in leisure activities, 11% in personal maintenance and less than 1% in work such as homework and chores (Carpenter et al., 1989). At different ages some activities become more popular. For example, television viewing peaked in the fifth and sixth grade for US children (aged 10–12), occupying 13% of their waking hours outside school (Larson, 2001).

Gender differences

Leisure activities reported in post-industrial countries have differed markedly by gender. Boys spent more time in organized sports and unstructured leisure with peers than girls (ABS, 2003; Mauldin & Meeks, 1990). Although girls spent more time than boys in adult supervised cultural activities they were also twice as likely

Table 14.1 Examples of classification schemes for out of school activities.

(Carpenter et al., 1989) clustered by (Posner & Vandell 1999)	(Hofferth & Sandberg 2001)	(Cooper et al., 1999)	(McHale et al., 2001)
LEISURE – structured[1]			
(1) Organized in home (2) Out of home group activities (such as scouts, special outings) (3) Non-sport extra-curricular enrichment lessons (such as music, dance) (4) Coached sports	(1) Inside structured (2) Sports (3) Church	(1) Extra-curricular, school sponsored (2) Structured – adult supervised	(1) Sports activities
LEISURE – unstructured[2]			
(5) Unorganised in home (6) Listening to music (7) TV – primary (8) TV – secondary (9) Video games (10) Outside unstructured activities (11) Interaction (12) Loafing	(4) Television (5) Reading (6) Outdoors (7) Visiting (8) Other passive leisure (9) Playing (10) Household conversations	(3) Television (4) Unstructured time	(2) Television (3) Reading (4) Outdoor play (5) Playing with toys and games (6) Hanging out
LEISURE – structure unknown			
(13) Pets (14) Shopping	(11) Hobbies (12) Art activities		(7) Hobbies
ACTIVITIES OF DAILY LIVING – including personal maintenance			
(15) Meals and snacks (16) Personal hygiene (17) Transportation/transit (18) Sleep	(14) Eating (15) Personal care (16) Sleeping	(5) Sleeping	
WORK			
(19) Chores (20) Miscellaneous (21) Academic – homework and reading	(17) Household work (18) Market work (19) Day care	(6) Student employment	

1 Structured leisure = primarily organized by an adult authority figure
2 Unstructured leisure = primarily organized by the child

to engage in unstructured activities like arts and crafts (ABS, 2003; Carpenter et al., 1989). The most common leisure activities for 7–12-year-old boys, in order of frequency, were playing video games, football, bicycling, television viewing and basketball (Harrell et al., 1997).

Social background differences

These differences may also impact on children's leisure time engagement. For example, children in dual parent families have been found to spend less time on household tasks than children from single parent families (Peters & Haldeman, 1987). Children of employed mothers and single mothers have been found to spend more time watching television and less time reading or sleeping than children from dual parent families (Hofferth & Sandberg, 2001; Timmer et al., 1985). Children of more educated parents watch less television, study more and devote more time to reading than children of parents with lower levels of education (Timmer et al., 1985).

Social and cultural expectations, and gender differences can influence the length of time devoted to studying outside school. While Taiwanese fifth graders (10–11-year-olds) spent 1.8 hours per day in adult assigned activities related to the school curriculum, Japanese children of the same age devoted just under an hour per day to studies, and US fifth graders spent just over half an hour per weekday on homework (Larson & Verma, 1999).

Time spent in productive, income generating or household labour tasks in developing nations and some agrarian communities represents a distinct contrast to time use patterns in western industrialized countries. In many post-industrial nations income generation is not an economic requirement for pre-adolescent children. However, time spent on schoolwork or structured extra-curricular activities that lead to income generation and higher occupational status may also be perceived as work rather than play (Bianchi & Robinson, 1997; Larson & Verma, 1999; Posner & Vandell, 1994). Cross-culturally there may be varying perceptions about time as a resource, which can either be used productively or squandered (Larson, 2001).

Social and leisure capital

The social capital resources derived from people's ties within communities has been postulated as leading to supportive and sustained engagement in health enhancing activities (Morrow, 1999). Parents can invest time by supporting their child's leisure activities through encouragement and scaffolding of supportive peer networks, and monitoring socialization experiences. In western nations, parental attendance and behaviour at sports venues is a popular means of acquiring social capital. Social capital can also be accumulated through volunteering (for example holding positions such as team manager or coach). Social ties with other participating parents, officials and team members can be nurtured, and promote long-term engagement in skill enhancing contexts.

A child's social capital is derived from multiple sources both within and outside the family. The size and composition of the child's family and the capital already acquired by other family members in specific leisure pursuits can impact on the acquisition of social capital generally and leisure capital specifically. The time invested by the parents in interacting, encouraging and creating opportunities for their child to be exposed to situations and people who can facilitate skill acquisition can also be considered as capital deposits.

The acquisition of leisure capital can be facilitated through early or increased exposure to activity in a maximally supportive environment. Physical resources such as money to purchase equipment, lessons, club membership, transport to leisure facilities and proximity to out of school activities will facilitate leisure capital attainment. Social conditions, including the family's ability to prioritize and timetable leisure activities, draw on coaching resources and network with others for transportation will impact on attainment of leisure capital. The child's human capital consisting of their innate strengths and acquired capital can facilitate positive outcomes later in life (Bianchi & Robinson, 1997).

Balance

Maintaining or restoring balance between the core occupational performance areas of work, play/leisure, self-care/maintenance and rest has been perceived as contributing to optimal mental and physical health (Christiansen, 1996). The concept of balanced time use is complex and multi-layered. The notion of readily quantifiable units of time distributed according to a predetermined formula across different occupational performance roles is appealing but simplistic. To move towards a deeper appreci-ation of the concept of balance, children's and parent's personal meanings and subjective experiences of activity engagement need to be considered. Perceptions of the costs and benefits of participation in out of school activity vary widely.

Culturally sanctioned ways of spending time have traditionally framed the temporal organization of daily patterns of activity engagement, including religious activity, secular and religious holidays and festivals. Changes to these time struc-tures have directly and indirectly impacted on how children spend out of school hours. For example, one of the results of the western Christian concept of Sunday as a day of rest and worship was the culturally sanctioned organization of time into clearly defined periods for rest and leisure related pursuits at the end of the working week. Declining numbers of Christian followers; the introduction of legislation to allow shopping and entertainment centres to open on Sundays; scheduling of extra-curricular activities and homework to be completed over weekends have meant that the boundaries between work, play and rest have been blurred. During the week the scheduling of extra-curricular pursuits, and possibly homework, until 10 or 11 pm, has meant that the daytime schedules of some children have lengthened well into the night.

Leisure

Leisure has been described as offering different kinds of experiences to play, such as involvement with human service activities, entertainment, passive forms of rest or relaxation and religious worship that can be associated with a more abstract state of being (Kraus, 2000). The essence of leisure for primary schoolaged children encompasses the sense of freedom to selectively engage or discontinue activity participation at any point in time and may include structured and unstructured recreational and cultural activities such as sports, hobbies and cultural pursuits (Mannel & Kleiber, 1997).

Leisure is conceptually different from work. One distinctive feature differentiating the two is the cultural perception that work is something one has to do, while leisure is something one chooses to do (Nakamura & Csikszentmihalyi, 2002). However, the boundaries between work and leisure can blur and overlap. For example, signing on for a season of football might originate as a self-determined leisure activity but evolve over time to be perceived as an obligatory work-like task. A complex interaction between individual and environmental factors at any stage of engagement can modify an individual's perceptions and motivations about activity participation.

To determine whether an activity is perceived by the child as leisure or work requires a close examination of individual motivation, beliefs, values and subjective experiences. Understanding the interplay between internal and external regulators of activity participation is an essential part of increasing our knowledge about leisure (Mannel & Kleiber, 1997; Ryan & Deci, 2000a). The self-determination taxonomy described by Ryan and Deci (2000b) and Wang & Biddle (2001) specifies the dimensions and the stages whereby motivation is increasingly internalized and an internal locus of control with autonomous pursuit of self-endorsed goals is adopted (see Figure 14.1). The perceived freedom of choice and inherent satisfaction in performing an activity is an integral aspect of playfulness as discussed in Chapter 9.

Intrinsically motivated activity engagement can be seen in many free play experiences where there is exploration and self-direction (Bundy, 1991; Burke, 1996). However, there is evidence that intrinsically motivated engagement can also occur at moments of intense absorption and creativity in more structured contexts (Grolnick & Gurland, 2002). When there is no need for external regulators, such as rewards or threats, to encourage completion of the task, children may move along the self-determination continuum from an extrinsically motivated to an intrinsically motivated state (Deci et al., 1999).

External regulation can be seen where there are pressures or rewards for consequences of the activity rather than for the inherent satisfaction of engaging in that pursuit. During out of school time there may be situations where a child's participation in adult organized activities is influenced by the use of external incentives, directives or threats to perform in certain ways. These external forces control the child's behaviour, while potentially inhibiting intrinsic motivation. This may lead to decreased persistence and creativity, and poorer problem solving over time (Deci et al., 1999; Sheldon & Elliot, 2000). Other factors that enhance or undermine intrinsic motivation include dispositional characteristics and an individual's reactions to, for instance, a coach's motivational orientation (Ryan & Deci, 2000b).

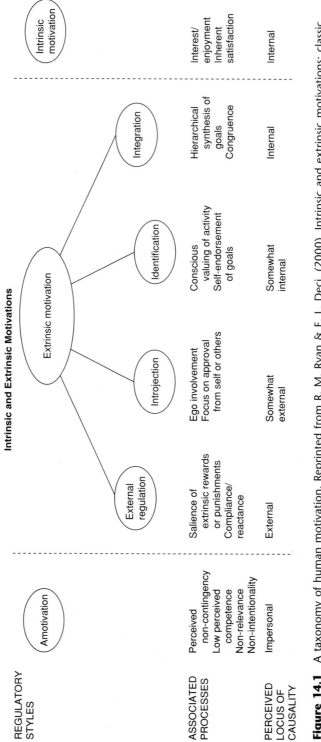

Figure 14.1 A taxonomy of human motivation. Reprinted from R. M. Ryan & E. L. Deci. (2000). Intrinsic and extrinsic motivations: classic definitions and new directions, *Contemporary Educational Psychology*, 25 (1), 54–67, with permission from Elsevier.

Table 14.2 The nine characteristics of flow (Jackson & Csikszentmihalyi, 1999).

Characteristics of flow	
(1) Challenge-skills balance	A sense that one is engaging in challenges at a level that is 'just right' (that is not overmatched or under-utilized) for one's skills or capacities.
(2) Action-awareness merging	There is total immersion in the activity so that action and awareness merge.
(3) Clear goals	There are very clear short-term goals that provide the focus for activity engagement.
(4) Unambiguous feedback	There is immediate and unequivocal feedback about the progress being made.
(5) Concentration on the task at hand	There is intense and focused concentration on what one is doing at that point in time.
(6) Sense of control	There is a feeling of personal control over the situation because one knows how to respond whatever happens.
(7) Loss of self-consciousness	There is loss of self-awareness in front of others.
(8) Transformation of time	Temporality is distorted so that time either seems to stand still or passes very quickly. Some children have described it as 'blinking out' or, after the event, as 'waking up'.
(9) Autotelic experience	The activity is rewarding for its own sake and is so enjoyable that the individual wants to repeat the experience again and again. Auto = self, telos = goal

Intrinsic motivation means engaging in authentic, self-authored and personally endorsed activities. When individuals are intrinsically motivated they have high levels of spontaneous interest, excitement, confidence, persistence and creativity. This leads to enhanced performance, heightened vitality, higher self-esteem and general wellbeing that provides opportunities for cognitive and social development, enjoyment and the autotelic experience of flow (Ryan & Deci, 2000b).

Flow is an intrinsically regulated state, conceptually similar to classical happiness described by Aristotle (Widmer & Ellis, 1998). The nine characteristics that have been described as integral features of a flow experience are described in Table 14.2. When individuals become deeply involved in activities that extend their talents, interests and abilities they are described as self-actualized (Rebeiro & Polgar, 1998). The long-term benefits of engaging in self-actualized autotelic activities may include skills enhancement, enhanced wellbeing, improved school performance, increased self-discipline and fewer behaviour problems (Foster, 2002).

A multidimensional model of time use: the SCOPE-IT model

There are multiple influences and reciprocal interactions between child and environment that can impact on developmental patterns of engagement in different activity contexts (see Figure 14.2). These can be visualized using ecological frameworks such as SCOPE-IT (Poulsen & Ziviani, 2004). This framework provides a graphic image of a watch-face, behind which lie the complex multifaceted processes that are involved in synthesizing incoming information from the environment (and individual) level factors to produce different patterns of engagement in occupational performance areas. The watch bands on each side represent the interlinking supports that provide the dynamic input into activity choice, effort and persistence from contextual and personal sources. On one side are environmental factors, both social and physical, that influence occupational engagement. On the other side are inputs from the child's physical and psychic background.

In many ways this conceptual framework represents what Humphry (2002) has termed a metaphor for organizing ideas about children's occupational behaviours, rather than a means for guiding practice. The SCOPE-IT model builds on the occupational frame of reference model for children and focuses on the dynamic relationships between the child, environment and occupations in a temporal context that incorporates the implicit assumption that the child is developing in a constantly changing world (Primeau & Ferguson, 1999). This model implicitly accepts the child as part of an open, living system continuously exchanging and being influenced by incoming information. At the same time, the significant influence of environmental factors, such as the social capital of the family, and the environmental supports and constraints for activity engagement are implicitly acknowledged.

Leisure-time activity choice, effort and persistence are influenced by child level variables on one hand and environmental variables on the other. Child level variables include biopsychological characteristics such as gender, chronological age, intellectual development and other physical, sensory or psychosocial attributes and skills. Environmental variables influencing leisure participation include the social and physical environmental factors that reciprocally interact with child characteristics to influence activity engagement. Four concentric circles of influence surround the child, with varying levels of penetration (Bronfenbrenner, 1979). Closest to the child is a proximal zone of influence consisting of a micro-system in which the child performs an activity with other actors in a specific place and time. Beyond this is a meso-system of interrelated micro-systems such as the home, school or community. At a more distal level are broader social influences, such as the exo-system containing the institutions of society, and the macro-system, where the values that drive societies historically evolve (Bronfenbrenner, 1979). Leisure time activity engagement is influenced by all four of these zones of influence.

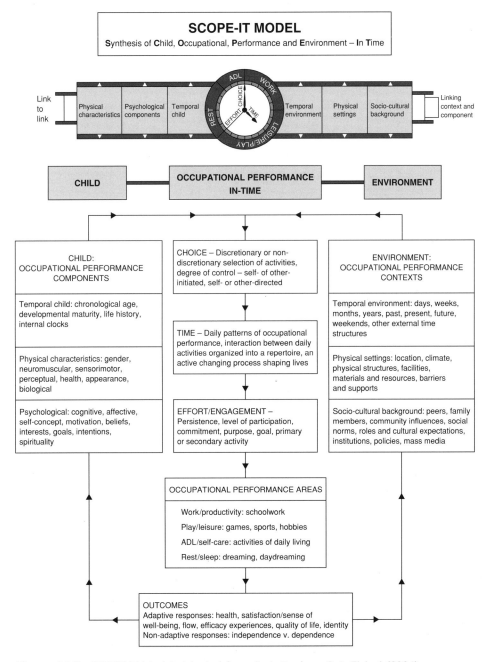

Figure 14.2 SCOPE-IT Model. Adapted from A. A. Poulsen, & J. Ziviani (2004). Can I play too? Physical activity engagement patterns of children with developmental coordination disorders. *Canadian Journal of Occupational Therapy, 71* (2), 100–107. Reprinted with the permission of CAOT publications ACE.

Healthy leisure

Identifying child and environmental factors that contribute to adaptive time use can positively influence mental and physical health of children (Mannel & Kleiber, 1997). Adaptive time use during leisure has been linked to overall wellbeing, with enhanced, positive feelings about oneself and one's world (Kaplan & Maehr, 1999). A wealth of socialization opportunities with peers and adults, as well as skill and knowledge acquisition can provide a buffering set of competencies that have been demonstrated to have powerful, sustainable effects on development (Larson, 2000).

Psychosocial benefits

An important and positive outcome of leisure time participation is healthy psychosocial outcomes. Participation in adult organized leisure activities has been found to be associated with higher teacher ratings of social competence and psychological maturity (Fletcher et al., 2003), greater levels of cooperative behaviour, improved peer relations and better school adjustment. Moderate, but not excessive, amounts of enrichment activities may confer emotional benefits on many children through the development of initiative and relational skills (Posner & Vandell, 1999).

Sports participation offers equal opportunities for physically competent children to participate, irrespective of social class, age, race, or gender. Participation in organized sport has been consistently linked with higher ratings of social competence and psychosocial maturity in the areas of work orientation and self-reliance (Fletcher et al., 2003).

Children who engage in structured pro-social activities, such as organized youth sports, religious activities, volunteer services, music or drama clubs, may be perceived by classroom teachers as having more positive attitudes to learning and better adjustment overall (Fletcher et al., 2003). The belief that adult organized activity contexts promote affirming relationships in safe, nurturing environments where there are positive role models for affiliative behaviours is a common perception of many parents, who consider leisure time as being 'learn and develop time' (Zeijl, 2000). There is evidence that 'hanging out' with peers during unstructured, unsupervised leisure time can be associated with delinquent behaviour in older children and adolescents (Osgood et al., 2001). Participation in adult monitored activities appears to have a protective effect when a sense of identity associated with the pursuit rather than with the popular peer culture forms (Larson, 2001). It has been proposed that positive identity formation, perceptions of competency in a leisure domain and development of constructive social networks provide important psychosocial benefits that increase resilience in adverse times (McHale et al., 2001).

Protective spread of activities

Children who engage in a broad array of leisure pursuits have the opportunity to explore and find areas of competence that provide a protective spread of activities which act as an emotional and social buffer in times of hardship. Studies of resilient children have found that having a broad range of interests in activities and hobbies can provide solace in adversity (Werner, 1993). This may be one mechanism that helps vulnerable children to cope with biological and psychosocial risk factors. There is also a belief that greater time invested in leisure activities may actually protect youth from exposure to risk and entrenched engagement in delinquent activities. While there is some empirical support for this view with older children and adolescents, there is limited evidence for younger children (Zeijl et al., 2001). Furthermore, there is some concern that high amounts of exposure to structured out of school contexts, particularly when associated with high amounts of external or internal pressure, may have negative impacts (Luthar, 2003). In balance, however, it would appear that moderate exposure to a range of enriching, safe, extra-curricular activities has the potential not only to offer positive psychosocial benefits, but also to provide protective benefits through skill acquisition and perceptions of accomplishment.

Competence enlargement

The most direct and measurable outcome of leisure time engagement is competence enlargement in educational, social, physical and cultural arenas (Zeijl et al., 2000). Most research about skill acquisition is in relation to participation in extra-curricular activities where structure and support are provided by adult figures who scaffold the acquisition of a range of physical and psychosocial competencies (Masten, 2002). There appear to be promising psychosocial benefits associated with investing time in extra-curricular programmes, particularly for children from low socio-economic backgrounds (Posner & Vandell, 1999). Higher academic grades, improved emotional adjustment and peer relations, as well as lower levels of conduct problems have been demonstrated when children from low-income families participate in formal, academically oriented, out of school programmes that are subsidized through the local community. These programmes have been identified as a positive way of reducing the social inequality gap, by offering tuition and adult supervision during the after school hours (Marsh & Kleitman, 2002).

Another positive source of after school activity is informal care by neighbours, baby-sitters or extended family members. This has some positive psychosocial and academic outcomes when exposure is not excessive. It has been found that there is a curvilinear predictive pattern with children, and particularly with girls, who are involved in no more than three hours per week of care. Girls who spend up to three hours per week in care showed better adjustment and academic gains than those who were unsupervised after school, or who spent large amounts of time in care (Pettit et al., 1997).

Community after school care can act in a positive way by increasing a child's exposure to developmentally beneficial activities in short bursts of time. The community neighbourhood is a context where healthy developmental outcomes for older children and adolescents are possible through exposure to stable, inter-generational, extended kin networks and opportunities for unstructured play, if safe environments are available (Lareau, 2000). In the local neighbourhood, children may develop friendships with a range of playmates and mentors and this may protect against loneliness and contribute to higher perceptions of social support, activity and friendships, as well as enhancing a sense of community.

At-risk leisure

Negative outcomes

Although most studies report a positive relationship between involvement in activities such as sport, drama and music and socio-emotional or cognitive gains, negative outcomes may be associated with over- or under-commitment beyond a certain threshold. Research aimed at investigating optimal thresholds for activity engagement is limited, however, at the current time. The threshold model of time investment has anecdotal and empirical support for a curvilinear engagement pattern, whereby there are diminishing returns past an optimal point of exposure (Marsh & Kleitman, 2002). For example, high levels of extra-curricular participation, defined as nine hours or more of structured out of school pursuits per week, have been associated with dramatic drops in achievement scores (Cooper et al., 1999). Displacement of potentially important developmental experiences such as schoolwork, extra-curricular activities and healthy behaviours, with supposedly less enriching activities such as television viewing or hanging out with peers has been associated with less advantageous outcomes (Safron et al., 2001).

Over-committed children

In recent times, concerns have been raised about the amount of time children participate in structured extra-curricular pursuits that have been thought to resemble work rather than play. Institutionalized play, purposive activity engagement and serious leisure, are some of the terms used to describe extra-curricular activity participation, where the focus is on involvement, perseverance and effort in acquiring knowledge, skills and dispositions (or habits) that can carry over into the corporate work world (Adler & Adler, 1994; Shaw & Dawson, 2001). In contrast, unstructured leisure time offers flexibility and 'wiggle room', where relaxation and ratcheting down to a slower pace of life is possible (Lareau, 2000). By de-cluttering the out of school timetable and reducing the number of structured extra-curricular arrangements, families can avoid time-binds associated with crunching deadlines. Increasing the amount of time to 'go slow' and engage in unstructured down time may be necessary to avoid excessive work-like leisure loads (Honore, 2004).

Claims that over-scheduling of extra-curricular activities can lead to performance pressure and stress related symptoms are often flagged in the popular press but these *must be* assertions have rarely been empirically tested. However, an association between excessive investment in accomplishments and maladaptive perfectionist strivings has been found to be associated with negative psychosocial outcomes for 11 and 12-year-olds (Luthar & Becker, 2002). Negative outcomes accrue when children adopt maladaptive perfectionist strivings to either beat others or meet self-imposed goals (Luthar, 2003). Similarly, negative outcomes can be observed when children spend time in highly competitive environments where the adults are perceived to be over controlling, over challenging or rejecting when a winning outcome has not been realized. Children in these ego oriented environments may drop out of leisure activity or withdraw concern for other perceived competitors. This can lead to antisocial activity, poor sportspersonship and cheating (Deci & Ryan, 2000).

When children have low perceptions of competency their motivational intentions become critical in predicting adaptive or maladaptive outcomes. If the child has a task orientation to increase skill levels and if the social climate also supports mastery, rather than rewarding superior performance based on other referenced evaluations, then positive outcomes such as persistence, enjoyment and progressive skill acquisition are facilitated. On the other hand, children with low actual or perceived ability who believe that beating others is more important than self-development may disengage after even one negative experience (Smiley & Dweck, 1994). In this way, perceptions of competency in combination with motivational orientations can act as powerful cognitions that drive helplessness.

Television viewing

Television viewing and other electronic media use are popular leisure activities that occupy the large majority of leisure time hours for children in middle childhood (Wells & Blendinger, 1998). They have attracted considerable research because of their passive, non-productive attributes as well as content related concerns for child viewing of aggressive or sexually explicit programmes (Larson, 2001). The demonstrated links between television viewing, sedentary lifestyles and unhealthy eating patterns are a significant health related concern. Television viewing, hanging around, daydreaming and doing nothing in particular have been considered default activities to turn to whenever nothing else is available and are unhealthy leisure pastimes when excessive preoccupation with these pursuits interferes with social interactions, physical activity patterns or other productive leisure interests (Huston et al., 1999).

The health consequences of long hours spent passively sitting in front of the television set have been well described (Posner & Vandell, 1999; The Royal Australasian College of Physicians: Paediatrics & Child Health Division, 2004). There has been a trend for children, particularly from lower socio-economic family backgrounds, to have their own television sets in their bedrooms, thus reducing the possible social benefits of parental interaction and monitoring of viewing behaviours (Posner & Vandell, 1999; The Royal Australasian College of Physicians: Paediatrics & Child Health Division, 2004). While educational television viewing has the potential to increase knowledge and encourage a broader understanding of the world, unfortunately time spent watching educational programmes declines rapidly between three to eight years of age and entertainment becomes the preferred viewing choice (Huston et al., 1999).

High time commitment to television viewing has been strongly linked to poor academic attainments (Williams, 1986). There is a curvilinear relationship between time spent viewing television and reading comprehension scores. It appears that reading comprehension scores increase with television viewing up to three hours a day, followed by plunges in reading comprehension when viewing exceeds this threshold (Doig, 1995). Watching more than three hours per day is more frequent for boys and children from lower socio-economic backgrounds. This is associated with increased computer game playing and movie viewing, less reading, lowered academic competence, decreased self-esteem and increased social isolation (Roe & Muijs, 1998). Less time spent watching television is found in families from higher socio-economic backgrounds and where parents have higher levels of education (Harding, 1997).

Computer use

More than two hours per day of computer use by males aged between nine and ten years has been found to be associated with a range of negative outcomes, including lowered general self-esteem, decreased academic achievement and increased social isolation (Roe & Muijs, 1998). Unmonitored access to computers, often in the child's own bedroom and therefore bypassing potential adult gatekeepers has been postulated as increasing a child's exposure to chat rooms, pornography and violent imagery (The Royal Australasian College of Physicians: Paediatrics and Child Health Division, 2004). Health organizations have stressed the need to monitor and develop guidelines for healthy use of screen based technologies.

The psychosocial health risks of exposure to harmful messages or pictures, the impact of marketing and consumerism, and possible exposure to sexual solicitation, are other issues to consider when evaluating associate developmental outcomes of participation in this out of school activity (The Royal Australasian College of Physicians: Paediatrics and Child Health Division, 2004). Moderate amounts of use may have socialization benefits for boys who use the computer for emailing, Internet, MSN, game networking and chat rooms. However, excessive computer use has been clearly linked to social isolation in large-scale studies of heavy users (Orleans & Laney, 2000; Roe & Muijs, 1998). It has been suggested that adult monitored use of chat rooms can facilitate the development of social networks for children with severe shyness, Asperger's syndrome, or severe illness (Bremer & Rauch, 1998).

Summary

This chapter has discussed the diversity of out of school activities engaged in by children and the many variables influencing engagement. A model of time use was presented to understand children's leisure ecosystems. The positive and negative outcomes of leisure engagement were discussed. Equalizing opportunity differences so that each child has equal access to a wide array of optimally enriching, learning experiences where competencies can be explored and developed is an essential first step in promoting healthy out of school time use (Scarr, 1996). Meeting current health guidelines for ensuring that children meet the basic requirements for daily physical activity means promoting safe and nurturing environments in which children can have regular access to lifestyle, recreational and organized physical activity options. Liaising with the leaders of formal physical and non-physical activity programmes to ensure that they are developmentally enhancing and age appropriate will contribute to skill acquisition in supportive environments.

Environment level interventions that focus on creating a mastery climate will help promote self-referenced learning and self-determined behaviours that are characterized by high levels of intrinsic motivation, effort and persistence (Brunel, 1999). This, in turn, will contribute to children's enjoyment and maximum participation in out of school activities.

Enjoyment is a major discriminator between continuous participation and disengagement from out of school programmes (Spray, 2000). Thus, finding activities and learning environments where enjoyable participation in self-regulated activities that promote development of skills, breadth of interests and competencies for each child is a key challenge for therapists and the families with whom they work. Consulting with parents, care-givers and children about out of school activities and activity contexts that are enriching is an important goal for those who seek to explore the possibilities of strength building in the out of school hours.

References

Adler, P. A. & Adler, P. (1994). Social reproduction and the corporate other: the institutionalization of after school activities. *Sociological Quarterly*, 35 (3), 309–328.

Australian Bureau of Statistics (2003). Children's participation in sports and leisure. In: *Year Book Australia* (Vol. 4177.0). Canberra: Commonwealth of Australia.

Bianchi, S. M. & Robinson, J. P. (1997). What did you do today? Children's use of time, family composition and the acquisition of social capital. *Journal of Marriage and the Family*, 59, 332–344.

Bremer, J. & Rauch, P. K. (1998). Children and computers: risks and benefits. *Journal of the American Academy of Child and Adolescent Psychiatry*, 37, 559–560.

Bronfenbrenner, U. (1979). *The ecology of human development: experiments by nature and design*. Cambridge: Harvard University Press.

Brunel, P. C. (1999). Relationship between achievement goal orientations and perceived motivational climate on intrinsic motivation. *Scandinavian Journal of Medicine and Science in Sports*, 9, 365–374.

Bundy, A. C. (1991). Play theory and sensory integration. In: A. C. Bundy, E. A. Fisher & E. A. Murray (Eds.), *Sensory integration: theory and practice* (pp. 46–48). Philadelphia: F. A. Davis.

Burke, J. P. (1996). Variations in childhood: play in the presence of disability. In: R. Zemke & F. Clark (Eds.), *Occupational science: the evolving discipline*. Philadelphia: F. A. Davis.

Carpenter, C. J., Huston, A. C. & Spera, L. (1989). Children's use of time in their everyday activities during middle childhood. In: M. Bloch & A. D. Pellegrini (Eds.), *The ecological context of children's play* (pp. 165–190). Norwood, NJ: Ablex.

Christiansen, C. H. (1996). Three perspectives on balance in occupation. In: R. Zemke & F. Clark (Eds.), *Occupational science: the evolving discipline*. Washington, DC: F. A. Davis.

Cooper, H., Valentine, J. C., Nye, B. & Lindsay, J. J. (1999). Relationships between five after school activities and academic achievement. *Journal of Educational Psychology, 91,* 369–378.

Deci, E. L., Koestner, R. & Ryan, R. M. (1999). A meta-analytic review of experiments examining the effects of extrinsic rewards on intrinsic motivation. *Psychological Bulletin, 125,* 627–668.

Deci, E. L. & Ryan, R. M. (2000). The 'what' and 'why' of goal pursuits: human needs and the self-determination of behavior. *Psychological Inquiry, 11,* 227–268.

Doig, D. (1995). Leisure reading: attitudes and practices of Australian year six children. *Australian Journal of Language and Literacy, 18,* 204–217.

Fletcher, A. C., Nickerson, P. & Wright, K. L. (2003). Structured leisure activities in middle childhood: links to wellbeing. *Journal of Community Psychology, 31,* 641–659.

Foster, E. M. (2002). How economists think about family resources and child development. *Child Development, 73,* 1904–1914.

Grolnick, W. S. & Gurland, S. T. (2002). The development of self-determination in middle childhood and adolescence. In: A. Wigfield & J. S. Eccles (Eds.), *Development of achievement motivation* (pp. 147–171). San Diego, CA: Academic Press.

Harding, D. J. (1997). Measuring children's time use: a review of methodologies and findings. *Working Paper 97–1.* Princeton, NJ: Bendheim-Thoman Center for Research on Child Wellbeing, Princeton University.

Harrell, J. S., Gansky, S. A., Bradley, C. B. & McMurray, R. G. (1997). Leisure time activities of elementary school children. *Nursing Research, 46,* 246–253.

Hofferth, S. L. & Sandberg, J. F. (2001). How American children spend their time. *Journal of Marriage and Family, 63,* 295–308.

Honore, C. (2004). *In praise of slow: how a worldwide movement is challenging the cult of speed.* London: Orion Publishing.

Humphry, R. (2002). Young children's occupations: explicating the dynamics of developmental processes. *American Journal of Occupational Therapy, 56* (2), 171–179.

Huston, A. C., Wright, J. C., Marquis, J. & Green, S. B. (1999). How young children spend their time: television and other activities. *Developmental Psychology, 35,* 912–925.

Jackson, S. A. & Csikszentmihalyi, M. (1999). *Flow in sports: the keys to optimal experiences and performances.* Lower Mitcham, SA: Human Kinetics.

Kaplan, A. & Maehr, M. L. (1999). Achievement goals and student wellbeing. *Contemporary Educational Psychology, 24,* 330–358.

Kelly, J. R. (1996). *Leisure.* Boston, MA: Allyn & Bacon.

Kraus, R. (2000). *Leisure in a changing America.* Boston, MA: Allyn & Bacon.

Lareau, A. (2000). Social class and the daily lives of children: a study from the United States. *Childhood, 7,* 155–171.

Larson, R. W. (2000). Toward a psychology of positive youth development. *American Psychologist, 55,* 170–183.

Larson, R. W. (2001). How US children and adolescents spend time: what it does (and doesn't) tell us about their development. *Current Directions in Psychological Science, 10,* 160–164.

Larson, R. W. & Verma, S. (1999). How children and adolescents spend time across the world: work, play and developmental opportunities. *Psychological Bulletin, 125*, 701–736.

Luthar, S. S. (2003). The culture of affluence: psychological costs of material wealth. *Child Development, 74*, 1581–1593.

Luthar, S. S. & Becker, B. E. (2002). Privileged but pressured? A study of affluent youth. *Child Development, 73*, 1593–1610.

McHale, S. M., Crouter, A. C. & Tucker, C. J. (2001). Free-time activities in middle childhood: links with adjustment in early adolescence. *Child Development, 72*, 1764–1778.

Mannel, R. C. & Kleiber, D. A. (1997). *A social psychology of leisure*. State College, PA: Venture.

Marsh, H. W. & Kleitman, S. (2002). Extra-curricular school activities: the good, the bad and the nonlinear. *Harvard Educational Review, 72*, 464–514.

Masten, A. S. (2002). Resilience in development. In: C. R. Snyder & S. J. Lopez (Eds.), *Handbook of positive psychology* (pp. 74–88). New York: Oxford University Press.

Mauldin, T. & Meeks, C. B. (1990). Sex differences in children's time use. *Sex Roles, 9/10*, 537–554.

Meeks, C. B. & Mauldin, T. (1990). Children's time in structured and unstructured leisure activities. *Lifestyles: Family and Economic Issues, 11*, 257–279.

Morrow, V. (1999). Conceptualizing social capital in relation to the wellbeing of children and young people: a critical review. *The Sociological Review, 47*, 744–765.

Nakamura, J. & Csikszentmihalyi, M. (2002). The concept of flow. In: C. R. Snyder & S. J. Lopez (Eds.), *Handbook of Positive Psychology* (pp. 89–105). New York: Oxford University Press.

Orleans, M. & Laney, M. C. (2000). Children's computer use in the home. *Social Science Computer Review, 18*, 56–72.

Osgood, D. W., Wilson, J. K., O'Malley, P. M., Bachman, J. G. & Johnston, L. D. (2001). Routine activities and individual deviant behaviour. *American Sociological Review, 61*, 635–655.

Peters, J. M. & Haldeman, V. A. (1987). Time used for household work: a study of school-aged children from single-parent, two-parent, one-earner, and two-earner families. *Journal of Family Issues, 8*, 212–225.

Pettit, G. S., Laird, R. D., Bates, J. E. & Dodge, K. A. (1997). Patterns of after school care in middle childhood: risk factors and developmental outcomes. *Merrill-Palmer Quarterly, 43*, 515–538.

Posner, J. K. & Vandell, D. L. (1994). Low-income children's after school care: are there beneficial effects of after school programmes? *Child Development, 65*, 440–456.

Posner, J. K. & Vandell, L. (1999). After school activities and the development of low-income children: a longitudinal study. *Developmental Psychology, 35*, 868–879.

Poulsen, A. & Ziviani, J. (2004). Can I play too? Physical activity engagement patterns of children with developmental coordination disorders. *Canadian Journal of Occupational Therapy, 71*, 100–107.

Primeau, L. A. & Ferguson, J. M. (1999). Occupational frame of reference. In: P. Kramer & J. Hinojosa (Eds.), *Frames of reference for pediatric occupational therapy*. Philadelphia: Lippincott Williams & Wilkins.

Rebeiro, K. L. & Polgar, J. M. (1998). Enabling occupational performance: optimal experiences in therapy. *Canadian Journal of Occupational Therapy, 66*, 14–22.

Roe, K. & Muijs, D. (1998). Children and computer games: a profile of the heavy user. *European Journal of Communication, 13*, 181–200.

Ryan, R. M. & Deci, E. L. (2000a). Intrinsic and extrinsic motivation: classic definitions and new directions. *Contemporary Educational Psychology*, 25, 54–67.

Ryan, R. M. & Deci, E. L. (2000b). Self-determination theory and the facilitation of intrinsic motivation, social development, and wellbeing. *American Psychologist*, 55 (68–78).

Safron, D. J., Schulenberg, J. E. & Bachman, J. G. (2001). Part-time work and hurried adolescence: the links among work intensity, social activities, health behaviors and substance use. *Journal of Health and Social Behavior*, 42, 425–449.

Scarr, S. (1996). How people make their own environments: implications for parents and policy makers. *Psychology, Public Policy and Law*, 2, 204–228.

Shaw, S. M. & Dawson, D. (2001). Purposive leisure: examining parental discourses on family activities. *Leisure Sciences*, 23, 217–231.

Sheldon, K. M. & Elliot, A. J. (2000). Personal goals in social roles: divergences and convergences across roles and levels of analysis. *Journal of Personality*, 68, 51–84.

Smiley, P. A. & Dweck, C. S. (1994). Individual differences in achievement goals among young children. *Child Development*, 65, 1723–1743.

Spray, C. M. (2000). Predicting participation in non-compulsory physical education: do goal perspectives matter? *Perceptual and Motor Skills*, 90, 1207–1215.

The Royal Australasian College of Physicians: Paediatrics & Child Health Division (2004). *Children and the media: advocating for the future*. Retrieved 15 June 2005 from http://www.racp.edu.au/hpu/paed/media/Guide_parents.pdf

Timmer, S. G., Eccles, J. S. & O'Brien, K. O. (1985). How children use time. In: F. T. Juster & F. P. Stafford (Eds.), *Time, goods, and wellbeing* (pp. 353–382). Ann Arbor, MI: Institute for Social Research, University of Michigan.

Wang, C. K. J. & Biddle, S. J. H. (2001). Young people's motivational profiles in physical activity: a cluster analysis. *Journal of Sport and Exercise Psychology*, 23, 1–22.

Wells, L. & Blendinger, J. (1998). *How middle school students spend their time outside of school: a longitudinal investigation*. Paper presented at the Mid-South Educational Research Association Conference, New Orleans, LA.

Werner, E. E. (1993). Risk, resilience, and recovery: perspectives from the Kauai longitudinal study. *Development and Psychopathology*, 5, 503–515.

Widmer, M. A. & Ellis, G. D. (1998). The Aristotelian good life model: integration of values into therapeutic recreation service delivery. *Therapeutic Recreation Journal*, 32, 290–302.

Williams, R. (1986). *The impact of television: a natural experiment in three communities*. London: Academic Press.

Zeijl, E., te Poel, Y., Dubois-Reymond, M., Ravesloot, J. & Meulman, J. J. (2000). The role of parents and peers in the leisure activities of young adolescents. *Journal of Leisure Research*, 32, 281–299.

Zeijl, E., du Bois-Reymond, M. & te Poel, Y. (2001). Young adolescents' leisure patterns. *Loisir et Société*, 24, 379–402.

INDEX

activities, 70, 99
  daily living activities (see also self-care), 93–4, 282
  discretionary, 93
  extra-curricular, 5, 96–7
  formal, 70
  informal, 70
  nondiscretionary, 93
  patterns, 79
  personal care attendants, 219
  structured, 25, 71, 78, 93, 94, 98
  unstructured, 93, 98–9
advocacy, 34–7, 56, 61, 82, 107, 127, 129, 183, 191, 211, 212, 218, 219, 236
  class advocacy, 36–7
  individual advocacy, 36
  skills, 37
after school care, 76, 291
Asperger's Syndrome, 167, 294
Assessment of Ludic Behaviours, 185
autism spectrum disorder (ASD), 48, 163, 164, 165, 167, 173, 201, 246
autonomy, 200, 219

balance, 14, 17, 92, 100–107, 125, 131–2, 280, 284
becoming, 115–16
being, 33, 115–16, 125–31
body image, 262

Canadian Occupational Performance Measure (COPM), 84, 153, 216, 218
carers, 5
child abuse and neglect, 26, 44, 120
child care, 24, 28
child-play-environment fit, 182–4, 189, 190, 195
child protection, 35
childhood disabilities, 25, 105, 130, 225, 241, 244, 248, 267, 272
Children's Assessment of Participation and Enjoyment (CAPE), 83

chores, 98, 261, 280, 281, 282
client centred practice, 123
clinical reasoning, 253
cognitive intervention for daily occupational performance (CO-OP), 123–5, 154
communication, 158, 177
  definitions, 160
  language, 159, 160
  nonverbal, 159
  skills, 159, 181
  social interactional perspective, 160–61, 164
  stages of, 161–3
community, 43, 47, 147, 274, 288, 291
  intervention, 106–107
  development, 106
  planning, 191
community capacity building, 28, 43, 47–8, 81, 82, 86
community consultation, 56
computers, 48–50, 103–104, 153, 164, 177, 182, 214, 215, 217, 204, 206, 246, 252, 294
contemporary society, 3, 7, 18, 22, 37

depression, 50, 166
development, 287
  affective, 118
  cognitive, 118, 159, 163
  physical, 117
  social, 118
developmental coordination disorder (DCD), 201, 272
diet, 263
doing, 33, 72, 115–22, 125, 262
disabilities, 25, 105, 130, 225, 241, 244, 248, 267, 272
divorce, 25
dynamic systems theory, 139

early childhood environment, 232
early childhood teacher/s, 230, 231, 232, 233

ecological systems theory, 96, 148
empowerment, 44, 47, 82, 131
environment, 3, 172, 177, 183
  barriers, 80–81, 85
  built environment, 42, 46, 75, 148
  cultural, 5, 41, 76–8, 147, 148, 191, 192
  economic, 78
  educational, 73
  environmental design, 53
  environmental factors, 42, 288
  evaluation, 50
  home, 5, 32
  interventions, 106, 295
  natural, 56, 59, 60, 75, 148
  physical, 5, 41, 53, 72, 74, 75, 80, 147,
    148, 181, 192, 222, 237, 245, 272
  political agenda, 72, 107
  school, 237, 288
  social, 3, 4, 41, 72, 75, 76–8, 80, 147,
    148, 187, 192, 194, 237, 247
  technological, 6, 103
  temporal, 248
  urban/rural, 76
  virtual, 48–50
evidence based practice, 123, 173
exercise, 263

family, 4, 22 102, 106–107, 236, 241, 262,
  274, 283
  composition, 22, 95, 102, 283
  culture/cultural context, 77, 202
  formation, 23
  function, 22
  income, 78–9
  intervention, 106–107
  life cycle, 27
  life, 24, 28, 131
  nuclear, 24
  patterns, 23
  routines, rituals, 30, 33–4, 74
  step/blended, 23, 24
  support, 26, 28
  types, 23
family centred care, 30, 32
family centred practice, 30, 33, 37, 202
family centred services, 31–2
fit, 41, 81, 146, 182, 187, 189, 195, 222,
  233–4, 245
flow, 125, 129, 149, 183, 194–5, 287
friends/ship, 158, 166, 168, 177, 234, 241,
  268, 292

geographical information systems, 51–2, 61

handwriting difficulties, 251–2, 272
health/health condition, 3, 6, 7, 8, 10, 11,
  12, 18, 23, 28, 31, 33, 34, 41, 47, 51,
  53, 56, 68, 70, 71, 81, 91, 96, 99, 100,
  102, 103, 105, 106, 115, 117, 121,
  124, 127, 132, 146, 170, 180, 201,
  207, 210, 211, 214, 261, 262, 263,
  264, 265, 266, 269, 272, 273, 284,
  294, 295
health promotion, 67, 96, 106, 107, 211,
  212, 267
home, 5, 32, 288
  programmes, 32, 34

identity, 15–16, 17, 98, 118–19, 120, 219,
  290
inclusion, 60, 73, 241, 248, 249
indigenous, 94
interactional model of occupational
  development (IMOD), 137, 141–2,
  154
interactionism, 137, 141, 154
  multiple determinicity, 144, 153
  multiple paternicity, 150
  staged continuity, 143, 153
International Classification of Function
  (ICF), 3, 7, 8–11, 18, 41, 68–70, 72,
  105, 123, 139, 202, 208–210, 211,
  213, 214, 223, 243, 251
  activity/limitations, 8, 18, 211, 215, 220,
    243, 251
  body functions/structures, 8, 10, 18, 211,
    214, 243
  children's version, 69–70
  contextual factors, 95, 213, 223, 243
  environmental factors, 8, 10, 18, 139,
    182, 214–15, 224, 251, 288
  participation/restrictions, 8, 18, 211, 215,
    220
  personal factors, 8, 18, 94, 139, 182,
    214–15, 223, 251
International Classification of Impairments,
  Disability and Handicap (ICIDH), 72
Internet, 6, 48–50, 103–104, 294

just right challenge, 178, 195

Knox Preschool Play Scale (PPS), 184, 185,
  186, 189

leisure/recreation, 93, 98, 99, 178, 280, 283, 284–7, 290, 293
  activity, 288, 291
  adult organized, 290
  benefits, 290–91
  competence enlargement, 291–2
  engagement in, 99, 106, 288
  extra-curricular, 280, 283
  gender, 281
  leisure capital, 283–4
  negative outcomes, 292
  out of school time/activities, 280, 281–2
  social capital, 283
  spread of activities, 290–91
  structured, 93, 283, 284, 292
  unstructured, 99, 284, 292
life satisfaction, 98, 219

Maslow's hierarchy of needs, 126
  being needs, 126
  deficiency needs, 126
  self-actualization, 126, 132
motivation, 263, 285–7, 293

nature, 56, 59
neighbourhood, 44, 56, 76, 79, 102, 147, 291, 292
  safety, 79, 102–103, 292

occupation, 11–12, 18, 28, 29–30, 72, 92, 116, 139, 146, 181, 223, 243, 244, 261
  evolution, 152–3
  family occupations, 32–4
  parenting occupations, 32
  spiritual, 128–30
occupation based intervention, 33
occupational balance, 14, 17, 92, 100–107, 125, 131–2, 280, 284
occupational behaviour, 136, 141, 153, 288
occupational challenges, 129
occupational competence, 136, 137, 139, 143, 146, 149, 151, 154
occupational deprivation, 42, 119
occupational development, 116, 136–54
  interactionist view, 138
  macro-occupational development, 151–3
  maturationist view, 138
  meso-occupational development, 141–51
  micro-occupational development, 139–41
  performationist view, 138

occupational (activity) engagement, 18, 25, 100, 115, 117, 132, 150, 158–9, 170, 181, 244, 280, 288
occupational environments, 143
occupational expectations, 146
occupational exposure, 144, 146, 149
occupational life course, 150
occupational opportunities, 153
occupational outcome, 145–6
occupational participation, 148
occupational performance, 28, 72, 75, 94, 105, 120, 122, 136, 145, 160, 223, 284
occupational performance components, 82, 122
occupational possibilities, 146, 153
occupational potential, 120
occupational pursuits, 243
occupational repertoire, 121, 132, 137, 141, 143, 145, 146, 147, 153
occupational science, 32, 91
occupational specialization, 152
occupational therapists, 159, 168, 170, 180, 182, 186, 187, 189, 191, 194, 195, 202, 215, 220, 222, 223, 224, 230, 232, 236, 245, 246, 247, 272
occupational therapy intervention, 11, 105, 116, 234–6, 243, 251–6, 252–6
  bottom up approaches, 122–5, 160
  evaluation, 251
  top down approaches, 122–5, 160, 251
occupational therapy role, 18, 119, 211, 224, 234, 241

palliative/terminal care, 130–31
parents, 236, 274, 295
  beliefs, 77, 262, 283
  dual parents, 24, 25, 283
  education, 95
  maternal employment, 95
  satisfaction, 31
  single parents, 23, 25, 102
  working parents, 5, 24, 283
parks, 44
participation, 11, 18, 29, 61, 67–8, 70, 78, 79–80, 115, 117, 139, 145, 160, 183, 202, 232, 244, 245, 247–8, 255, 262, 263, 265, 267, 272, 280, 290
  barriers, 86, 105
  elements of, 71
  facilitators, 86

participation (*cont'd*)
  family participation, 32
  recreation/leisure, 70
partnership, 30, 32
person environment occupation (PEO), 79,
    81–2, 136, 142, 144, 149, 180, 182–4,
    189, 195, 211, 288
  macrolevel practice, 82
  microlevel practice, 82
physical activity, 6, 51, 70, 74, 76, 92, 99,
    103, 261, 263, 269, 272, 273
  active transport/commuting, 45, 74,
    269–71, 274
  benefits, 262
  curricula, 264–5, 267, 271, 273
  determinants, 262
  fitness, 264, 272
  games, 265
  lifestyle, 265, 295
  motor skills/programmes, 267, 272
  organized sport, 262, 281, 290
  physical education, 264, 267
  physical inactivity, 6, 76
  promotion, 273
  recess, 268, 272, 273
  recreational physical activity, 264, 274
  safety, 269, 270
  school based, 267
  school sport, 265–6
  transport, 45
play, 49, 53, 57, 81, 125, 139, 148, 158,
    163, 168, 261, 268, 281, 284, 291
  activities, 194, 195
  assessment, 184–9
  barriers to, 182, 189, 194
  definitions, 178–80
  environments, 178, 192–4
  episode, 179
  equipment, 194
  functions of, 180
  materials, 194
  occupational supports, 177, 178
  participation, 183, 184, 189
  partner, 187, 194
  play occupations, 140, 181
  role of player, 177–8, 181, 241, 242
  sociodramatic, 163–4, 191, 194
  street play, 46
  supports, 189, 194
  threats to play, 177
play history, 185

play spaces, 44, 46, 53, 59, 76, 191
play style, 177
playgrounds, 44, 45, 57, 269, 273
  environments, 59
  equipment, 57–9
  inclusive design, 59, 60
  safety, 57, 269, 273
  school, 235
playfulness, 177, 179, 184, 185, 186, 284
playscapes, 177
  virtual, 177
policy
  government/public policy, 22, 86, 107,
    192
  social policy, 96
Preferences of Activities (PAC), 83

quality of life, 96, 98

relaxation, 146, 292
resilience/resiliency, 75, 105, 130, 290–91
rest/sleep, 93, 99
restoration, 59, 61, 126, 292
roles, 11–18, 28, 29, 158
  familial, 12–14
  occupational, 12–14, 29, 42, 115, 119,
    170, 171, 182, 222
  personal sexual, 12–14, 29
  role change, 15
  role competence, 16, 18, 180
  role conflict, 17
  role disruption, 17
  role dysfunction, 16, 17
  role engagement, 30
  role importance, 14–15
  social, 29, 119

schedules, 25
  children's schedules, 5, 28
  family schedules
school, 72, 74, 93, 98, 223, 261
  academic functioning, 231
  buildings, 245
  classroom/school rules, 245, 248, 268
  curricula, 242, 249–50
  environment, 241, 246, 250, 261
  inclusion, 60, 73, 248, 249
  instructional materials, 245
  intervention, 252–6
  learning/classroom environment, 225,
    232, 233, 234, 242, 244, 245, 246

models of transition, 227–32
occupation based assessment, 242
readiness, 224, 227, 230–32, 236, 262
routines, 243, 244, 247, 251, 255
social adjustment, 231
student/learner, 226, 236, 241, 242, 243, 246, 256, 261
teacher expectations, 248
transition/s, 222, 224–8, 232, 236, 241, 242
School Assessment of Motor and Processing Skills (SCAMPS), 252
School Function Assessment (SFA), 52, 252
School Outcome Measure, 252
SCOPE-IT, 280, 288–9
screen based activities, 6, 49, 92–3, 103–104, 263, 281
television, 6, 44, 49, 50, 75, 79, 92, 93, 94, 102, 103, 104, 126, 164, 227, 281, 292, 293–4
self-care, 200, 272, 280, 281
assessment, 202, 208–210
basic activities of daily living (BADL), 200, 203–205, 216, 243
instrumental activities of daily living (IADL), 200, 206–207, 216, 217, 218
instruments, 208–210
management/intervention, 211, 212, 216, 217, 218
needs, 200
routines, 200
self-carer, 201
self esteem/efficacy, 115, 117–19, 130, 219, 226, 262, 287, 294
skill acquisition, 14, 18, 96, 122, 124, 130, 170, 177, 227, 228, 235, 262, 284, 291, 295
social skills, 104, 158, 164–6, 177, 181, 242, 247, 268
acquisition deficit, 166
assessment, 167–9
cognitive behavioural, 172
conversation skills, 165, 168, 172
deficits, 166–7, 174
emotional motivational, 172
fluency deficit, 166

intervention, 167–73
macro-level, 165–6, 170
micro-level, 165–6, 170
performance deficit, 166
social competence, 159, 164–5, 181
training, 170, 173
socialization, 15, 16, 118, 146, 290, 294
sociocultural beliefs, 153
speech pathologists, 159, 168, 170, 172
spirituality, 127–32
psycho-spiritual integration, 128
spiritual qualities, 130
strengths based/perspectives, 81–2, 86
support
formal, 26–8, 47–8
informal, 26–8, 47–8

Test of Environmental Supportiveness (TOES), 53, 55, 191
Test of Playfulness (ToP), 185, 186, 187, 189
time budget, 70, 93
diaries, 93, 281
time use, 91, 92, 94, 95, 96, 102, 105, 280, 281, 283, 284, 288, 290, 294
classification systems, 281
patterns, 283
surveys, 281
Transdisciplinary Play Based Assessment, 185
transition, 14, 15, 25, 26, 44, 70, 141, 151, 177, 222–37, 241, 242

universal design, 42
Universal Design for Learning (UDL), 250

virtual toys, 49
volunteering, 283

walking school bus, 271
wellbeing, 12, 18, 26, 28, 31, 33, 41, 50, 51, 68, 70, 71, 91, 96, 100, 105, 115, 121, 124, 127, 131, 166, 211, 220, 287, 290

zone of proximal development (ZPD), 186